FIX YOUR OWN PAIN WITHOUT DRUGS OR SURGERY

Jolie Bookspan, Ph.D.

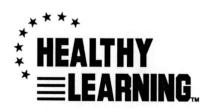

Prior to beginning any sports medicine, rehabilitation, or physical activity program, including that described in this book, individuals should seek medical evaluation and clearance to engage in activity. The information and materials presented in this book are in no way intended to be a substitute for medical counsel and advice. It is important to note that not all sports medicine, rehabilitation, or physical activity programs are suitable for everyone and some programs may in fact result in injury. Activities such as those detailed and depicted in this text should be undertaken only if they are consistent with advice and guidelines provided by a qualified medical and/or health/fitness professional. Individuals should discontinue participation in any sports medicine, rehabilitation, or physical activity program that causes pain or discomfort. In such event, medical consultation should be immediately obtained.

ISBN: 978-1-58518-984-7
Library of Congress Control Number: 2006927177
Book layout: Deborah Oldenburg
Cover design: Brenden Murphy
Text photos: Jolie Bookspan and clipart.com © 2005 Jupiterimages Corporation
Author photo: Robert Troia
Illustrations: Jolie Bookspan and Todd Sargood

Healthy Learning
P.O. Box 1828
Monterey, CA 93942
www.healthylearning.com

Dedication

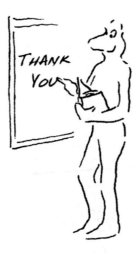

To my grandmother. To her the highest things in life were learning and Jack LaLane.

To my mother, who I promised when I was four years old that I would find the cure for back pain.

To my saint of a husband, Paul, who supports me in all I do and tries all my cures. You are my hero.

To all of my students and patients.

Acknowledgments

Thank you to the expert reviewers who examined, checked,
and made sure this book is healthy.

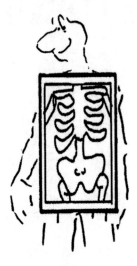

Alan Berg, Ph.D. M.D. Geritrition and House Call Doctor.
Philadelphia County Medical Society Practitioner of the Year, 2000

Lt. Col. Keith E. Brandt, M.D., MPH. EMEDS. Military medicine

Major Kelly J. Fripps, United States Air Force, Flight Commander, Primary Care Teams

Catherine Ratzin Jackson, Ph.D., FACSM. Sports medicine and nutrition

David Hsu, Ph.D., M.D. Clinical and research neurologist

Richard G. Ruoti, Ph.D., P.T., CSCS. Physical therapy

Audrey Tannenbaum, M.Ed., A.T.C., CSCS,
Athletic trainer and Maccabean Games triathlon gold medalist

Foreword

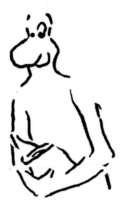

This book is for the millions of us who wake up every morning with hot pokers jabbing in our spine, shoulders, knees, and more. It is for the millions of us who have tried many remedies over and over without success, often succumbing to the surgeon's knife to little or no avail (this from a surgeon!). Using simple techniques, Dr. Jolie Bookspan is able to carefully lead the sufferer through a program that almost miraculously relieves pain, strengthens muscles, and provides a return of confidence.

Dr. Bookspan is a career research scientist, widely acclaimed for her work in human physiology and sports medicine. Her methods to reverse pain and injury are gems of common sense management.

Dr. Bookspan is known in scientific circles for successfully debunking traditional, yet ineffective or wrong ideas. For that reason, some of the finest clinicians in the field have compared her to Galileo for changing the "held paradigm." She is known as a careful and brilliant researcher who has found the reasons why things were not working, and changed the paradigm to a simpler and more effective one. She has done so with a regimen that is successful, not available anywhere else, and best of all, self-empowering.

Even in those conditions thought to be only correctable by surgery, her program offers distinct benefits of decreased pain and physiological and psychological well being. I have had patients come to me asking about their particular problems with back pain in relationship to 'fitness for diving' - asking if their condition warranted a cessation in their favorite sport. Referrals to Dr. Bookspan brought about almost miraculous alterations in the courses of the patients (somewhat to my surprise, I must admit!) with remission of pain.

One person in particular who had just about reached the end of his rope, was on increasing doses of narcotics and was considering risky surgery. Dr. Bookspan placed him on her regimen and he is now off of pain medication, is enjoying his retirement from the military for the first time in years, and is back scuba diving. No wonder Harvard School of Medicine clinicians have named Jolie, "The St. Jude of the Joints."

—Ernest S. Campbell, M.D., FACS*

*Retired, board-certified general surgeon. Prior to his retirement, he had been president of the medical staff, chairman of the Department of Surgery, and a member of the Board of Directors at Brookwood Medical Center in Birmingham, Alabama. A fellow of the American College of Surgery, Campbell's memberships have included the American Medical Association, American College of Physician Executives, Southern Medical Association, Medical Association of the State of Alabama, Southeastern Surgical Congress, Birmingham Clinical Club, Birmingham Academy of Medicine, Birmingham Surgical Society, and the UHMS Webmaster, Author Diving Medicine Online www.scuba-doc.com.

Contents

Introduction

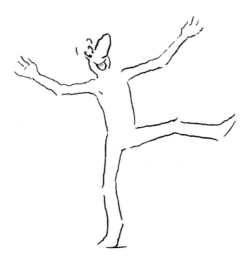

"Doctor! It hurts when I go like this!"

"Then don't go like this!"

This joke is often played out in real life. Whatever activity means the most to you—you may love to play tennis or go running—when your back, shoulder, or knee hurts, you may have been told, "No more tennis." "No more running." Often, it may not be one activity you lose, but your active and independent life as pain slowly robs you.

This philosophy is called: "Limit the patient to limit the pain." It does not always fix the problem. It can create a cycle of decreasing activity and decreased ability to do the very activities that could help you recover, and keep you in the physical shape you need for healing, mobility, and health.

Someone who swims or plays golf may get shoulder pain from bad shoulder-stretching practices or poor movement patterns during their sport or daily life. Instead of finding the cause of the problem, they are told to give up their sport. They may be given shoulder exercises, but pain returns when they return to activity because they have not retrained how they move. They may give up tennis or swimming because of the overhead arm actions, but use the same harmful patterns in hundreds of everyday. overhead motions like combing hair and putting away groceries. The pain continues and no one understands why. They may be prescribed anti-inflammatory medication, which may not help as much as hoped because their pain is not inflammatory in nature. Or it helps, "a little but not enough," so they take more. Then more. Or the medicine helps, but they don't want to spend their life on medication, or it goes off the market. Or the medicine causes stomach pain so they take new medicines for the new problems. Each new medicine causes more strange aches. They gradually restrict more activity. They may finally go for surgery, but the pain persists or returns because they never fixed the cause. Worse, it was not necessary to quit their favorite activity in the first place.

I worked years in the laboratory studying what works and what doesn't. I applied the answers in my clinical practice with patients, watched how patients live and move during their house-call appointments, and studied how my hundreds of students move in my martial-arts, rehab, yoga, and training classes, and sit in my academic classes every semester. Their pain went away with the methods I developed. Physicians started calling, asking how I did it. They said that their office exercise handouts weren't working and asked if I would write new handouts to give their patients. Requests grew. I expanded them into articles, then this book—each time looking for better ways to make it all work.

This book is for everyone who hurts and wants to stop hurting. It's for everyone who wants to prevent injuries for themselves and others. It's for everyone who wants their life back. This book will teach you the concepts of how pain often develops and continues. With that knowledge, you can apply simple techniques to stop the causes of pain—and keep pain from coming back. You will be able to evaluate claims of the many products and exercises out there and make your own decisions. People are often told to, "Just live with it." This book shows you: "You don't have to just live with it."

Each chapter has real stories about patients who fixed their own pain. Some of the photos are examples and others are real patients. Their stories show what they did, why things worked and why they didn't work. Many of the names are real and unchanged from patients who wanted to serve as examples—good and bad.

Chapters include information on pain the way you experience it: "Lower-back pain," "neck pain," "tight shoulder," and "repeated ankle sprains," rather than only technical diagnostic categories. Everything is in "plain English," the way I explain things to my own patients, family, and students. Each section includes things to try, step-by-step instructions, and how to retrain your muscles for healthy movement on a daily level, rather than doing a bunch of exercises or "therapy." This book can't cover everything, but covers common problems that are often missed—with simple solutions you can do yourself.

"Fitness" isn't a set of exercises. Real fitness teaches you how to move in daily life—which has been my mission in my sports medicine practice. I use the patient's regular activities as part of their rehab. We look at how they move and how to fix injurious habits. I show them how to properly use the injured area during their daily activities to strengthen, and to avoid harmful patterns. Many of the exercises are techniques I developed by combining the best properties of existing exercises, cutting away parts that were harmful, extraneous, or not effective, and then applying them to your real life.

The goal is not only to get people back to all of their activities, but also to surpass where they were before pain took their lives away. Often, when people realize they don't need to give up their activities and can learn healthy ways to do them, their eyes light up, they straighten their body, and announce some dream they previously thought they had to give up. One lady asked me if bicycling was all right for her curved back. I showed her that you can slump over handlebars, or hold your back in healthy position. "In that case," she said, "I will bike across Europe! I always wanted to do that." "Africa!" said another lady. "I always wanted to go to Africa."

If you want your life back, I will show you how. You don't have to live with pain.

A Patient Comments

I had been suffering for nearly five years from lower-back pain that had slowly taken over my life. I tried chiropractors and exercising on my own and with trainers. After starting with Dr. Bookspan, I eliminated my lower-back pain. I feel it's been a privilege to have worked with Jolie personally. She has an incredibly vast knowledge of the technical and mechanical operation of the human body. More rare, and remarkable, is her knowledge of human motivation and its effect on exercising and health. I also learned, more importantly, that exercise does not mean suffering in a tedious or boring routine. Jolie makes it enjoyable, not an obligation. Working with her is not about doing what you're told; it's learning about the body, practicing, strengthening, and miraculously, enjoying it.

—*Thomas Devanney, architect*

1

No More Neck and Upper-Back Pain

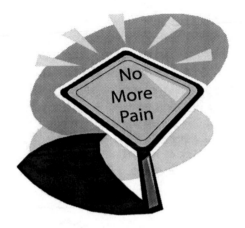

- Muscular Neck and Upper-Back Pain
- Kyphosis
- Tight Upper Back
- Herniated Cervical Discs
- Impingement
- Osteoporosis

The most common causes of neck and upper-back pain—even disc pain and muscular pain that have gone on for years—are easily correctable. This chapter shows simple techniques you can use to stop the cause of the pain and keep it from coming back.

Muscular Neck Pain

Jada's neck and upper back hurt most of the time. The pain made a diamond shape up her neck, across her shoulders, and down her upper back. Sometimes after long hours at her desk, the pain went down her arm. Jada pointed at her arm, jutting her chin forward for emphasis. "My doctor told me the pain was from using my computer. He said I have to choose my job or my health." Jada was frightened. I asked her why she had to choose. She said her neck hurt when she used the computer. She worked from home and it was her only job. She had spent a lot of money on an ergonomic desk but the pain continued. She pushed her chin forward even further and told me how she didn't know what she would do.

Jada was holding her neck at an angle so that her head was forward of her body—a common bad posture called a "forward head." A forward head is an

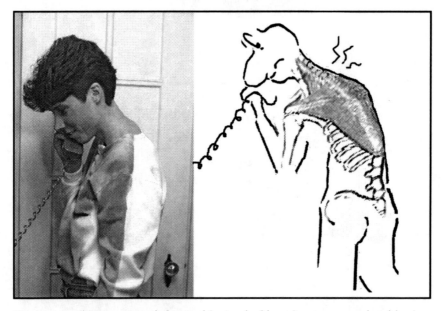

Figure 1-1. Tilting your neck forward instead of keeping ear over shoulder is called a "forward head." A forward head hangs the weight of your head and neck on the diamond-shaped neck and upper-back muscles, making them hurt.

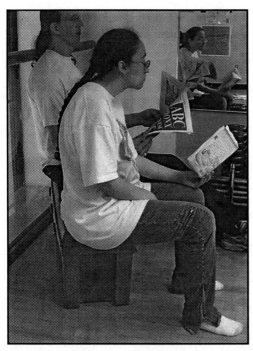 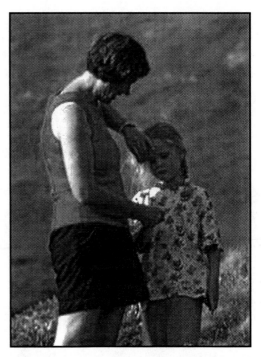

Figure 1-2. A "forward head" (right) is a bad posture that causes much neck and upper-back pain. Fix this posture by keeping your chin in with your ears over your shoulders (left). Are you sitting with your head forward right now as you read this?

Figure 1-3. Do you let your head hang forward during regular life activities? Keeping healthy neck position doesn't mean to never look down, just not to hang the weight of your head forward. Keep chin in.

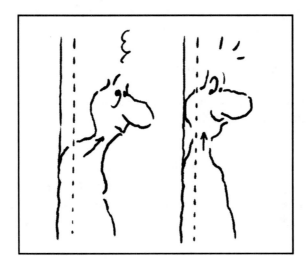

Figure 1-4. On the left is the forward head. On the right is the exercise of bringing in the chin to a comfortable and straight position. Figure 1-5 shows how to apply this exercise during real activity.

overlooked (but major) source of neck and upper-back pain. When your head and neck jut forward, the weight of your head doesn't rest over your spine, but hangs forward, making the muscles and discs miserable in the back of your neck. Of the many people coming to see me for neck and upper-back pain year after year, the forward head is the most common cause of their pain. People with neck and upper-back pain who stop the forward head usually feel the difference from that moment onward.

Jada said her doctor sent her for physical therapy. I asked her what they showed her. "*This!*" she said, forcing her chin inward and downward so much that it made her have two chins. "They say I have to do this 10 times a day."

"That's called the 'double-chin' exercise," I told her. "What else did they say?"

Jada's chin flopped to her forward head posture with a clunk. "Nothing," she said.

I explained to Jada that her neck and shoulders weren't hurting from the computer. She could use the computer without pain by repositioning her head instead of letting it hang forward.

Repositioning the head doesn't mean that you never look down or up, but that you don't let the weight of your head hang forward. It is not a matter of strengthening the area through an "exercise." The double-chin exercise is not supposed to be done just as an exercise 10 times. It is used to learn how to hold your head and neck in all the time instead of letting it hang forward. The pain will start subsiding as soon as you no longer cause the pull on the back of your neck.

Using Bad Posture When Trying to Stand Straight

Many people are so tight that they crane their neck or arch their back (or both) when trying to correct the forward head. They get more pain trying to stand straight (Figure 1-6).

Craning the neck means pinching it back, with the chin and face lifted. Craning the neck is surprisingly common. It is a big source of neck and shoulder pain. Many people crane their neck to look up, to drink water, to reach overhead areas, and even to eat. Check yourself to see if you jut your chin forward or hunch your shoulders up during daily life.

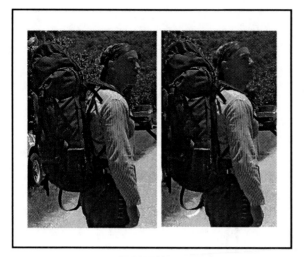

Figure 1-5. Keep your head from hanging forward in all of your activities, not just as an exercise you do 10 times.

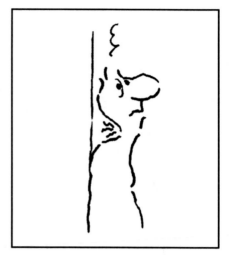

Figure 1-6. Are you so tight that you crane your neck to look up, or pull your head back trying to stand straight?

How to Check Neck and Upper-Back Pain and Positioning

The wall stand is a test to see if you can stand comfortably in straight healthy position (Figure 1-7). When standing with your back against a wall, if you can't touch the back of your head without craning your neck or arching your back, you are too tight to stand straight. You probably have a forward head and tight muscles.

- Stand near a wall, with your back toward but not touching, the wall.

- Back up until something touches. If your hips touched first, you may stand bent because of tight muscles in the front of the chest and hip (Figure 1-7, far left).

- Did your upper back touch first? You may arch or lean backward (Figure 1-7, second from left).

- With your heels, hips, and upper back touching the wall, is the back of your head still forward of the wall? (See Figure 1-7, second from right.) Can you bring the back of your head against the wall without raising or dropping your chin, or arching your back?

If you can't keep your heels, hips, upper back, and the back of your head comfortably against the wall, you are too tight. Tilting the neck and upper body forward during the day creates neck and upper-back pain, as well as a surprising amount of mystery shoulder pain and impingement. Not being able to straighten out is usually the reason for pain that occurs when you try to lie flat on your back, too. If your head doesn't comfortably reach the floor and your lower back has to arch up when you try to lie flat, tightness may be pulling you into a strained position.

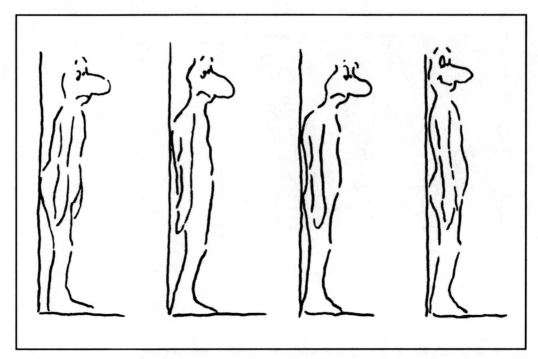

Figure 1-7. Can you stand comfortably straight against the wall (far right) or does your head come forward in various slouches (first three figures from right)?

Another interesting way to see if your chest is tight is to put your arms comfortably at your sides, and note the direction of your thumbs. Do they face inward toward each other? (See Figure 1-8.) The thumb-in position is not the normal position of the arms. When your pectoral (chest) muscles are tight, the tight muscles rotate your arms inward, turning your thumbs toward your body.

Fixing Neck and Upper-Back Pain and Positioning

To restore the chest muscles to a healthy resting length, do the pectoral stretch (Figure 1-9) and the trapezius stretch (Figure 1-10).

Pectoral ("Pec") Muscle Stretch

- Face a wall and lift one arm up, with the elbow bent, as if "in a stickup" (Figure 1-9).

- Turn your feet and body away from the wall. Use the wall to gently brace your elbow back as you turn. Feel the stretch in your chest, not in your shoulder capsule.

- Keep head and back posture in line. Don't let your back arch or your chin jut forward. Hold just a few seconds and then switch arms.

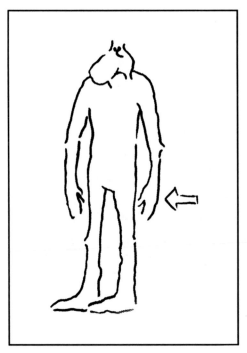

Figure 1-8. If your thumbs face inward, it is often the result of a round-shouldered position.

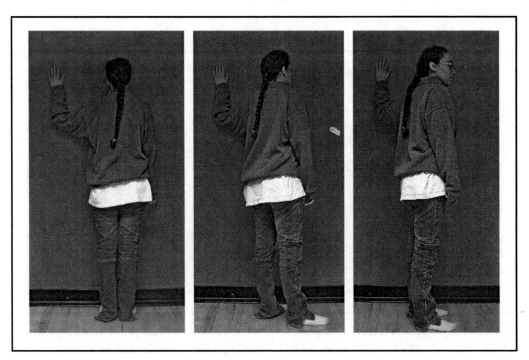

Figure 1-9. Pectoral (chest muscle) stretch

- Drop your arms by your sides and look at your thumbs again. If you got the stretch from the chest muscles, your thumbs should face forward now.
- Try the wall stand again. It should be easy to stand straight (Figure 1-7, far right).

Trapezius Stretch for the Side of Your Neck

- Put one hand behind you, as if in an opposite pocket (Figure 1-10).
- Tip one ear toward your shoulder. Don't round or hunch forward.
- Breathe in. Then while breathing out, slide your hand down the side of your leg to your knee. Feel a nice stretch along your entire side. Keep the back of your head against the wall to tell where straight positioning is.
- Hold a few seconds then breathe in and out and switch sides. Don't force. No need to hold for long periods, just a few seconds on each side.
- Try the wall stand again and note that it is now easier to stand straight (Figure 1-7, far right).

When to Do the Pectoral and Trapezius Stretches

Use the pectoral and trapezius stretches (Figures 1-9 and 1-10) first thing in the morning to set your muscles in a healthy position to start the day without the forward rounding that injures and brings on pain. Repeat several times a day to restore the muscle length that makes it possible to stand in healthy straight position.

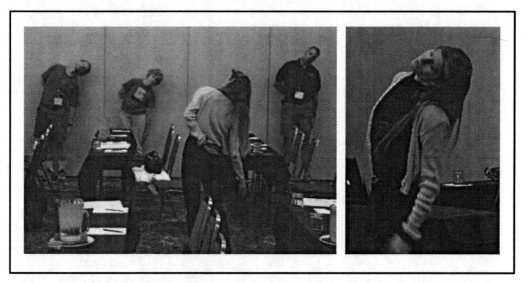

Figure 1-10. Trapezius stretch. Tilt the neck and body, sliding the hand to the knee. To learn straight position, keep the back of your head against the wall.

The double-chin exercise that Jada was given is a commonly prescribed exercise for the forward head. It is often misunderstood. In the double chin, you pull your chin in and back, without lifting or dropping your chin. Many people are told to do it 10 times every hour. Then they go back to going around all day with their head forward, wondering why their neck still hurts, or they force their head back, causing more pain.

- The double-chin exercise is not something you "do 10 times" then stop. It is something you do once. Use it to relearn proper head position, and then keep your head in place.

- Keep your chin in, not stiffly or tightly that it hurts, but easily so that your ear is above your shoulder, not forward of it. Don't make a new pain by forcing good posture.

- Pull from your head, chin, and shoulders. Don't just arch your lower back.

- Check your body positioning with your back against a wall often during the day, to see if the back of your head touches comfortably.

Using Ordinary Objects to Stretch Your Upper Back

- Lie on your back over a comfortable pillow or rolled towel between your shoulder blades. Let your shoulders drape back.

- Lie backward over a ball, bench, bed, firm pillow, or other raised surface, and let your upper back drape backward over the edge (Figure 1-11). Don't let your neck pinch back and don't do this stretch if you have neck injury, glaucoma, or other reasons not to turn upside down.

- Make sure the stretch comes from your upper back and shoulder, not just by arching your lower back or letting your neck crane back unsupported.

- While lying head down, let your arms stretch overhead to add a nice shoulder stretch (see Figure 3-10).

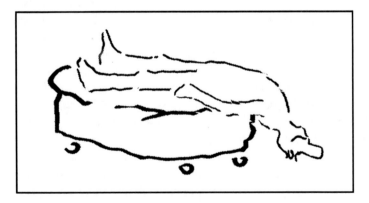

Figure 1-11. Find comfortable ways to safely stretch.

Muscular Upper-Back Pain

Mario worked at his desk much of the day. He was told that his pinching, burning upper back was from stress. He went to a chiropractor three times a week but the burning and pinching pain came back each day when he went back to work. Sometimes his upper back felt numb and the top of his shoulders tingled, but a neurological check showed "nothing wrong." He stretched his back several times a day by bending forward, and by pulling his arm across his body in front. He pulled his chin down to his chest and his knee up to his chest. He was fitted for orthotics and slept on a heating pad at home. He had an ergonomic chair. He called me asking what stretch he could do for his upper-back pain.

When I arrived for Mario's house-call appointment at his office, he was sitting at his expensive ergonomic desk, rounded over his computer. The flexibility of his back was excellent. In fact, his back was so stretched that it easily rounded, which became the comfortable position for him to sit. His chest had shortened so much that it easily rounded inward to match his rounded back. I asked Mario what standing up straight would mean to him and he arched his lower back to swing his shoulders back, with his upper back still rounded forward and his neck stiffly pulled back.

"That looks like no fun," I said.

"Yeah," he said. "That posture stuff is for the birds. Can you show me that stretch now? The guys said that I should lie on my back and bring both knees to my chest, but I can't do that at work." I told him that was just as well since the last thing he needed was more forward rounding.

I explained that sitting with a rounded back was a common cause of numb and painful upper back. Letting your head and upper back round forward hangs their weight on the upper-back muscles and joints. When you slouch forward, it keeps back muscles overly stretched, which weakens and strains them. Strained muscles can tighten in "knots" or spasm, trying to protect themselves, which changes their muscle chemistry. All of the chronic forward bending creates an overstretched, weakened upper back, and a shortened, contracted chest. The back rounds and the chest tightens until you are too rounded to sit or stand up straight. This creates a cycle of rounding, which causes pain and tightening, which promotes more rounding. The pressure of your own body weight rounding forward on your neck and upper-back muscles and discs over years of poor sitting, standing, and bending habits is enough to injure your neck

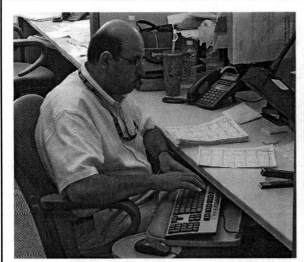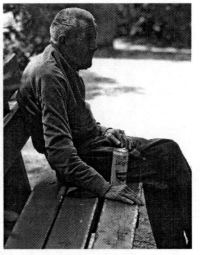

Figure 1-12. Many people sit with their upper back and neck rounded forward for much of the day, which is a common source of upper-back pain.

as badly as a single accident. The problem is reinforced by more forward rounding during stretches and exercises.

Mario said his doctor told him to strengthen his back, so he did crunches and lifted weights by bending forward. To "balance" that out, he used a weight machine for his chest, bending his arms together in front to contract the front of the chest. The chest machine was not balancing out the back exercises as he thought. It was more forward rounding, which he didn't need.

Mario felt worse, but his doctor told him it was normal to feel worse before he felt better. I told him there was no need to feel worse. It was the forward bending. Crunches, bending forward, and chest exercises also do not strengthen the back. To strengthen a muscle, you need to contract it. Contracting the back muscles pulls you to the back, a movement called extension. His back needed extension exercise. As soon as we retrained Mario's bending habits, and replaced his forward bending exercises with upper-back extension (Figure 1-15), he began feeling better.

Exercises to Strengthen and Retrain Neck and Upper-Back Muscles

Neck and upper-back pain exercises are misunderstood. People often injure their neck all day then hope to fix it with a few exercises. They don't understand when this does

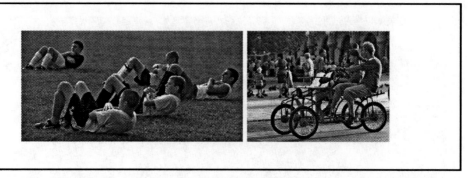

Figure 1-13. After sitting rounded all day, do you exercise with your upper back rounded?

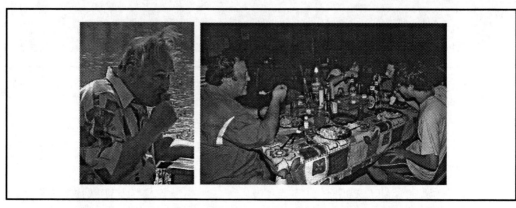

Figure 1-14. Forward rounding is a common bad habit when eating. Forward rounding for so much of the day is a common source of upper-back, neck, and shoulder pain.

not work. They lie on the floor to do exercises, then stand up and walk away with no use of the positioning or strength they just practiced. The key is what you do all day. Try upper-back extension (Figure 1-15a). See how you feel the next day, then increase to at least 10 to 20 at a time.

Upper-Back Extension

Most people stretch their back by forward rounding but never strengthen the back and neck muscles that hold the back and neck upright. Upper-back extension is an important exercise to strengthen at the same time that you practice moving your back in the other direction. It also unloads the discs that are pushed outward by forward bending

- Lie face down on the floor. Hands and arms should stay off the floor in any comfortable position.

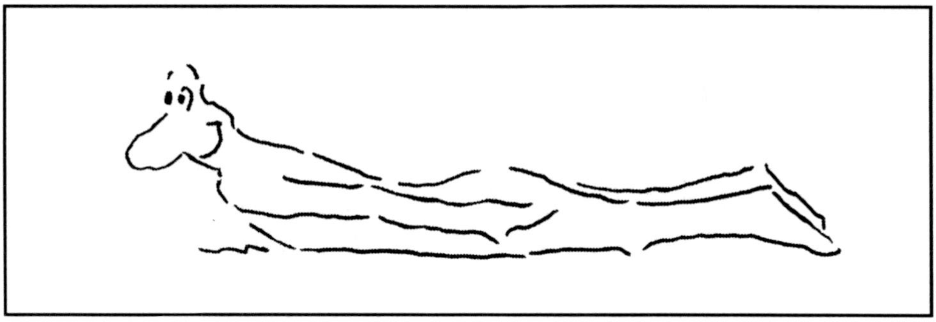

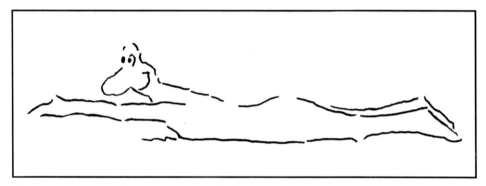

Figure 1-15a. Upper-back extension

Figure 1-15b. Upper-back extension with hands overhead for more exercise and range.

- Gently lift the upper body without using your hands. Don't force it.
- Don't crane your neck; keep it straight. Lift using your upper-body muscles.
- If you are debilitated by injury or illness, start first by resting on your elbows and letting your shoulders move down and up. Keep your head from drooping down or craning backward. Use your muscles to hold your head up comfortably. Work up to pushing up and down with your hands. It doesn't matter where you position your hands. Be comfortable. Progress to lifting up without hands.
- Increase by holding hands in front of you (Figure 1-15b). Try lifting your body up more to one side than the other.

The Point Is to Stop Rounding Forward

When propping on elbows, be sure to reverse the forward rounding in the upper back. It is common to push up from the lower back, folding on the lower vertebrae, leaving the upper back still rounded forward (Figure 1-16, top). Instead, let the entire upper back stretch to the back (Figure 1-16, bottom).

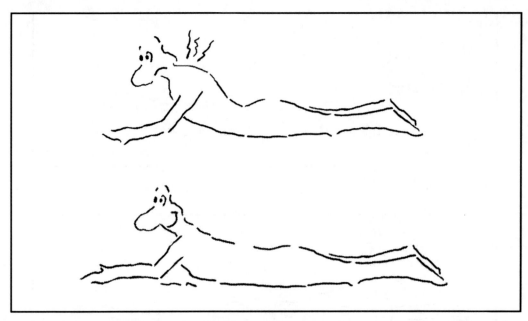

Figure 1-16. The point of upper-back extension is to reverse forward rounding. Don't keep the upper back rounded (top). Let the upper back reverse and stretch back (bottom).

Ellen's upper back was overly-rounded, a posture called "kyphosis." Kyphosis originally meant the small normal amount of rounding in the upper spine that helps shock absorption. Kyphosis later came to mean too much rounding. Ellen's kyphosis was pronounced. She regularly went to yoga and exercise classes where the most common stretches were bending forward to touch toes, both sitting and standing, and sitting cross-legged and rounding down to touch head to feet (Figure 1-17). When the yoga class stretched backward by lying face down and pushing up in upper-body extension, Ellen's upper back stayed rounded, and only her lower back extended backward. Her upper back stayed in this overly rounded position when she stood, walked, and exercised.

We worked on straightening Ellen's upper-back posture. To make it possible to stand straight, we needed to stretch the chest muscles that had become pulled forward and tightened. Once the chest muscles were reset to normal resting length using the pectoral stretch (Figure 1-9) and the trapezius stretch (Figure 1-10), Ellen could stand straighter. To reverse the rounding of her upper back, and retrain the upper-back muscles to pull back, we practiced extension exercises, with the reminder that the exercise isn't just for lying on the floor (Figure 1-16), but also for standing and sitting, too (Figure 1-18).

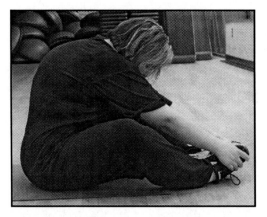

Figure 1-17. Ellen's pronounced upper back rounding and pain was worsened by forward bending (flexion) stretches. Instead, she needed back-extension exercise.

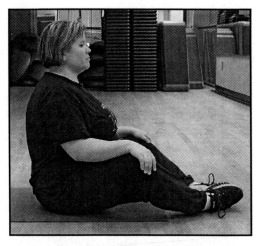

Figure 1-18. Although told that her upper back rounding was the permanent shape of her bones, it was a postural habit. Through repositioning exercises over a short time, she restored fairly good upper-back positioning.

Tight Upper Back

Ardella never used a computer but her upper back and neck hurt most of the time. Her posture looked beautifully straight. Her neck and upper back were tight as a brick when I touched her shoulder. I rubbed her upper back gently with my thumbs.

"That's where it hurts," she shuddered. "My doctor said it was fibromyalgia and prescribed antidepressants." I reassured Ardella that many things make the area tender. One of them is just being tight.

"Oh, I'm tight all right. I go for massage, but it can be painful." She said that over the winter she couldn't get out of the house for three days to renew the antidepressant and felt better without it. I told her I heard that often. She looked at me with interest. I told her that the people who come to me hurt a lot, and are unhappy about hurting. I told her it sounded normal to me that they don't enjoy an unhealthy situation. Several have told me they felt worse on the anti-depressant but didn't know that was the problem until they stopped taking it.

I reminded Ardella to get out in the sunlight. You need sunlight in your eyes to feel better. Sunlight helps depression. Sunlight also makes your body produce vitamin D, which strengthens bones and joints in combination with exercise. Many people feel achy without enough vitamin D. I opened the blinds so that her place would be brighter and more cheerful. We agreed that the sunrays she needed most can't get through the glass windows.

"Go outside every day in the sunlight," I told her. "If you can't get outside, call me and I'll come get you. It's that important." In the newly bright living room, I showed her the pectoral stretch and the trapezius stretch (Figures 1-9 and 1-10). She said both stretches made her back better, but she still didn't want anyone to squeeze the area.

To start mobilizing her upper back, we tried upper-body extensions (Figure 1-15). Ardella could not lift up from the floor. Suddenly she shuddered saying it hurt. We needed to add an exercise to soothe and mobilize the muscles that had gone so long without stretch or movement. We did lunges (see Figures 3-6 and 4-6). With one foot in front and one in back, we dipped up and down several times without moving the feet. Lunges made a difference to her neck, even though the lunge doesn't exercise the upper body. The muscular activity warmed the body and helped her feel more able to move. After the lunges, she was able to reach more easily for the trapezius stretch, and to do upper-body extensions with no pain if she pushed off the floor with her hands.

Next, since it is important to teach muscles how not to tense up, I asked her to squeeze my hand, then release it. I told her to think of her muscles squeezing then relaxing in the same way. I asked her to practice breathing in without tightening, then relax her muscles even more as she breathed out. We practiced "untensing" as we did the upper-body extensions again: breathe in and lift up, breathe out and lengthen her muscles on the way down. We went on to try lower-body extension (Figure 2-12). Each exercise helped her feel better about getting moving and using muscles instead of tensing them. Merely breathing deep isn't enough. You need to consciously unclench the area and let it move.

She had other painful areas, and we worked on fun movement for each. We practiced getting groceries from the shelves, chopping vegetables, and other functional activities around the house, without tensing her shoulders. Doing exercises for rehab won't help if you go back to unhealthy movement the rest of the day. When I left, I squeezed Ardella's shoulders and it felt good to her. It was nice to see her smile. Over the next weeks, she did her pectoral and trapezius stretch (Figures 1-9 and 1-10) every day, and used lunges (Figure 4-6) and extension exercises (Figure 1-15) to get moving more easily. She felt better each day, until the tender spots didn't come back. On follow-up, she told me that retraining her upper body to not tighten and use the new healthy ways to move for regular activities made the difference.

Do Not Exercise in Ways that Damage Your Neck

Many people hurt from hanging their head, neck, and upper body forward. They ride stationary and regular bicycles with head forward and back rounded. They sit on exercise, weight, and rowing machines with their back rounded. Then do many exercises for their back pain with more forward bending—toe touches, knee to chest, crunches, and shoulder stands. It is important to strengthen the muscles that pull your upper back and neck the other way.

Strengthening and stretching are crucial, but alone will not change positioning or lifting habits. Many contribute to the original problem of over rounding and bad posture. A far more effective use of back exercises and stretches is to retrain movement and positioning while strengthening and restoring functional muscle length. Strengthening has no effect on posture if you don't apply the strength the rest of the day to control joint angles during activities.

Ira's neck and upper back hurt all the time, but it wasn't her fault that she rounded forward. After an accident years before, where she woke up in a surgical unit with rods in her upper back, she had been in constant pain. They had made the rods too curved so that it forced her upper back to round. She said she constantly felt like she was about to tip forward. When I asked her to lie on her back, she looked a little like a baby turtle rocking on a rounded shell. We worked on upper-body extension exercises (Figure 1-15) and stretching the

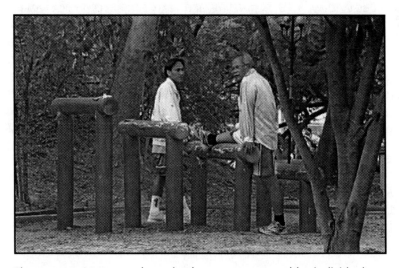

Figure 1-19. Most people notice bent posture on older individuals (right). Do you see it in young people, too (left)? Poor upper-back positioning isn't from aging.

chest with the pectoral stretch (Figure 1-9) and the trapezius stretch (Figure 1-10). At first Ira had to crane her neck to move at all. She realized that she was craning a great deal because her neck was the only place she could move, which is a problem with surgically fixing an area of the spine. Damage often grows in surrounding areas over the years of having to do double movement in compensation. Through her dedication, it was only a short while to make the upper back more mobile, even with the rods. We didn't want to destabilize anything; we just wanted to get controllable movement. Her pain diminished considerably and she said she was happy to be able to help herself.

Herniated Cervical (Neck) Discs

Dave was a drummer in a hard rock band. He was tall, tattooed, and dressed in leather. His skin was pale from the pain of three large herniated discs in his neck. He had empty hollows where the muscles of his neck and shoulders used to be, before the herniated discs pressed so much on the nerves that they could no longer send signals to his muscles. One arm hung strangely weak by his side. He had a nationwide tour starting in two weeks. He and the band and all their heavy gear would crowd for two months into a van. Could I help him? I gave Dave the good news that a disc injury is not a life sentence. Disc degeneration or slippage (herniation) can usually heal, like a sprained ankle, if you understand what is happening and take simple corrective action. It is important to understand how a disc herniates; then it is easy to see how to help it. Between each neck bone is the disc, like a tough cushion. When you hold your head up, each neck bone sits on top of the neck bone below it, and each disc between the bones is pressed from all sides at about the same pressure. When you bend your neck forward, the neck bones bend closer together in front and open farther in back. The disc is squeezed in front and (like a water balloon that you squeeze in front) squeezes a bit out in back (Figure 1-20).

Over years of letting the weight of his head hang forward on his neck for drumming, when walking around during normal life, and the thrashing head movement of hard rock music, Dave had pushed the discs in his neck outward. It didn't help that he often did a shoulder stand exercise where you lie back and lift legs in the air above you with the weight of the body on the bent forward neck (Figure 1-21).

Dave's discs were herniated far enough out of his spinal column that they pressed on nerves that went out the side of the spine to the arm, sending pain down his arm. The discs were pressing in on the spinal space enough that it hurt to cough, laugh, or even raise enough pressure to speak loudly.

"First we need to get the pressure off your discs," I told him. "Can you stand with your back against the wall and the back of your head touching?" Even though Dave's three herniations were large, he could almost do this. Sometimes, a disc sticks so far out from between the vertebrae that the person has to bend forward because standing up pinches the disc. The vicious cycle is that bending forward presses the discs further to the back. I showed Dave the pectoral stretch (Figure 1-9), and the trapezius stretch (Figure 1-10). These two stretches help reset the chest and shoulder muscles to healthy length, allowing you to stand straighter without strain. He stood against the wall with the back of his head touching. He said he could feel the pressure subside. I explained

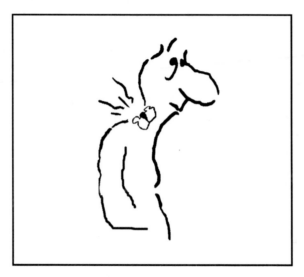

Figure 1-20. The forward head can pressure neck (cervical) discs outward over years, degenerating and herniating them.

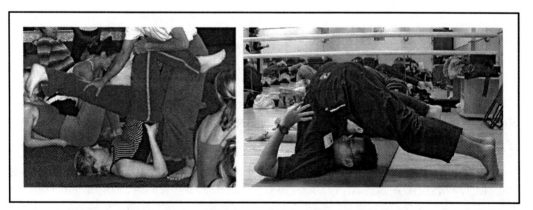

Figure 1-21. The shoulder stand, or "plow," forcibly pressures neck discs and overlengthens the structures that hold the neck and discs in place.

that just not hanging his head forward would go a long way to stop pushing the discs out so they could heal.

We checked around his house for places where he needed to prevent the forward head that was so hard on discs. We practiced how he worked at his desk. We worked on head positioning during the weightlifting he needed to restore his strength for his shrunken arm and shoulder, and for all the gear he would need to carry on the tour. First, we did all weightlifting lying flat on the floor. In this way, his neck was supported, he practiced straight neck positioning, and his shoulders were in line. So if a weight fell out of his weakened grip, it would not damage anything. We worked on upper-back extensions (Figure 1-15), then on how to stay positioned to practice and play drums. I tried to sound sympathetic, saying I understood that we had to preserve his musicianship while retraining healthy position. "Hey, I'm not a musician," he laughed. "I'm in a *band*!" Dave was smart with a sense of humor and a drive to help himself. It was easy to work with him. He checked in with his neurologist at the one- and two-week mark when he had to leave for the road trip. The neurologist pronounced him recovered enough to make the trip as long as he was careful. I was glad and worried. They carried all their own heavy gear and did all their own set up on a bumpy and strenuous two-month tour, traveling in a van with little headroom for Dave (who was over six feet tall). I asked him to phone me from the road if anything went wrong. All was quiet for a month. Then the call came.

"Dave, are you all right?"

"Yeah, neck is great. Our guitarist broke his ankle."

I asked when this happened and he said a week before. The ankle pain was getting worse fast and they were in a different city from the hospital where they were seen. "Find a hospital and make sure his cast is not too tight. Everything else okay?"

"Yeah, we're cool. The band is calling me 'the old man' because I keep getting on them about how they're lifting the equipment with their head forward."

How Long Does It Take to Stop Cervical (Neck) Disc Pain?

Using everything presented here, you could begin to feel the difference as soon as you try the two easy stretches—the pectoral stretch (Figure 1-9) and the trapezius stretch (Figure 1-10)—and apply them to reposition your head and upper body (Figure 1-4). Use the repositioning for everything you do. Even jobs that many people think

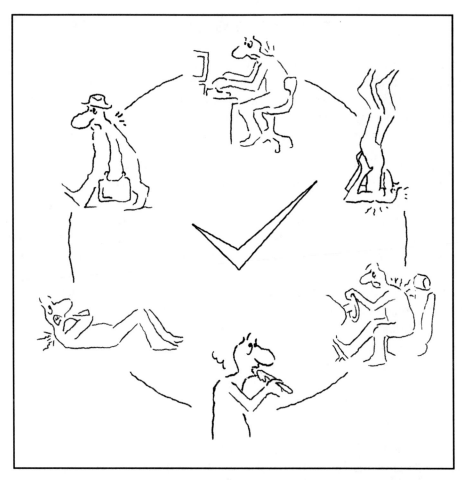

Figure 1-22. Sitting, standing, and living with your neck and head forward is a major cause of neck and upper-back pain, and can eventually push cervical (neck) discs outward (herniate them).

require craning the neck and upper back forward, such as playing the violin or other musical instruments, can be done with healthy positioning without sacrificing quality of the music.

It takes years to hurt a disc and only days for it to start healing once you no longer are injuring it. Stop damaging your muscles and discs with bad bending, standing, and sitting habits and you can heal. It is like learning any other new skill, and it will fix your neck pain—free. If you are not feeling better right away, check what you are doing compared to what you have read in this chapter. Make sure that something else isn't contributing to your pain. It is usually not difficult to start feeling better quickly and get your life back.

A Quick Overview of Osteoporosis

Three main sites of osteoporosis are the hip, wrist, and upper back. A main factor in osteoporosis is lack of exercise—no matter how much calcium you eat. The physical pull of muscle on bone during exercise makes bones thicken. Lack of exercise in youth can mean you do not build enough bone. In later years, lack of exercise leads to accelerated bone loss. Exercising, even late in life, can still build bone and stop loss.

A forward-rounded upper-body posture can increase risk of what are called crush fractures or wedge fractures. The front of the upper-spine vertebrae, already thin and weak from bone loss, crushes under body weight. The newly-compressed front of the bone gives it a wedged, triangular shape. The upper back rounds further. Regular exercise with healthy upper-body position, including upper-back extension exercise (Figure 1-15), can be important to avoiding this serious injury. It is not necessary to do forward rounding to get exercise. Instead of doing abdominal crunches, use the abdominal exercises in Chapter 2 that teach how to hold healthy position while getting more abdominal exercise than with crunches (Figures 2-30 through 3-38). Regularly check upper-back position with the wall stand (Figure 1-7) and lie on your back flat to make sure you are not developing or promoting a forward-rounding upper-back posture. Chapter 2 on lower-back pain has a section on hyperlordosis that shows how to strengthen the core and abdominal muscles without the forward rounding that can endanger an upper back compromised by osteoporosis.

Some prescription drugs reduce bone density, such as the anti-convulsant phenytoin (Dilantin), chemotherapy agents, prednisone (and other oral medicines called corticosteroids for rheumatoid arthritis), allergy, chronic obstructive pulmonary disease, and asthma, and others. Sadly, when periods stop in young women (amenorrhoea), the women are often told to stop exercising and are treated with corticosteroids—both of which decrease bone density. Exercise is beneficial to build bone density.

Nutrition to prevent osteoporosis is more than just eating calcium. Without enough vitamin D, calcium is not well used. Smoking and drinking alcohol are both directly toxic to bone cells. Antacids reduce calcium absorption. Antacids that contain aluminum increase calcium excretion. Excessive dietary phosphorous is bad for bones. Meat, cola drinks, and soda have high phosphorus content. Animal protein, even the animal protein in dairy, increases urinary calcium loss. Get protein from vegetables as much as possible. If you use protein powder, use vegetable powder without dairy or whey. Don't load up on unfermented soy in protein drinks, powders, bars, and commercial products. The high phytic acid content blocks minerals like zinc and calcium. Fermented soy, like tempeh, miso, natto, soy sauce, and tamari reduces phytic acid, and has benefits that unfermented soy does not have. Broccoli has more calcium per calorie than any other food. A cup of navy beans and two corn tortillas has more calcium than a cup of milk.

Spinach, seaweed, tofu, almonds, tahini, and sunflower seeds are high in calcium. Sesame seeds are high in calcium and have more iron, per ounce, than meat. Exercise lets you use more of the calcium you eat.

Analine took a stretch class. She was only 59, but was sick, thin, and weak from many medical troubles. Her thin back was already rounded stiffly. Her doctor wisely sent her for exercise. Analine and her husband enrolled at one of the adult continuing education classes on stretching. The young, cheerful teacher was certified through a major fitness organization. During the first class, they breathed deeply and bent over from a stand to touch their toes. They sat and bent forward to touch their toes. They brought chin to chest, and knees to chest, and sat on their knees, draping their body over the knees with the head to the floor in a position called "child's pose" (named for the way babies and young children often sleep). They sat with legs apart and leaned forward to each leg. They sat with knees bent out to the side and feet touching, rounding forward to bring head toward the feet. Each stretch came with the instruction not to force, to breathe, and to "listen to the body." At the end of class, while lying face down, they pushed up on hands "to stretch the other way." Analine's upper back stayed rounded forward. Then they stood and brought one arm over the front of the body to stretch the back of the shoulder, then the other arm, and bent over from a stand to the floor one more time "to relax." They hugged themselves to end class.

The next week, Analine's husband came alone to class. He thanked the teacher, saying Analine wanted the teacher to know how much she enjoyed class. She was looking forward to coming back, but was home resting after suffering "unexplained" crush fractures at home. He was in class to learn what we did so he could show her at home. How do I know all this happened? Because I was sitting next to Analine in class and was standing with the other students at the beginning of the second class when her husband came in alone. I hadn't said anything through the whole first class. I was trying to avoid many of the stretches for myself without annoying the teacher. But I hadn't wanted to intrude on another teacher's class and be rude by stopping Analine. It still haunts me.

What Else to Check

Sometimes the cause of neck pain comes from common medications: cholesterol-lowering medicines called statins, some prescription allergy medicines, prescription acid reduction medicines, erectile enhancing drugs, the calcium channel-blocker drug

---

verapamil, the antibiotics erythromycin and clarithromycin, some HIV medications, some anti-anxiety and antidepressant medicines, prescriptions for constipation and irritable bowel, and others. It used to be thought that muscle and joint pain only came with overdose. It is now known that body and joint pain is a common side effect of these drugs. Doing a few stretches does not change that. It is better to solve the cause of the original problem than take drugs that cause new problems.

Check with your doctor to make sure that neck pain is not from the less common causes of cancer, infection, thyroid problems, inflammation of the esophagus, meningitis, fractures, or problems with blood supply.

What to Do Every Day to Stop Neck and Upper-Back Pain

- Before getting out of bed in the morning, don't sit on the bed rounding your back. Lie face down. Prop gently on elbows, not so high that it strains (Figure 1-16). Make sure the upper-back stretches backward; don't keep rounding forward. It should feel good and help you straighten out. Keep the neck straight (not pinched back), with your chin in, lifting from the front of the chest. Get out of bed without sitting.

- Do the pectoral stretch and the trapezius stretch (Figures 1-9 and 1-10) to establish healthy muscle length. Then you can stand in a comfortable straight position throughout the day without being so tight that you are pulled into bad posture, or having to strain for good positioning.

- Check yourself during the day with the wall stand test (Figure 1-7). Use walls, elevators, and doorways.

- Double-chin exercise (Figure 1-4). Pull your chin inward without straining your neck or arching your back. Keep the new, healthy position all the time, which will be easy and more natural after learning the stretches and principles in this chapter. Don't make it stiff or forced, since doing so will only increase neck and shoulder tension.

- Lie on your back to relearn what straight position feels like. If you can't lie comfortably without a pillow under your head, your neck and chest are tight. The pectoral and trapezius stretches (Figures 1-9 and 1-10) should restore needed length to lie flat comfortably. If rounding is serious, use a pillow if necessary, gradually decreasing the size of the pillow over days of restoring muscle length with the pectoral and trapezius stretches. Don't lie flat if pain worsens or goes down your arm.

- Upper-body extension (Figure 1-15). Lie face down. Lift arms and upper body. Gently lower. Contract upper-back and shoulder-blade muscles. Try three to five to start. See how you feel, and then increase. Work up to at least 10 to 20 at a time.

- If shoulder tightness contributes to neck and upper-body pain, read Chapter 3. Try the shoulder/scapula mobilizer (Figure 3-12). Hold arms outstretched in front with elbows straight. Curl shoulders forward as if trying to touch your shoulders together in front, gently, without bending your elbows. Then arch backward as if trying to touch shoulders together in back—again, without bending elbows. Make the shoulders move a lot. Alternate back and forth a few times to loosen (mobilize), and determine where neutral posture is. Then repeat this with hands against wall to practice preventing stiffness and stress while driving and computer use.
- Use a hand mirror to see your profile sideways in a big mirror. Notice your neck positioning. Reposition to a healthy, relaxed position with your chin in.
- Retrain your exercise habits and mindset away from conventional exercises that curl the neck and upper back forward for stretching and strengthening.
- Walk lightly when walking, moving, and taking the stairs. Use muscles for shock absorption instead of clumping each foot down heavily.
- Don't just "do exercises." Learn the principles of healthy neck placement and apply them to all you do. Instead of memorizing "rules" and buying expensive ergonomic chairs, pillows, and beds, make healthy motion part of your enjoyable life.
- Watch other people's head and neck tilt when they drive, sit, exercise, talk on the phone, eat, and walk. You may easily see where their neck and upper-back pain is coming from.

Computer, Desk, Driving, and Television

- Raise your computer monitor if it is too low. Use a low shelf or phone books.
- Move the keyboard off the "below desk" tray and back up on the desk.
- Raise your television up higher. Stop sitting hunched over and forward to watch.
- Move desk and car seats closer in. Sit leaning back, not forward. How are you sitting right now?
- See the section on healthy sitting in Chapter 2 (Figures 2-45 through 2-57).

What to Avoid

- Omit sit-ups, "crunches," and forward bending exercises. These exercises add to an already over-rounded back and neck. The section on lordosis in Chapter 2 gives better abdominal exercises (Figures 2-30 through 3-39). Chapter 9 provides effective hamstring stretches that don't force the back and neck into rounded position.

- Don't droop or jut your head and neck forward when sitting and standing—which doesn't mean to never look down, or to force your head back into straight position. It means not to flop the weight of your head forward onto the joints of your neck. Keep your chin in, lightly, without strain, including when looking up and down.

- When you pull your chin in, don't do it by arching your back. The postural change needs to come from your upper body, not by creating another strain on another part.

- Avoid neck circles. The neck bones aren't shaped to roll. Don't pull your neck to the side with your hands, which compresses the spine instead of stretching the muscles. Instead, use the trapezius stretch (Figure 1-10).

- Don't stretch so that it hurts, pinches, or strains. Stretch to where it feels good and releases tightness.

- Don't think you have to live your life "on eggshells," constantly holding yourself rigidly straight. Restricting movement to limit pain isn't healthy and isn't fun.

When to Notice Necks and Upper Back

- Common times for uncomfortable jutting neck position are when drinking, looking upward, reaching upward, kissing, looking downward, eating, sitting, bicycling, putting on contact lenses and makeup, sitting in a car or bus wearing a wide brimmed hat, playing a musical instrument, and brushing teeth. Keep chin in softly without strain.

- When you lie on your back without a pillow under your head, does your head crane backward or your chin jut upward? If you are too tight to lie flat, you are too tight to stand up straight without the poor neck positioning that adds to neck pain. Use the pectoral stretch and the trapezius stretch (Figures 1-9 and 1-10) to reestablish healthy muscle resting length.

How to Get Natural Neck and Upper-Back Exercise from Daily Activity

- Stand and move all the time without letting the upper back round forward and you will exercise the muscles and prevent your upper body from getting straight in the first place.

- Hold your upper-body weight up on your muscles, not slumped down on your neck and upper-back joints. It's free exercise.

- Sit without rounding. It may be natural to let your weight sag, but it is also "natural" to wet your pants. Learn healthy comfortable control.

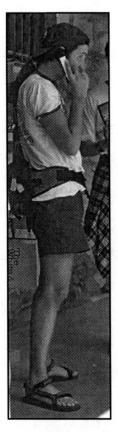

Figure 1-23. Notice if you jut your neck forward in everyday activity. Healthy position in real life is the key to a pain-free neck—not just doing exercises.

No More Neck and Upper-Back Pain

Neck and upper-back pain are not mysterious "conditions." Many people spend their day sitting, working, walking, and driving in rounded position, hunching over the computer, lifting and bending wrong all day, walking so heavily that they jar their neck with each step, then exercise and stretch bent over forward. Many people do physical therapy or exercises, but are not aware that stronger muscles will not automatically give good positioning, make you stand and move properly, or make up for all the things you do the rest of the day to hurt your neck. It is no wonder that people have pain even though they "do their exercises."

Many people want pills, shots, treatments, and even surgery, to relieve the pain, but don't simply hold their own head up. Neck and upper-back pain are easy to understand and fix yourself. Instead of doing a bunch of rehabilitation exercises and then going back to injurious habits, stop the pain by no longer damaging yourself with unhealthy mechanics. Then you will have no need for pills or surgery, and your neck can heal. Good positioning burns calories, strengthens, and is a free, natural workout. How is your neck and upper-back positioning right now? Use your muscles to stand, sit, and bend in healthy, comfortable position for all daily life.

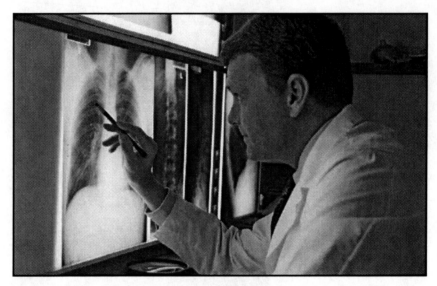

Figure 1-24. Can you tell the cause of the neck pain in this photo? (Hint: The pain isn't in the person in the x-ray).

2

No More Lower-Back Pain

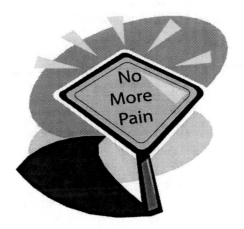

- Muscular Lower-Back Pain
- Herniated Disc
- Sciatica
- Hyperlordosis
- Swayback
- Facet Pain
- Spondylolisthesis
- Stenosis
- Long Sitting, Lifting, and Carrying

Back pain is often made to seem like a mysterious, long-term condition that you need special devices and beds, uncomfortable exercise plans, restrictions on activity, and medicines or surgery to relieve. Many people are told to stop their favorite activities and to accept pain and ongoing treatments as part of life. A cycle of pain, unhappiness, and reduced activity continues, which is tragic because most back pain is simple and easy to reverse. The good news is that back pain is not a normal part of getting older. It's not because we walk upright on two legs or as a result of simply bending wrong one day. Bed rest and inactivity can make back pain worse. Abdominal crunches are not a good remedy for back pain. Surgery is almost never needed. Muscular lower-back pain can start subsiding as soon as you begin the simple principles in this chapter. You don't need to "learn to live with pain."

Muscular Lower-Back Pain

Bill came to me with the story I hear almost every day. "I do crunches and stretch my hamstrings every day but my back is still killing me." Bill had been to physical therapy, "work hardening," a pain clinic, massage therapy, Pilates class, chiropractors, and was getting acupuncture. His pain would come and go, year after year. He bought a special chair with lumbar support for his desk and an expensive adjustable mattress. His x-rays were normal except for some arthritis, for which his doctor prescribed over-the-counter anti-inflammatory drugs for everyday use, and a prescription "for bad days." "They told me I had to live with this just like everyone else. I'm just getting older."

Bill described his several visits to the orthopedist, neurologist, and a specialist called a physiatrist (fizz-EYE-a-trist), which is a physician of physical medicine and rehabilitation (PMR). They checked his muscle strength by pressing the inside and outside of each leg, then the top and bottom.

"They said my strength is in normal limits," Bill told me. "But I know it is worse than it used to be. I used to be in shape, but this pain is taking its toll. I can't do things like I used to. They wanted to see how far I could bend over. They said my hamstrings were tight, and gave me hamstring stretches. They had me lift my legs while lying down. They measured my leg length. It seemed that they did a lot. They sent me to physical therapy. There I did the same crunches and hamstring stretches I do anyway, but the heat and cold packs felt nice. They taught me a stretch where I bring my knees to my chest while lying on my back, then bend my knees to each side. They showed me another stretch to do after sitting for long periods where I bend over in the chair with my chest over my knees. They said that no one knows what causes back pain or how to fix it, so just try to say active. I try but how can I when it hurts like this? They said to get a firmer bed. Do you know what those things cost? They asked me a lot about my emotional state and if I wanted to talk to a support group or a shrink. When my insurance ran out, they told me there wasn't any more they could do for me."

I asked Bill to move a trashcan out of the way for us. He bent right over from a stand and lifted it. I asked Bill to show me how he stretched and exercised. "First I stretch," he said. He bent over from a stand with straight legs to touch his toes. Then he bent over from the waist to pick up his dumbbells and lifted the weights in a bent-over position to show me the rows for his back. Then he bent over with straight legs to put the weights down again. He sat on the floor and bent his hip, lifting his legs from the floor. "Here is my Pilates. It's supposed to strengthen my core." He stood and bent over to pick up his shoes, then flopped down heavily in his chair and leaned forward. "I do everything, and have been to everyone, and no one knows why my back hurts."

How You Get Muscular Lower-Back Pain

You know you shouldn't bend wrong, but you do it. Every day. All day. Bending over from the waist and hip puts hundreds of pounds of pressure on your lower back, no matter whether you keep your back straight or round. You bend over wrong picking up socks, petting the dog, for laundry, trash, making the bed, looking in the refrigerator, picking up shoes, and all the dozens (even hundreds) of times you bend every day (Figure 2-1). You work bent over your desk or bench. You drive bent forward. If you go to the gym you probably lift weights bent over, stretch by touching your toes, exercise by crunching forward, then bend over wrong to pick up your gym bag to go home. No wonder your back hurts.

People often try to stay active to help their back but do activities with unhealthy bending habits (Figure 2-2).

Many of the common exercises people do for their back are more forward bending, like toe touches and crunches. They may do back rehab exercises but not be aware that strong muscles will not automatically make you sit or bend in healthy ways, or make up for all the things you do the rest of the day on the job and home to hurt your back (Figure 2-3). On exam, the diagnosis is often written off as "stress." They wonder why they still get pain even though they "do their exercises." Many people with back pain wind up in surgery, or long-term pain, not understanding why their physical therapy or exercise program, or pills, or yoga "didn't work."

The relentless pull of bad mechanical use of your body every day will eventually strain, squash, tear, degenerate, and injure you in the same way that parts in your car that are rubbing, tilting, or not seating properly will cause early wear and tear. Many people won't stand, sit, and bend properly even knowing this will fix most (or even all)

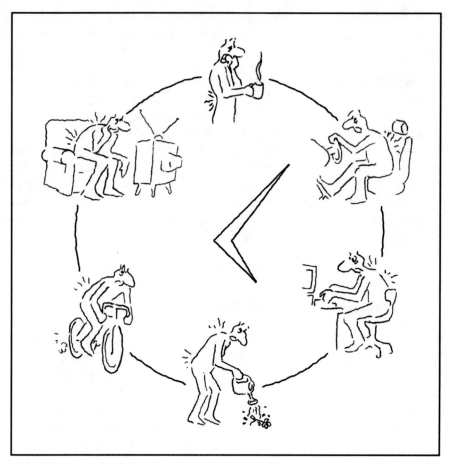

Figure 2-1. Most people bend with damaging position many times every day. It is a common cause of back pain.

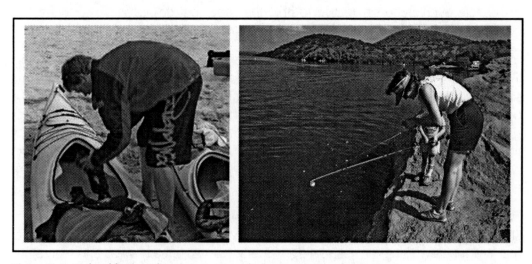

Figure 2-2. Unhealthy bending is common during recreational activities.

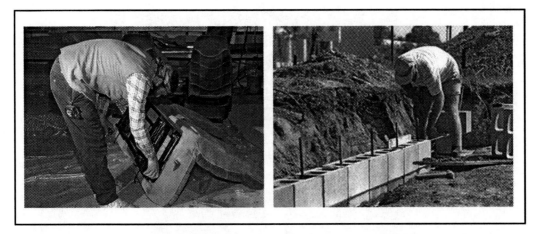

Figure 2-3. Back-pain programs commonly include strengthening exercise but strengthening doesn't make you bend properly, which is why many strength programs fail to stop pain.

of their pain. First, they don't like this idea. Slouching is easier than using muscles to support your body. Next, most people are so tight and weak that they can't stand or bend properly; it doesn't feel natural. Many people are so tight that standing up straight hurts. A third and unfortunate reason is that bad posture is so pervasive that people think it is normal, even desirable or "cool" to stand and bend with poor positioning, or that posture doesn't matter much (Figure 2-4).

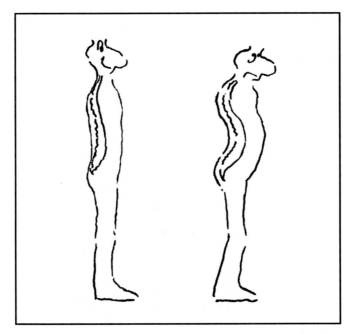

Figure 2-4. Unhealthy positioning is often thought of as normal, relaxed, even cute or desirable, rather than harmful.

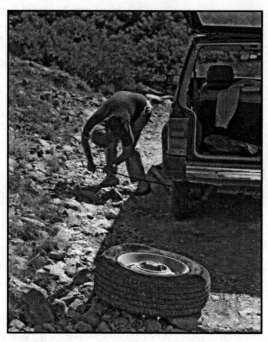

Figure 2-5

If you can't stand with your back against a wall with your heels, hips, upper back and the back of your head comfortably touching, without raising your chin or arching your back, you are too tight to stand up straight. After spending so much time bent forward, it is no wonder that people get too tight to straighten out. In turn, the tight, weak muscles pull you into slouching positions, further tightening and weakening your muscles.

Bill didn't want to hear about "that posture nonsense."

"My doctor told me that good posture was fine and good but wouldn't stop my back pain. Why should it? It only makes my back hurt more to stand up straight anyway." I told him it was true that the way many people strained, arched, and tensed to stand "straight" made more pain.

I showed Bill how he was too tight to stand straight with his back against the wall (Figure 1-7). His head and upper back were forward of the wall, his thumbs pointed inward at each other because of his rounded shoulders (Figure 1-8). "Man, I look like I'm still sitting in my recliner at home. I stand like a gorilla," he said. I agreed that most people bent forward all day, sat bent, and rarely straighten out. I told him that the stretches and exercises I would show him wouldn't just stretch or strengthen, but would retrain his muscles so that he could stand and move with healthy positioning. That's the difference between straining to stand awkwardly straight (and calling that "straight posture"), and being able to move in healthy, comfortable ways.

I took a wooden ruler between my hands and started to bend it so much that it looked like it would snap. Bill stared at the bend in the ruler.

"Where will it break?" I asked.

"Right where you're bending it, of course."

"Bill, this is your back."

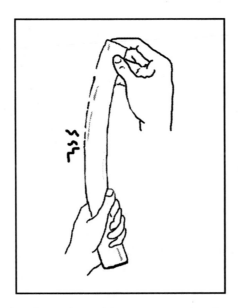

Figure 2-6. When you bend a piece of wood between your hands, you can see which area will be strained to the breaking point. Can you imagine the same thing happening when you sit and bend with your back rounded?

Exercises for Muscular Lower-Back Pain

Back-pain exercises are misunderstood. People often injure their back all day then hope to fix it with a few exercises. They don't understand when this does not work. They lie on the floor to do exercises and then stand up and walk away with no use of the positioning or strength they just practiced. It is like eating butter and sugar all day, then doing ten minutes of exercises and wondering why it doesn't 'work." Plenty of muscular people have terrible posture and lifting habits and the back pain that comes with it. Strengthening and stretching are crucial but not the whole answer. The key to back exercises is using them to retain how you position your back all the rest of the day.

Squat

You know not to bend wrong to pick things up, but you do it—every day, hundreds of times a day. Instead, bend your knees. You already know that. But most people won't bend right because their legs are too weak or they bend in ways that hurts their knees. Bending right keeps your body weight off the knee joint and on the thigh and hip muscles, strengthening the musculature, which helps the knee. Properly done, the squat retrains bending habits and gives you free leg and back exercise at the same time during all the many things you need to bend and lift (Figure 2-7).

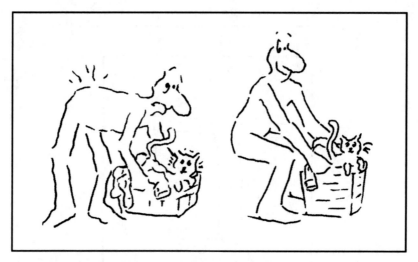

Figure 2-7. Instead of bending wrong and making your back hurt (left), get free leg exercise by bending in a healthy way (right). Keep heels down and your weight back to protect back and knees. Don't stick your behind out.

Many people won't bend right to save their back because it hurts their knees. Keep your weight back toward your heels, not forward through your knee.

- Keep heels down. Shift your weight back to your heels.
- Keep your knees back over your feet, not forward of the feet. When you bend your knees, look down and see if you can see your toes. If you can't because your knees are in the way, your knees are forward.
- Don't let your behind stick out in back when bending. Keep hip tucked under, but not so much that you round your back. Stay straight.
- Use a mirror to practice positioning until it becomes a normal bending habit.

Figure 2-8 shows the concepts of healthy squatting and Figure 2-9 shows how to apply it in real life.

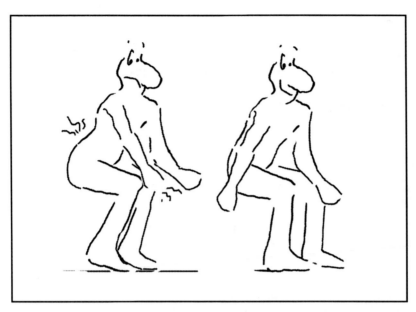

Figure 2-8. Don't let knees come forward, heels lift, or your behind stick out with your back arched (left). Keep knees back, heels down and weight on heels. Keep hip tucked under until your back is straight (right).

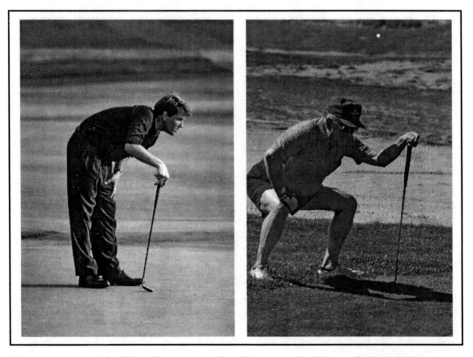

Figure 2-9. Instead of bending over and making your back hurt (left), bending knees is good for your back and strengthens knees (right). Keep weight back toward your heels to keep knees from coming forward.

Standing Lunge

Another healthy way to bend for all the many times you bend every day is to lunge with one leg in front and the other in back (Figure 2-10). Instead of doing ten lunges as an exercise, then going back to bending badly all day, use the lunge along with the squat for all the times you bend. Don't hold yourself rigidly. Bend right as a comfortable habit.

- Stand up with your feet apart.

- Slide one foot comfortably back, keeping foot straight not turned out.

- Bend knees to lower enough to retrieve objects from the floor. Keep your torso upright easily, not stiffly. If this is too much, start with dipping a few inches.

- Don't let your front knee come forward. Keep front knee over ankle. If your front knee comes forward, it will send your weight through your knee joint.

- Don't stick your behind out in back.

- To use the standing lunge as a hip stretch and leg strengthener, keep the upper body completely upright, not leaning forward to back. Tuck the hip to prevent the behind from sticking out in back. Dip toward the floor up and down many times (Figures 3-6 and 4-6). Increase the exercise by holding hand weights. When you put the weights back down, don't bend over wrong. Use the lunge you just practiced.

The lunge can be a great exercise to strengthen your legs and practice healthy bending. You already know you should use your legs like this to bend and lift. Now you will be strong enough to do it.

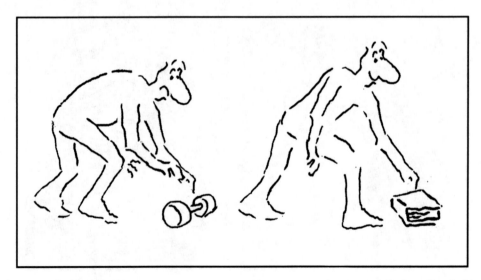

Figure 2-10. Use the lunge, not as an exercise to do 10 times, but as a daily bending habit. Don't round your back or let your front knee come forward (left). Keep your torso as upright as you can, with back straight and front knee over ankle (right).

Upper-Back Extension

Upper-back extension is an important exercise to strengthen your back at the same time that you practice moving your back in the other direction (Figures 2-11a and 2-11b). Upper-back extension contracts overstretched back muscles and unloads vertebral discs, which are pressured outward by forward bending.

- Lie face down on the floor, or a bed or bench if that is easier.
- Lift hands and arms up, holding them at your sides or wherever comfortable.
- Gently lift upper body without hands. Don't force.
- Keep your neck straight. Don't crane. Just lift using upper body muscles.
- Progress to lifting your upper body with arms held out to the side, then up in front of you (Figure 2-11b). Roll your shoulders back and use the upper-back musculature.

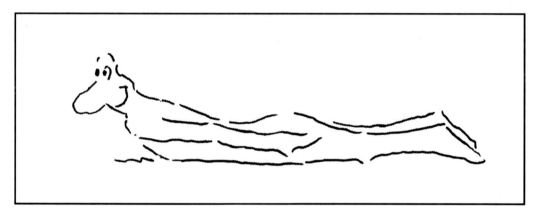

Figure 2-11a. Upper-back extension

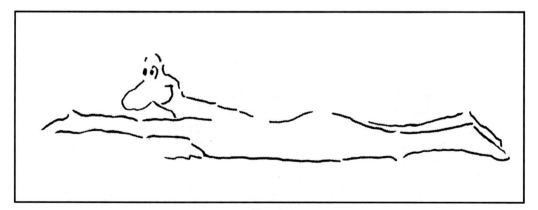

Figure 2-11b. Upper-back extension with arms out in front

Lower-Back Extension

Lower-back extension is another important exercise to strengthen the back and practice extending the hip (Figure 2-12). Lower-back extension unloads the discs that are pressured outward by forward bending.

- Lie face down, hands under your chin or wherever comfortable.
- Gently lift both legs and keep your knees straight.
- Don't yank or force. Don't pinch the lower back. Just use the lower-body muscles.

My patients often ask me if there is a special belt or device they can wear that will stick them or signal them when they bend or exercise wrong. I tell them they already have one—it's called their back. If they have pain, it is a good signal that something is not right. They can use this helpful warning to stop damaging themselves before they make things worse.

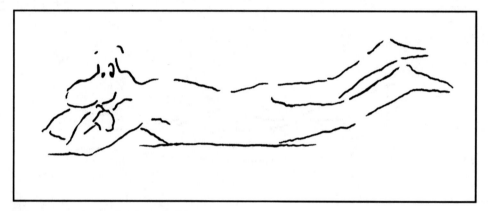

Figure 2-12. Lower-back extension

Maura was a bodybuilder with back pain. "They told me to strengthen my abs. Can you believe this joke? I already do 500 crunches a day." She was glorious with muscles and probably could bench press the doctor. She was also doing straight-legged dead lifting, and an exercise called "good mornings"—both of which involve bending over with straight legs and lifting a heavy weight. Maura told me she does them to work her back and leg muscles. I explained to her that it is true it works the muscles, but at the price of slowly (or quickly) harming the lower back.

"Maura, you know not to bend wrong to pick up a package. It doesn't become magically healthy by calling it dead lifting."

"No," she said. "I tighten my abs to protect my back to do it. And I keep my back straight."

I explained, "Unfortunately, as much as we all used to hope that would work, it doesn't as much as hoped. Using back muscles to lift upward instead of rounding helps keep pressure off the discs, but your lower back is still the lever point of hundreds of pounds of pressure from your upper body alone. Adding your barbells is compounding the injury. It works the muscles, but pushes the discs and other structures outward. I can show you the math of how the leverage works to multiply the forces on the lower back where it pivots, it's simple enough." Maura didn't want to see the charts and math.

I told Maura it didn't mean she had to giving up lifting. I would show her other exercises that would make her able to lift and do more than before. In weightlifting competitions, what is called the dead lift is not done bending over with straight legs, but with upright torso and bent knees. Straight-legged dead lifting and "good mornings" are examples of something that "works" in one way but still has unhealthy effects. Like smoking to lose weight, they "work," but are unhelpful for other reasons. Often several factors go into evaluating the overall worth of an exercise. I gave her extension exercises (Figures 2-11 and 2-12) that would contract her back muscles without the forward bending that was making them hurt so much. By bending right for household activities, she would get the equivalent of doing hundreds of lunges and squats a day. Her legs would look great and get a more sleek, athletic, and symmetrical look from the natural exercise than from isolated and artificial gym exercises.

Maura told me that previously the pain was a miserable aching from the strained muscles, but had recently added a new feeling of pressure. We had caught her just as she was beginning to herniate a disc.

What to Do Every Day to Stop Lower-Back Pain

- First thing in the morning, don't sit on the bed. Instead, turn face down (Figure 1-16). Prop low on elbows. Don't push so high that it strains. It should feel good and help you start the day straightened out. Keep neck straight, not craned or pinched backward. Stretch back through the upper back, not just folding the lower back. Get out of bed without sitting.

- Right after getting out of bed, do the pectoral (chest) stretch and the trapezius stretch (Figures 1-9 and 1-10). These stretches help you start the day standing straight so that you don't go around bent forward. The gentle side-to-side bending of the trapezius stretch helps discs heal by moving oxygen in and wastes out.

- During the day, check your standing position using the wall stand (Figure 1-7).

- Upper-body (upper-back) extension (Figures 2-11 and 2-11a). Lie face down. Lift upper body and gently lower. Try three to five lifts to start. See how you feel, then increase. Work up to at least 10 to 20 at a time.

- Lower-body (lower-back) extension (Figure 2-12). Lie face down. Lift legs, keep knees straight, and gently lower. If lifting both legs is too much, try one at a time. Progress to both. Contract back and behind muscles. Try three to five to start. See how you feel, then increase. Work up to at least 10 to 20.

- Squat or lunge for every time you lift and bend, Figures 2-7 and 2-10. Keep torso upward and shoulders back. Don't use bad knees as an excuse to wreck your back. Bending right strengthens knees. Chapter 5 gives more fun and healthy bending techniques that help knees.

- Raise your computer monitor up if it is too low. Use a shelf or phone books.

- Move the keyboard off the tray below the desk back up on the desk.

- Move your television higher. Stop rounding your back to watch.

- Move desk and car seats closer in. Sit back, not forward. Don't worry about having to keep feet on the floor or hold your body at specific angles. Just get the concept of healthy back positioning.

- Hold a push-up position (Figure 2-33). If you can't comfortably hold a straight body position without sagging, your back muscles are so weak and untrained that it is no wonder that you sag and hurt when walking around all day.

- Don't just "do exercises." Make healthy motion part of your enjoyable life.

What to Avoid

- Avoid exercises that add to rounding and tightening in the forward position. Omit sit-ups, "crunches," leg lifts to the front, and forward-rounding hamstring stretches.

- Don't round forward to carry a backpack or other load. Use your muscles to stand straight.

- When you sit down, don't flop in your seat. Use leg muscles to decelerate and sit lightly. It's free leg exercise.

- Don't complain that moving right is work. It's free exercise. It's like learning any other new skill, and will fix your lower back pain at no charge.

When to Notice Your Lower Back

- The most common times to round the lower back are when sitting and bending. Watch other people's back positioning at work and home. Watch in the gym when they are doing exercise for their "health." See where their lower back pain is coming from.

- Count how many times you bend each day. For most people, it is many dozens (even hundreds) of times. Imagine the injury to your back by bending wrong that many times each day.

- Stand sideways to look in a mirror at your positioning. Use a hand mirror to see yourself in the big mirror.

No More Muscular Lower-Back Pain

The majority of muscular lower-back pain is the result of unhealthy standing, sitting, and bending habits that accumulate damage over time without your feeling it, just as smoking one cigarette at a time eventually can cause trouble. Even when pain comes suddenly, or starts after an accident, pain was almost always brewing from many simple bad habits. The sudden onset is like a heart attack developing over years that suddenly occurs with one more aggravation. Stop the cause of the injury, and you can prevent and stop the pain that results. Just as after a sprained ankle, you can heal from back pain without surgery and regain your life, better than before.

Sciatica, Degenerating Discs, and Herniated (Slipped) Discs

A herniated (or "bad") disc, or pain down the leg (sciatica), can be painful and frightening. Despite the fact that herniated (slipped) discs, degenerating discs, and sciatica usually can heal quickly and easily, people are often told it is a difficult and long-term condition. They are told to accept and live with pain and reduced ability. They may stay on pain and anti-inflammatory drugs for long periods. Their pain comes and goes even after acupuncture, strengthening, therapy, surgery, massage, and chiropractic. It is common to hear that back pain is mysterious and that no one knows why discs herniate or why sciatica occurs. However, disc pain is usually simple to understand and fix, without surgery, prescription medications, repeated treatments, or special beds and equipment. Disc injury is not a life sentence. Disc degeneration or slippage (herniation) can heal and stop hurting, if you let it, no differently than a sprained ankle. Stop damaging your discs with bad bending, standing, and sitting habits and your discs can heal. It takes years to herniate a disc, and only days to weeks to let it heal it by using the techniques in this section.

Mike was sent to me by his yoga teacher. They had tried for months to stop his pain with stretches, exercises, deep breathing, herbs, four kinds of massage, acupuncture, and meditation. He had been diagnosed with a herniated (slipped) disc. His doctor told him that nothing could help a disc except surgery. Mike described it as a ball of pain and pressure right in the buttock. It spread over his hip, sometimes so painfully that he could feel the outline of his hipbones. It went down one leg in a hot, thin line. He hurt most in the morning, but the pain didn't stop enough during the day to give relief. Sitting hurt more than standing. He wanted to play basketball again but couldn't even cough without pain. He had heard that once he had a disc injury, he would always have trouble, and that no one knew why discs herniate. I told him that doesn't have to be true. Just like other injuries, this injury was not a condition or disease, but an injury and could heal.

What Are Discs?

Vertebral discs are tough, fibrous cushions between each of your vertebrae (back bones). You also have two discs in each knee. A knee disc is commonly called a meniscus. You even have a little disc between your lower and upper jawbone at your temporo-mandibular joint (TMJ). Discs are living parts of your body. They do many things, like absorb shock and keep your bones from grinding against each other. They are not much like soft jelly donuts, as commonly said. The outer covering of your discs is tough and fibrous and firmly attached in between each vertebra. It doesn't easily slide around. That's a good thing, since discs take a lot of pounding. But after many years of bad bending and lifting, they can finally start to fray and break down.

How Discs Herniate

The pressure of your own body weight unevenly distributed on your discs over years of rounded sitting, standing, and bending habits is enough to injure them as badly as a single accident. Years of forward rounding from slouching, bad lifting, and bending squashes and degenerates your discs in front and pushes them outward toward the back. The discs eventually break down (degenerate) and push outward (herniate or slip) (Figure 2-13). Think of braces on your teeth. After years of pushing, things eventually move.

Chronic forward bending (flexion) from rounded lifting and sitting also overstretches the muscles and long ligament down the back, which weakens the back and makes more room for vertebral discs to protrude (Figure 2-14).

Mike had done all the usual things that herniate a disc. He sat bent forward hours a day at his desk, he bent over from a stand to do laundry, feed the dog, pick up around the house, and for dozens of daily activities. At the gym, he bent over to pick up his weights, did straight-legged dead lifting, bent wrong to put the weights back down, then bent over from a stand to touch his toes in yoga class (Figure 2-16). The exercises the yoga teacher gave him for his pain matched the ones given by his own doctor: stretch hamstrings by sitting bent forward to touch his toes. They said that to balance the bending forward, he should lie on his back and bring knees to chest. This is not the opposite of bending forward. It is more bending forward at the hip and back. I worked with

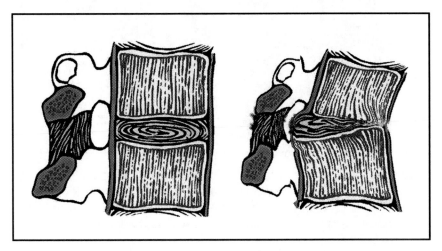

Figure 2-13. On the left is a side view of a normal disc between two vertebrae. On the right is a disc that has been pushed outward (slipped or herniated) from years of bad forward bending.

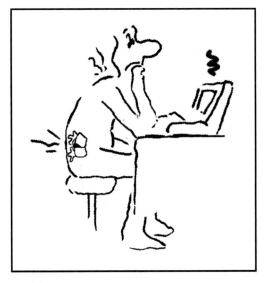

Figure 2-14. Like sitting on the front of a balloon, squeezing it in front makes it bulge out the back. Forward bending gradually pushes discs outward, which is the herniation process.

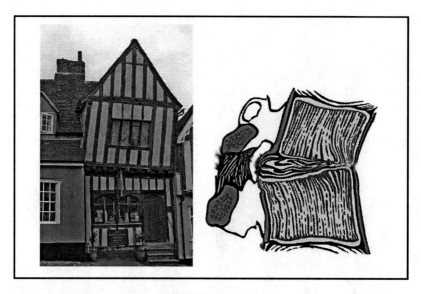

Figure 2-15. Sitting with lower back bent forward pressures the discs in the lower back until they can eventually push outward enough to degenerate and herniate. It is easy to see the forces pushing structures outward in a tilting house (left). Can you imagine it in your own back (right)?

Mike to help him understand that years of forward bending had pushed the disc out of place. He said that his back never hurt when he was doing those exercises before. I told him it was like smoking and eating junk—the damage accumulated over time. In between each time that Mike abused his back with bad bending and lifting, his back was industriously trying to repair the harm. It would have been great if it hurt each time to warn him but the body is strong and uncomplaining until you damage it more than it can repair. Mike said he had heard that all it takes is a sneeze to herniate a disc. He thought discs were so fragile and that he would always be in peril from the slightest move. Now he understood that discs were tough workers that only give out from a sneeze after years of being beaten into it.

Mike asked why it hurt so much first thing in the morning. I explained that overnight your discs have been trying to heal after getting pushed out of place all day. They absorb moisture and plump back up compared to the compression they get all day under your body weight. That's why you're taller first thing in the morning. Astronauts get a little taller in space without gravity compressing each disc in their spine. Since a herniated disc is already swollen and occupying space that doesn't belong to it, the extra plumping up pushes more on surrounding nerves, making it hurt more in the morning. That was why it was so important not to sit rounded on the bed, but to lie face down propped on elbows. The discs have just healed a bit overnight. You don't want to undo the gain by doing the bent forward posture that pushes them out in the first place.

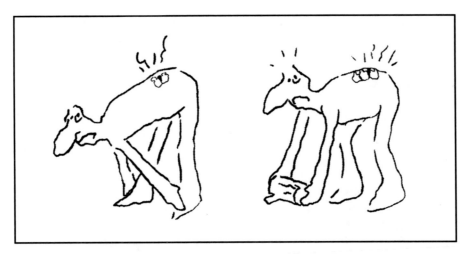

Figure 2-16. Forward bending to stretch or lift weights may feel good and work the muscles, but pressures discs outward.

I showed Mike the upper-back extension and lower-back extension exercises (Figures 2-11 and 2-12). I asked him to hold off on doing forward bending for the week and just do extension exercises. Then we'd see how he was doing. He phoned the next day to say he was feeling better. Mike felt encouraged that he could stop injuring his discs and that they could heal.

At the one-week check-in, Mike said that he had first gotten better but was worse again and didn't understand it. We went over everything he was doing. After much talking, it turned out that Mike did his extension exercises then went back to all the forward bending exercises because he thought that "more would be better" and he had to do "both sides." I reminded him that discs don't like to be pressured to the back. He needed to give the disc a chance to heal first. He said he understood and was confident he knew what to do, even though he thought the extension exercises were hard. His back muscles were not used to contracting to the back. I checked with him the next day and he was better. Several days later he phoned saying it was all "gone to heck," as bad as when we began.

"Mike, are you bending over when you walk around or to lift weights?"

"No," he assured me. We went over the list. Again it turned out that he was doing hamstring stretches several times a day by sitting and leaning forward, and of course, his yoga by bending over from a stand.

"Mike, remember that study I told you about? The one they did in 1964 that stuck electrodes in people's discs and found that the highest stress you can put on them is to stand and bend over, and the other highest stress you can put on discs is to sit leaning forward?"

"Yeah, I know. But I read that stretching your hamstrings helps your back."

"Mike is it helping?" There was silence. I asked him, "Mike are you bending forward right now? Where are you?" The background noise and his on and off silence was strange.

"I'm on the freeway."

"Mike, hang up. Call back when you're not driving. And stop driving hunching forward."

A week later Mike called and said the pain was almost gone, except in the morning. I asked him if he were turning over to face down instead of sitting. He assured me that he was. With further questions, I found he was then lying down and pulling his knees to his chest. "Mike, why are you pushing your discs back out again, especially first thing in the morning? He replied that it was common knowledge to bring knees to chest first thing in the morning to fix back pain. I told him that was not for disc pain. He promised to omit that one and just turn face down.

Three days later, Mike called saying he was completely pain free, except when he sat. We went over again how sitting bent forward, rounding forward, and flopping down into his chair dozens of times a day with no deceleration from his legs was forcefully compressing and jarring his discs. "Mike, use your muscles. Are you using the lumbar roll?" (See Figure 2-50.) He said he was. When we investigated that further, he was keeping the roll on his chair, but rounding against it (Figure 2-52). Many chair backs are rounded and, if you relax against the back of these chairs, you will sit rounded. The point of the roll is to pad the space in the chair so that you sit up, leaning your shoulders back above the roll, not rounding against the roll. The section on long sitting later in this chapter explains more. We were able to whittle down injurious factors week by week. I started him on lunges, push-ups, and other exercises to get him doing real movement again. He was worried that he might start to hurt again. I told him he knew what to check for if he did.

Mike called a week later and asked if drinking vinegar cured disc pain. I told him it didn't that I knew of. He said that his nutritionist told him to try it the day before and he hasn't hurt since then. I asked when was the last time he hurt before that. He said the previous week. "Mike, don't forget that you've been working to fix your pain. It's common to try many things out of desperation. When pain goes away, if a black cat walked in front of you, you'd think it was the cat, or if you ate an apple you'd think it was the apple. That's how 'snake oil' cures get sold."

"Oh," he said. "Do apples work, too?"

What Does L-4, L-5, and S-1 Mean?

To know which disc is which, we name them. You have five lower-back bones, called lumbar vertebrae. The names of the lower-back bones are L-1 ("L" stands for lumbar), L-2, L-3, L-4, and L-5. The first vertebra of your sacrum is S-1. The disc between your last lumbar vertebra and your sacrum is named "L-5, S-1" because it's the disc between those two bones. Your disc named "L-4, L-5" is the one between the last two lumbar vertebrae. You hear about these two discs more than others because those are the two where people usually put the most stress with bad bending and sitting habits.

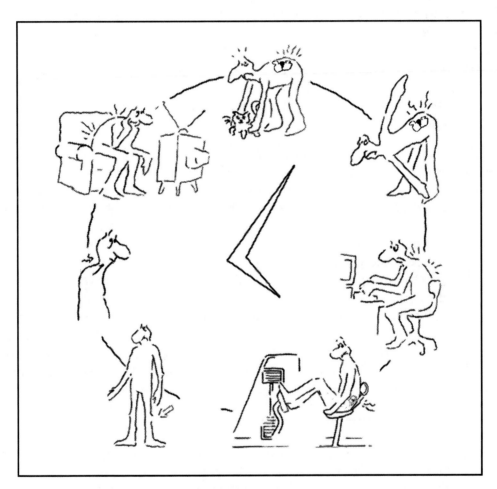

Figure 2-17. Hunching and bending forward all day pressures your discs until one day they finally break down (degenerate) and press outward (herniate). Standing with your hip bent or turned out shortens muscles around the nerves in your legs, which can also make nerve pinching and pain. These problems are easy to avoid and fix.

Why Does Pain Go Down One Leg? What Is Impingement and Sciatica?

It takes years of bad bending habits to make a disc start to break down (degenerate) or push a backward until it finally bulges out of place. When the disc is damaged, that can hurt. If you are lucky, you will get this small warning sign—some small pain or pressure in the side or middle of your back, top of your hip, or right in your behind. By fixing positioning when sitting and bending, and doing extension exercises (Figures 2-11 and 2-12), you can stop disc damage and pain, and keep them from coming back.

If you let more time go by with damaging sitting and body-positioning habits, the disc can begin to push outward and press on nearby structures like nerves. That process is called impingement because the disc impinges on (presses against, or takes up the space of) the nerve, which spreads more pain to other places. After years of damaging the disc, you may suddenly feel pain shoot like electricity when bending wrong just one more time, or reaching for something small. Sometimes, the disc is so ready to give out, you may be just standing or sitting, thinking you have done nothing at all to bring on the sudden bolt of pain.

Discs don't usually protrude straight back. Their path is blocked by a long, tough, band running down the back of your discs called the posterior longitudinal ligament. Such blocking is good because that helps keep them in place and protects your spinal cord, which lies behind the discs. Since the disc can't bulge straight back, if you keep pushing it out, it has to go somewhere and squeezes out sideways. The long nerves going out of your spine to your legs are also on the side. When a disc bulges against these nerves, pain extends down your leg. The most common nerve to be pushed on by bulging discs in your lower back is the sciatic nerve. Your sciatic nerve works both for feeling and movement of your leg—which means if you squeeze it, it will hurt and may also reduce function in your leg. In the most serious cases, discs can protrude directly backwards against your spine, disrupting your ability to move from that level down and to control your bowel and bladder. As you heal your discs, the pain starts moving away from the leg and more to the back, which is called "centralizing." Centralizing is a sign that things are healing. Eventually, the centralized back pain goes away, too.

Grete's daughter, Anni, called me about the back-pain workshops I ran. Anni said that her mother had pain for over 20 years and, since she was a nurse, would be able to benefit from the information. The next workshop was in two weeks. Grete didn't call. A week before another workshop two months later, Grete left a message that I had to call her back to explain the class before she would come to it. She was at work at the time and said I must phone her at home. I called and left her a message with class content and my Web site so she could read the syllabus, course information, and articles explaining what we do. She phoned back saying she needed to talk to me before taking the

---

workshop. When I called she announced, "I am a nurse. I have a herniated lumbar disc at L-4 and L-5 and I have degenerative disc disease at levels L-3, L-4, and L-5. I have sciatica that radiates down my leg. I do exercise and have taken many treatments and I don't understand what you could possibly do for me that I haven't already done." She didn't take a breath. "I don't see how you can say that you can help my pain when you don't even know me. You can't just give everybody the same treatment." I told her that the goal of the class was to find what was causing the pain so that we could help it. She repeated, "I told you, I have herniated discs and sciatica. I don't see what you can do that I haven't already done." I explained that what we try to do is find the cause. For example, sciatica is not a cause, but a result of something that makes the disc or something else press the nerve. We go over the things that are the usual causes. She repeated that sciatica caused her pain.

"I understand," I told her. "But that is still a result. We will practice stopping the things that cause the sciatica. Don't worry. We won't just do a bunch of exercises."

"You are very negative," she yelled and hung up on me.

When I arrived to teach the workshop that weekend, Grete wasn't there. I noticed another woman, Donna, sitting uncomfortably and shifting in her seat. Then she stood up and leaned weakly against the wall. Often people come to the workshops in pain, but this was a lot of pain. I said that it seemed a shame to launch into teaching about how you get back pain while she was standing there suffering. Tears streamed down her face. I asked if I could make her more comfortable before starting class. She nodded. I helped her lie on the floor of the classroom, face down, propped on elbows (Figure 1-16). "This is the only way I can sleep," she said. She had been diagnosed with two herniated discs. Her doctor had her on Neurontin (a nerve medicine) and gave her several injections into the area. They did many tests and sent her to physical therapy. For as long as her insurance lasted, they did electrical stimulation, heat, ultrasound, and traction. They told her to swim, which made things worse. They gave her exercises and a hamstring stretch that involved sitting with one leg bent and stretching over the extended leg. She tried it but the pain was too much to sit in that position let alone reach over the leg. She did all the other stretches they gave her for up to an hour a day. She used her prescribed lumbar roll, but sitting was excruciating. Standing in my class after months of all these treatments and medicines, the pain was so great that tears fell. I explained to the class how extension (propping backward) can be helpful for disc pain because leaning forward is often the cause of the outward pressure on the discs—which is part of why people with disc pain and sciatica hurt a lot when they sit. Lying on the floor, propped on her elbows in back extension, reduced the painful outward force on Donna's injured discs. I asked her if the pain was lessened. She smiled and we started class.

Disc Degeneration Is Not A Disease

An unfortunate situation is that someone with a slipping or degenerating disc, or sciatica from any reason, is often told they have "degenerative disc disease" or simply "disc disease." But it is not a disease. It is misnamed. A hurt disc is a simple, mechanical injury that can heal if you just stop grinding it and physically pushing it out of place with terrible habits. It will heal and stop pressing on nerves. The disc pain and sciatica will go away. It is simple and depends a great deal on how you hold your body when sitting, bending, and exercising.

Discs Can Heal

A herniated disc is not a permanent condition. It is an injury that can heal. Discs need movement to help healing. Bed rest does not help this. Joints are not very vascular, which means that they don't have a high blood supply. The way they move food in and waste out is through movement. The side-to-side movement of the trapezius stretch is one example of a good way to move your discs and joints of your back. The upper- and lower-back extensions are another good way to more in ways that feed and mobilize discs.

After taking the "No More Back Pain" workshop, Donna kept me posted with her progress. The extension exercises helped her greatly. She weaned off the Neurontin with no side effects fairly quickly. She still had pain with sitting, which we determined was from rounding against the lumbar roll. I showed her how to use the roll so that she kept the small inward curve of the lower back when sitting, instead of sitting rounded with pressure on the discs. That weekend Donna was able to make a business flight carrying bags and sitting for long periods without aggravating the pain. She used her scarf and sweater as a lumbar roll because the airline no longer gave out pillows. It seemed that things had turned the corner. Days later, she contacted me she had been in a collision and her air bag deployed. All of the pain was back. In the emergency department, they took an x-ray. They told her there were no findings on the x-ray. They touched her spine until she told them the area where it hurt. Then they asked her get up and see if she could walk. They left her lying in pain for the afternoon. Donna asked them to lower the gurney in the emergency room so she could roll on her stomach and do her extension exercises. She was discharged from there with nothing for the pain and no instructions for exercise. She couldn't get an appointment with her regular doctor for another month at the earliest. With nothing more than what she already knew from our work, she again reduced her pain and the injury was able to heal. One week later, she attended a stretch workshop I gave. She looked good, with color in her smiling face. She got up and down from the floor repeatedly for the three-hour workshop. She was bending and moving—carefully, but fairly easily, and most importantly, with almost no more pain in only a short time since we started.

When Sciatic Pain Isn't From Discs

You can get pain down your leg even when scans show your discs are not involved. Tight muscles in the lower back and hip from years of poor positioning and keeping your hip bent (which shortens the muscles) can also press on the same nerves, mimicking sciatica. Sometimes, the pain may only go down to the knee, not all the way into the little toe. One way tightness like this happens is standing and sitting with your feet turned out—duck foot. The muscles that turn your leg and feet outward are in the back of your hip. They fasten sideways from the back of your hipbone to your upper-leg bone. The sciatic nerve passes behind (and, in some people, through) one or more of these muscles, mainly the piriformis muscle, a little pyramid-shaped muscle. When these muscles tighten from years of walking, sitting, and standing with your hip bent and your feet turned out, the tight muscles can press and add to sciatic pain. Pain can also go down the front of your leg when different nerves are pressed.

When "Disc" Pain Isn't From Discs

Often, a person may be in great pain from simple damaging bending and movement habits. They may go for an x-ray (or other imaging scan) and the scans show a degenerating or herniated disc. The pain may not be from the disc, but from the strained, achy muscles from bad habits. Just like car tires that are mid-life but perfectly good, some wear shows on exam. The disc wear is often unrelated to the pain, but the pain is falsely ascribed as disc pain. The person is told they have disc disease and often told that it is a life-long problem with little to relive it but surgery or pills. The pain continues from the poor mechanics, not the disc. This situation is no mystery. Change the bad habits to change the pain.

When Surgery Doesn't Help

Sometimes when people have pain from simple damaging habits, their scan shows a disc with wear. It might not be the disc causing the pain, but they go for surgery for the "bad disc." Their pain persists or returns because they never corrected the bad mechanics that caused the pain, or they herniate another disc for the same reasons they herniated the first one—bad sitting, bending, and all the other habits that they did not change.

I got a call from a physician that his office partner "had two successful disc surgeries, and now had a third herniated disc and was considering surgery." They wanted a referral. I told them that was not successful back surgery. It was like saying you had two successful appendectomies and now had problems again.

Impact

People are often told to give up impact activities once they have disc pain. They dutifully give up activities they love and need for exercise, instead of learning how to move using their muscles for shock absorption. They still walk around with such poor shock absorption that just walking is higher impact than if they ran, or even boxed, with good mechanics. Use leg and truck muscles to walk softly and decelerate with each step during all the activities you want to do.

Getting In and Out of Chairs

Do you flop down in your chair, jolting your spine? Use your leg muscles to decelerate. It's free squatting exercise for all the many times a day you get into and out of your chair. Don't stick your hips out in back or lean your upper body forward. Use your thigh muscles. Can you get out of your chair without needing your arms? Work on leg strength and balance.

Sleeping

You don't need special beds, chairs, and desks. You can slouch in unhealthy ways in an expensive ergonomic chair, and sit well on a garbage can. How you sit is up to you. If your bed is too hard, it is possible for that to be painful. An inexpensive foam "egg crate" pad on top can help. You don't need a hard bed unless you find that to be comfortable. It is not necessary to buy an expensive mattress. Remember that the majority of the non-Western world sleeps on a straw mat or a foam pad—with no pain. A foam pad instead of a mattress is inexpensive and has the added advantage that a person moving on one side transmits no motion to the other person. A twenty-dollar foam pad often does better than a thousand-dollar special "no bounce" mattress.

People often are told to never sleep on their stomach, or never on their back without a pillow under their knees. This advice does not address the cause of the problem. One contributor to not being able to sleep on your back without upper-back pain is tight chest and neck muscles. The pectoral stretch and the trapezius stretch usually reverse this problem (Figures 1-9 and 1-10). Another common reason for not being able to lie flat without lower-back pain is tight muscles in front of the hip (Figures 2-42 and 2-43). Stretching the hip through extension stretches (Figures 4-6 through 4-13) lengthens the front hip muscles allowing a comfortable flat position that does not arch and pressure the back. The main thing to do is get your muscles back to normal resting length in the daytime so that you can lie comfortably at night, using the daily habits and stretches in this book. For now, get sleep whatever way you are comfortable. People with pain have enough trouble sleeping without being more uncomfortable with rules about positioning. Change your waking habits to healthy ones. Then sleeping will straighten itself out.

If you spend much time in bed reading or watching television, or sleep sitting up, don't sit rounded. Instead of rounding the upper body up on pillows, put another pillow under the lower back to keep a small, inward curve to prevent pushing discs outward (Figure 2-50). Don't round against the lower-back pillow (Figure 2-52). The section on healthy sitting later in this chapter shows how to sit in comfortable and healthy ways.

Don't Exercise in Ways that Damage Your Discs

People exercise for health, but often exercise in unhealthy ways. Many exercises done "for their back" involve forward bending: toe touches, knee to chest, leg lifts, and crunches. Don't stretch by bending over. Many people are surprised to find that they injure their back doing forward yoga stretches. You wouldn't pick up a package that way. It is not really a surprise. Use other yoga poses that don't involve pushing discs outward, and extension stretches.

When sitting to lift weights, remember that sitting is harder on your discs than standing. Sitting rounded multiplies damaging pressure. A common exercise injury occurs when sitting rounded on weight machines (Figure 2-18). After years of unhealthy sitting position, pushing against a leg press or other resistance can become too much for the discs, sending pain into the lower back and leg.

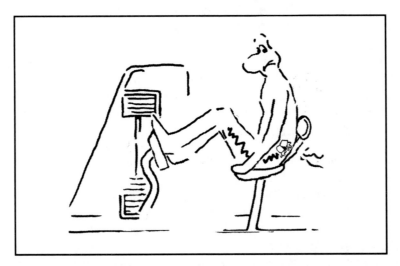

Figure 2-18. Don't let your lower back round to raise or lower the weight. Lift up and sit straight or lean back. Push your upper back, not your lower back, against the seat.

Exercises To Stop Disc Pain

Strengthening and stretching are important, but will not change positioning or lifting habits, and so cannot "cure" disc pain. Many exercises contribute to the original problem of rounding and bad bending. Look around the gym to see people hunching and bending over to lift things, pressuring discs outward.

Back exercises are supposed to be used to retrain you how you hold your body all the time. Doing exercises for disc pain is not like getting a shot of penicillin or going to confession. It does not "fix" bad habits the rest of the time.

Use the squat (Figure 2-7) and lunge (Figure 2-10) for every time you bend: to pick things up from the floor, look in the refrigerator, use the dishwasher, and drink from the water fountain. You get free exercise and retrain bending habits to stop back pain at the same time. Keep knees over feet, not slumping forward, which is hard on the knees. Don't worry about holding a straight and rigid posture. The point is natural, easy, and healthy movement. Use upper- and lower-back extension (Figures 2-11 and 2-12) every day to strengthen back muscles while reversing the forward-bending pressure that pushes discs outward. To rest, lie face down propped on elbows in an extension stretch. Lie this way propped on elbows first thing in the morning. Don't sit rounded on the bed. Stretch backward over things (Figures 1-11, 3-10, and 4-10). Try extension exercises slowly and gently at first. Understand the concept of what they are supposed to achieve. Don't just "do a bunch of exercises." Do the *purpose* of the exercise, not the exercise.

Steve was an active photographer running his photography business and school in Thailand. Several highly-qualified orthopedic surgeons in three countries had told him that the only remedy for his degenerated and herniated lumbar disks was surgery and pain medication for life. "Nothing to be done about it, so get used to the idea. Perhaps a pain clinic can teach you how to manage the pain better." They convinced him to resign himself to a life of surgery followed by chronic pain, limited physical activity, and continuous medication. It was not a bright future. He was taking pain medications many times every day and wasn't happy about it.

I showed Steve the obvious pressure he was putting on his discs by bending, standing, and sitting in all the ways he already knew he shouldn't do. To remind him how to move with healthy mechanics, I told him to watch how other people injure themselves through their own body weight. Steve came back excited. He said he saw others who were complaining about the same back pain he was experiencing, bending, sitting, and standing badly—in general, living their physical lives in an unhealthy way. Once he started moving his body in healthy ways, he was no longer putting the pressure on the spinal discs. The pain stopped and the discs started to heal. The exercises he had been given by the surgeons seemed correct in theory but incorrect in practice. He needed to stretch his back muscles, but not by bending over touching his toes. As much as discs need movement to heal, that was creating more outward pressure on the discs. He needed to strengthen his abdominal muscles, but not with stomach crunches that exacerbated the problem in his back and created more problems in his neck. He began paying attention to positioning when standing, how he stood up from a chair, when he reached, and how he got out of bed in the morning. He told me that, with repetition, it became ingrained and he didn't have to think about it again. He was thrilled that he didn't need to go to the health club or gym for any of it. He said that his health is something he gets to do built-in, all day, every day—not just two hours a day twice a week. He mailed me at the holidays: "On the seventh day of Christmas, my true love didn't give me any pain meds for my back. None. Zip. Zilch! Zero. Nada! From 200mg of Tramadol per day, plus 40mg of piroxicam per day and still having pain, I am down to zero. Not even an aspirin. It's a Merry Christmas, indeed. Thanks. Steve."

What to Do Every Day to Stop Disc Pain

- First thing in the morning, don't sit on the bed. Turn face down (Figure 1-16). Prop low on elbows. Don't push so high that it strains. It should feel good and help you start the day straight. Keep neck straight, not craned or pinched backward. Try to stretch back throughout the upper back, not just folding the lower back. Get out of bed without sitting.

- Right after getting out of bed, do the pectoral (chest) stretch and the trapezius stretch (Figures 1-9 and 1-10). These stretches help you start the day standing straight so that you don't go about your day bent forward.

- During the day, check your standing position using the wall stand (Figure 1-7).

- Upper-body (upper-back) extension (Figure 2-11). Lie face down. Lift upper body and gently lower. Try three to five to start. See how you feel, then increase. Work up to at least 10 to 20 at a time.

- Lower-body (lower-back) extension (Figure 2-12). Lie face down. Lift legs, keeping your knees straight and gently lower. If lifting both legs is too much, try one at a time. Progress to both. Contract your back and behind muscles easily, not tightly. Lift; don't yank. Try three to five to start. See how you feel, then increase. Work up to at least 10 to 20.

- Squat (Figure 2-7) or lunge (Figure 2-10) for every time you lift and bend, instead of bending at the waist. An average person bends hundreds of times a day. Imagine the pressure on your discs bending wrong hundreds of times a day. Imagine the free leg exercise and calories burned from bending right.

- Take breaks lying face down, lightly propped on elbows. If this pinches your lower back, the front of your hip is probably tight. Chapter 4 shows good stretches for the anterior hip (Figures 4-6 through 4-8 and 4-10 through 4-14).

- Walk lightly. See if you make noisy steps on the floor or stairs and, if so, lighten up. This doesn't mean walk on tiptoe. Use normal movement, using muscles for shock absorption.

- Sit down lightly. Use leg and hip muscles for deceleration instead of flopping down, jarring your spine.

- Hold a push-up position (Figure 2-33). If you can't comfortably hold straight body position with your head up and back straight without sagging, your back muscles are so weak that it is no wonder that you let your back round and sag all day.

- Use your muscles, not joints, to hold you up. It's free exercise. Sit, stand, and bend without rounding. It may be natural to let your weight sag, but it is also natural to wet your pants. Learn healthy, comfortable control. Remember that positioning is a voluntary muscular exercise. No need to be ramrod-straight or hold muscles tightly. That only makes more tightness and pain.

- Don't just "do exercises." Make healthy motion part of your enjoyable life.

Computer, Desk, Driving, and Television

- Sit without rounding

- Raise your computer monitor if it is too low on the desk. Raise your television higher. Stop sitting hunched over and forward to watch. Sit against the chair back. Lean the upper back backward; don't round against the lower back.

- Move the keyboard off the "below desk" tray and back up on the desk.

- Move desk and car seats closer in. Sit back, not forward. How are you sitting right now? See the section on healthy sitting later in this chapter.

What to Avoid to Stop Disc Pain

- Don't bend over wrong to look in the refrigerator, get the laundry, pick things up, or for all the hundreds of times you bend.

- Avoid exercises that add to disc pressure by bending forward with your weight on your back. Omit sit-ups, "crunches," exercises that bend forward at the hip, supposedly to strengthen the core, and forward rounding hamstring stretches. These only add more tightening in the front of the body. Better core exercises without forward bending are next in the lordosis section of this chapter.

- Don't round forward to carry a backpack or other load. Use your muscles to stand straight. The lifting and carrying section later in this chapter shows fun ways to carry more without pain.

- Don't do things that increase pain. Stretch to where it feels good and relieves tightness, not where it pinches, tightens, or strains.

- Don't worry that you have to live your life "on eggshells" holding yourself rigidly straight. Restricting movement to limit pain isn't healthy and isn't fun. Stay active. Learn the principles and apply them, instead of memorizing "rules" and buying expensive ergonomic chairs and beds.

- Don't complain that it's hard. It's free exercise. It's like learning any other new skill, and will fix your disc pain.

When to Notice the Lower Back

- The most common times to round the lower back in unhealthy ways are when sitting, bending, bicycling, and exercising.

- Watch other people bending wrong to pick things up. Notice such movements at the gym during exercises that are supposed to be for people's health.

How to Get Natural Disc Health during Daily Life

- Standing, moving, and sitting well instead of rounding forward will give free, all-day, functional strengthening for the entire back, and stop the outward pressure on the discs.

- Bending with legs and an upright torso gives free, functional strengthening and balance exercise for the back and the legs at the same time. Good bending moves the body, which is needed for disc health, while preventing the pressure that degenerates and pushes discs outward.

- Instead of letting body weight slump downward, flattening discs between each spine bone, pull upward to stand and sit up taller. Doing so gives more space between each vertebra. It's free traction. Astronauts return from floating in space temporarily taller. The lack of spinal compression temporarily restores disc space. Then they return to previous height. Hanging from an overhead bar or between two counters or other supports temporarily gives some traction. Don't go back to flattening discs when you stop hanging and walk away.

No More Disc Pain

Disc herniation and degeneration are not mysterious "conditions." Many people spend their days degenerating and pushing their discs outward by forward bending and slouching habits. You don't need strange exercises, pills, or surgery. The cure is not just strengthening, because that does not change the bending habits that injure discs. The cure is not removing the discs because you need the discs. Removing discs predisposes you to lack of shock absorption, arthritis, and more pain. The cure is not fusing the vertebrae or getting rods in your back because that can create a life of poor mobility and added strain on nearby spine segments. Many people with spinal fusion wind up getting more surgery. The cure is not stopping activity. That is harmful to the entire body. Address the cause of the pain. If you retrain simple body positioning to stop the disc damage, then you will have no need for pills or surgery and the discs can heal.

The point of exercise and physical therapy is missed when exercisers don't learn to consciously use their muscles the rest of the day for standing, sitting, bending, and shock absorption. Positioning is the same as brushing your teeth—a simple health activity. Make health part of real, daily life—not a separate activity you have to change clothes to do. How is your body positioning right now? Sitting, standing, and moving in healthy ways for real life all burn calories, strengthen, and are a free workout. You don't have to live with disc pain.

Lower-Back Pain from Lordosis, Arching, Swayback, Facet Pain, Spondylolisthesis, and Stenosis

A slight inward curve belongs in the lower back. It is needed for shock absorption and to prevent the disc degeneration that comes with rounding the low back. But sometimes a little knowledge is a dangerous thing. People hear that they need an inward curve, so exaggerate it. Other people let their body weight slouch downward as a regular habit, pressing the lower back into an overly-arched position. Letting the lower back arch too much pinches and folds the lower back under your upper-body weight. Much "mystery" lower-back pain results that often does not show up on scans. Tilting the hip forward, sticking the backside out, and leaning the upper body backward all increase the normal arch to a painful one (Figure 2-19, right). This kind of pain can go on for years while people try one cure after the next. If you need to bend forward or bend your knees to relieve a backache, it is likely that overarching is involved in the pain.

It is simple to stop the pain by using your own muscles to move your back into a less arched and more normal position during everything you do. Pain from overarching the back is the easiest of all back pain to fix.

Many people think that abdominal muscles have some mysterious role in back pain, and that somehow, making them stronger or pressing them in some way will do something to stop back pain. But abdominal muscles work the same way every skeletal muscle in your body works. They move your bones. Your biceps muscle bends your elbow. Your hamstrings bend your knee. Your abdominal muscles bend your spine forward. When your back is overly arched backward, you can use your abdominal muscles to bring your spine forward enough to restore healthy position. To see how the abdominal muscles are involved in solving lower-back pain, try the following:

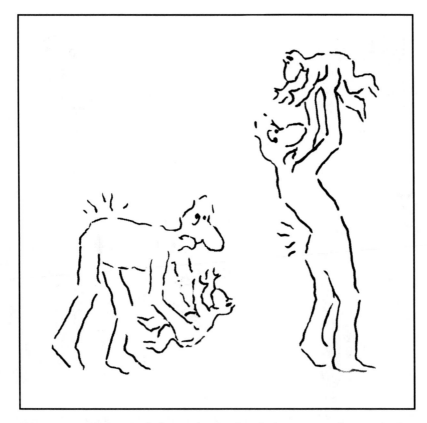

Figure 2-19. Most people know that back pain is common from rounding forward when sitting or bending (left). A major hidden cause of back pain is arching backward when standing and reaching overhead (right).

- Stand up and put one hand on the front of your hipbone where your abdominal muscles begin (close to the bottom of your pants' zipper). Put your other hand on your ribs where your abs end (Figure 2-20, center).

- To see what happens when you don't use your abdominal muscles, still holding your ribs and hipbone, arch back and let your ribs lift and your abdomen curve out. Let your weight relax back. The distance between your hands increases (Figure 2-20, left). This shows how slack abdominal muscles allow your back to arch. Your upper-body weight presses down onto your lower back. You may feel a familiar pressure. (Don't do this if it hurts).

- Draw your hands closer together until your back straightens (Figure 2-20, right). This movement is the key to understanding how shortening (using) your abs moves your spine and hip away from arched position. The discomfort from the arching should disappear.

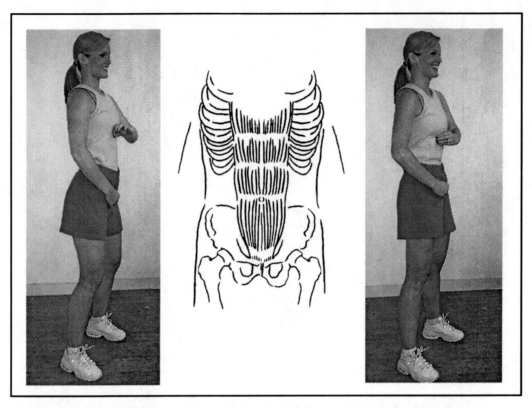

Figure 2-20. Your abdominal muscles attach from ribs to hip (center). When abs aren't working enough (left), the ribs lift and the back arches. Hands are far apart showing lengthened abs. Shorten your abs (hands move closer together, right) to tip your hip under and pull ribs down, reducing the arch and the pinching low back pressure.

Ken worked security at a medical university where I taught. He was a big, jovial guy. I enjoyed his big greeting and wave every day. He was previously a police officer who had been increasingly off duty from constant back pain. A series of doctors told him he was getting older and that being on his feet all day and being heavy were unavoidably hurting his back. They told him the pain was the price we paid as humans for standing on two legs. He was first put on light duty, and then disability. He took the security position, wanting to stay "in the field." He had been to physical therapy where they gave him crunches, pelvic tilts, and lists of things he should not do any more (like never lift anything heavy, jog, or sit on anything soft). Ken was no complainer. He obeyed. He was a big guy and they told him to lose weight. Without being able to lift weights or go for his usual run, he gained weight and became more sedentary. Activity aggravated his back anyway, but the awful ache continued even without going out to have any fun. He took the medicines they prescribed and something to help his stomach that was upset by the medicines. The company provided him a soft mat to stand on for his security post. I walked past him every day at work. He had that "leaned back, big belly, big guy" look. Big guy, big smile—but with his face in that recognizable pained expression.

One day I asked, "Ken, does your back hurt?" He was surprised. He had never mentioned it, and wanted to know how I knew. "Ken, you arch your back and lean back when you stand. It's not rocket science. When you arch like that, you bend your spine backward too much in the lower back. The weight of your upper body pinches it at that folding point."

He was surprised. He said he was taught to "stand tall and lift his ribs." The other guards standing with him agreed that they had heard that also: "Shoulders back, chest out, lift ribs." They did it "when they remembered," thinking it was good posture, but it made their back hurt and it was too much effort so they stopped. For people who slouch forward, with sagging ribs, they need to lift their ribs to a straight, not downward position. But lifting their ribs too high pinches the back into an arch. I showed Ken that he was arching his back to bring his shoulders back and that lifting his ribs was also tilting him backward so that his lower back was being almost crushed by arching back on it.

I showed them all where the abdominal muscles go from the hipbones to the bottom of your ribs. When you don't use your abdominal muscles to pull your ribs down and forward enough, the ribs lift up and you arch your back. Your weight falls on the arch. When you use your muscles to pull your spine out of the overly-arched position, the pressure stops. Ken tucked his hip and pulled his upper body forward so that he was standing straight. I smiled. "Hey, you look taller."

Ken's mouth opened. "It stopped. The pain stopped." This is why I like this method so much. It is simple mechanics to pull your body weight off the lower back, stopping the pressure right there.

Ken asked me if that was all there was to it. I told him that it was pretty much the concept in a capsule and it was good to keep it simple. Ken remembered all the crunches and pelvic tilts he was given in physical therapy. "No wonder they didn't help. When I stood up again, I just went back to leaning back. This is like doing them standing up!" I told him that was exactly the idea, that you use your abdominal muscles when standing, not by tightening them, but just moving your spine away from arching under body weight.

Not long after, I didn't see Ken at work. "He quit and it's your fault!" The guards told me that Ken could jog and lift weights without back pain. He had missed so much for so long. Ken was so overjoyed that his back pain was gone (and his life was back) that he took his benefits and left on a cruise.

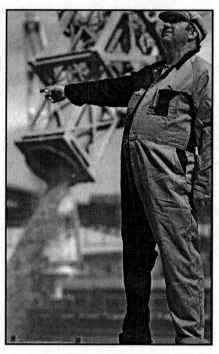

Figure 2-21. A common cause of lower-back pain
is leaning or arching backward when standing.

What Is Lordosis?

Sometimes people with back pain are told they have a "condition" or "disorder" called lordosis. They think this "condition" is something anatomic, unavoidable, or that it "just happens" to them, like the flu.

Technically the word "lordosis" originally meant the normal inward curve of the lower back. It has commonly come to mean too much inward curve, allowing the back to sway and arch. Lordosis and hyperlordosis often are used interchangeably to describe the same overly-arched position. Too much lordosis, or hyperlordosis, creates much lower-back pain. A small, inward curve belongs in the lower back. But preserving the small arch does not mean tipping the hip forward or allowing the upper body to lean backward, increasing the arch and compressing the lower back under body weight. Many people allow the overly-arched, hyperlordotic posture during daily life and during exercise, particularly when standing, lifting, and carrying.

If you need to bend over forward to relive an achy back, it is likely that arching contributes to the pain. Many restaurants and pubs have a footrest at the foot of the bar. Many people who stand for long periods feel better when they put one foot up on the rest. The reason for this is putting one foot up bends the back away from an arched

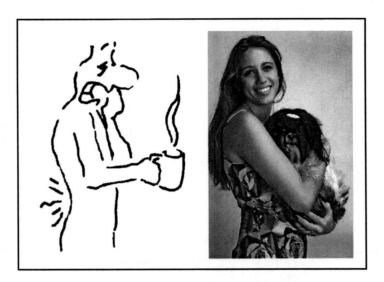

Figure 2-22. Overly-arched, hyperlordotic lower-back posture is not normal, even though it is common. Tipping the hip forward or leaning the upper body backward overly arches and compresses the low back. It is the cause of much "mystery" lower-back pain.

position. Instead of needing to do this with a footrest or bending your knees, just tilt your hip under you using your own abdominal muscles. Then you can also stop pain for regular life without a footrest.

Hyperlordosis (now commonly interchanged with the term lordosis) is usually completely controllable by using your muscles to simply move your spine and pelvis to reduce the large arch, and leave only a small inward curve to the lower back. You can see that it is not "tightening" that makes you stand with good posture, it is just voluntarily moving your spine.

How to Stop the Pain of Arching (Lordosis or Hyperlordosis)

Overly arching your back is not a condition but a posture that causes much lower-back pain. Stop the pain it by moving your spine and bringing your ribs back down to straight position, as if starting a "crunch," and tilting the hips back so that you reduce the arch in your back.

Some back-pain treatment centers use the concept of moving the pelvis to help stop pain, teaching this as a set of exercises of "pelvic tilts" or "pelvic clock," moving the pelvis as an exercise while lying down, sitting, or standing. Instead, the key to reducing pain on an ongoing basis is to take the idea of positioning the hip and spine during all activities, not just during the exercise. Moving the spine into healthy position for normal, daily posture is a different way of thinking about use of torso or "core" muscles to stop the cause of lower-back pain.

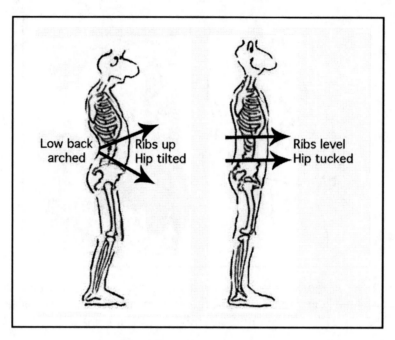

Figure 2-23. Pressure and pain often comes from hyperlordotic arching (left). Tuck hips and pull ribs to straight position (right). Don't tighten; just move the spine. Use this new good position all the time to stop pain.

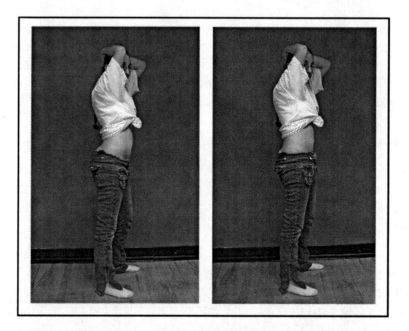

Figure 2-24. How to tuck the hip: On the left, the lower back is arched and the waistband of the pants tilts down. On the right, the hip is tilted back under, reducing the arch and the pressure in the lower back.

What Are Facets? What Is Facet Pain?

Your facets are the joints of your backbones (vertebrae). They are smooth, flat little surfaces that got their name when the people who originally named anatomical parts thought they looked like little faces. Sometimes they're called zygapohysial (z) joints, which just means the place where the vertebrae fit together. When you let your body weight arch, your lower back pinches backward, and pressures and jams those joints and the soft tissue around them, which is a common source of lower-back pain. The most usual treatment for facet pain is injections. However, it is simple to stop the cause of the pain by using not arching without need for injections.

Commander McKean saw the chain of military and civilian specialists who gave him exercises for back pain. He did them faithfully while the pain continued year after year. In twenty-five years of daily pain, he had been to five pain clinics, had surgery, and been prescribed narcotics that he was told would be a regular prescription, as nothing else was stopping the unremitting pain.

His scans and x-rays showed a herniated disc and facet injury. Facets are the joints of the vertebrae. He was told he had a condition. For ten years he went for facet injections on a regular basis—a standard treatment for facet pain. They gave him crunches and other forward bending to strengthen his "core." He was strong and muscular. But the pain continued. I showed him that the cure for facet pain is not facet injections, or strengthening core muscles. The key is stopping the cause of the pain, meaning the arched lordotic position that drops upper-body weight on the facet joints (the joints of your vertebrae). Use this concept for everything you do. The commander was doing the exercises prescribed to him by the pain clinics and therapy centers, but the exercises included bending over to stretch his hamstrings, pressing knee to chest, and other forward-bending exercises, which were all pushing the herniated disc further outward (see disc information in the previous section of this chapter). He was lifting weights and doing push-ups and other exercises for his core. The arched-back position that he had been taught to use was hurting his facet joints and causing pressure and aching in his lower back. No one told him to reduce the large arch of his back when standing. He was a tough guy. He was tough enough to 'handle" the pain on a daily basis, but smart enough to know did didn't have to. I showed him how to tip his hip under until it was straight, so that his back did not arch when standing. He said the best part was no longer waking up in pain.

What Do Abdominal Muscles Have to Do with Lower-Back Pain?

You've heard that developing your abdominal muscles will help your lifting, posture, and your back pain—so why isn't it working?

Christine's mother was a dressmaker. When Christine was a child, her mother made her dresses longer in the back to "make up for her big behind." She told me they both knew it was her posture, not her size, and joked that if she ever stood properly, her dresses would all be too long in back. But she didn't stand properly because she was told that her "swayback" was "just the way she was" and there was nothing she could do about it. She came to me with back pain that that been ongoing for years. She had been in physical therapy and had been given crunches. They didn't fix her lordosis, but made her neck hurt. They told her that she needed to press her navel to her spine and tighten the buttock muscles. She tightened when she could, wondering how she could learn to walk around all the time with her abdomen tight and her behind clenched the way they taught her.

Many people have heard the traditional saying that using your abdominal muscles means "sucking them in," "tightening them," or "pressing your navel to your spine." But you can't move or breathe easily that way. If you bend your arm, you don't tighten your muscles, you just move your arm using your arm muscles. Abdominal muscles work the same way. Abdominal muscles connect your ribs to hips along your front and sides. When you use your abs, they pull your ribs and hips closer, bending your spine.

When you stand up and don't use your abdominal muscles, you allow your ribs and hips to be too far apart. Your lower back sways, exaggerating the normal inward curve. Arching like this drops the weight of your upper back on your lower back, grinding away your soft tissues and discs, and irritating the joints (called facets) where each vertebra attaches to the next. Much facet pain commonly results from this simple bad-positioning habit.

When do people arch like this? When they stand up. When they look up. When they reach up. When they carry a load in front of them, like a laundry basket, chair, or baby. Many people can't pull their shoulders back or drink a glass of water without arching their back. Much back pain results but it is just an easily-changed bad posture.

The way your abdominal muscles work in everyday life is to keep your spine from overly-arching back or to the side, which does not come from strengthening the abs. It only happens when you use your abs to prevent arching back. Abs control posture and stop the strain of dropping your body weight on your lower back in this way. It is also

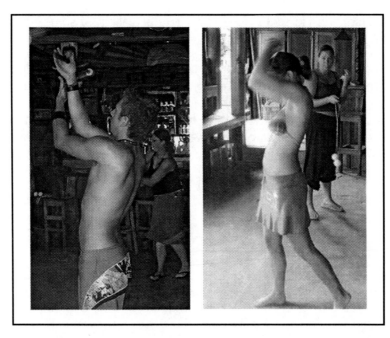

Figure 2-25. Many people arch their back to reach up. You are not supposed to let your back slump into an arch like this. The arching rests upper-body weight on the lower back, making it hurt.

not tightening your abs that helps your back; it is using your muscles to move your spine out of an overly-arched (and into a healthier) position.

Antoine had cerebral palsy. Sometime around his birth, there was damage to parts of his brain that controlled his muscles. Some people with cerebral palsy have a form called "athetoid cerebral palsy" where muscle tone in their body keeps changing from tight to loose, giving them uncontrolled or writhing movements. Antoine had the spastic form, which made his body stiff. Tight muscles in his hips and legs turned his legs inward. It was hard for him to bend and walk. He had surgery to lengthen tight muscles so that he could walk better. Even then, his gait was stiff and forced. Tight facial muscles made his speech labored. Tight back muscles pulled him like an unseen hand into a large hyperlordotic arch. Over his lifetime, the arching pressed on the joints of his vertebrae. He was headed for back surgery for his damaged facet joints.

I showed Antoine the technique of reducing the lower-back arch (Figures 2-23 and 2-24) as if he were starting a crunch. I told him to pull forward until he was straight. He pulled. It was hard work but he pulled and pulled, and then—with startled eyes—he looked down at his body standing almost normally for the first time. He said, "Ho-ly cow!" (He actually said something a little stronger.) "Look at me!" I was looking.

"Antoine, you got speech therapy to control your speech muscles for others to understand you, and physical therapy so others could read your writing. This is for you." It would be more work for Antoine (than for other people) to use his abdominal muscles to keep him from being thrown backward into his familiar and unwilling arching. But it was hard work just for him to walk and speak. This necessary muscular activity was the same he needed to improve his health and mobility.

"So, this will give me free ab exercise?" he said slowly. "Six pack is mine! Look out, ladies!"

If You Don't Believe that "Tightening" Is Not How to Use Your Abs

Try the following:

- Tighten your abdominal muscles, as commonly taught. Press your navel to your spine. Tighten the entire area and hold. Now try to breathe in. Note that tightening would not be possible or useful for daily activity.
- Next, stand with arched posture. Tighten your abs and surrounding musculature. Note that posture does not change.
- Stop tightening. Tuck your spine and hip to remove the lordotic arch, straightening your posture. See that "using your abs" means using them, like any other muscle, to move your body.

Instead of lying on the floor and hunching forward, train your abdominal muscles to work the way you really need them, which is standing up. By using your abdominal muscles to hold healthy spine positioning during all activities, you get free exercise and abdominal training that benefits your life and helps your back. Simply strengthening abdominal muscles will not help your back. Using abs to keep healthy torso posture is how it works.

Aren't You Supposed to Stick Your Behind Out?

Alma had back pain as a teen. She was heavy and held her back in the arched posture that was a popular way of standing in her neighborhood. She had learned to hold her behind stuck out in back like that from her friends who learned it from teen fashion magazines. She didn't lean or arch her back. In fact, her upper body rounded forward a bit. But her back still arched from tilting her hip to stick it out in back. She went to her doctor who told her she had a problem with her back—that she was "a swayback." The doctor told her it was a disease or condition, she couldn't remember which, and that she needed to lose weight. It frightened her that she had something in her back that was permanent. Her friends told her she just had "a big butt."

Her doctor had told her to lie on the floor and do pelvic tilts. I asked Alma what else the doctor told her. She said the doctor said there was nothing much else she could do for her condition except to strengthen her abs. I asked her what the doctor said the tilts would do. She said she wasn't sure, but the doctor said it would strengthen the area and make it better somehow but that it was her heredity to have a curved back and nothing more could be done. She said the tilts were so mild she didn't know how it would strengthen anything, but she did them. I asked her if the doctor told her to do anything when standing up, which is when her back assumed the arched posture. She said, "No, the doc said there is nothing you can do."

Alma was smart and her face suddenly brightened. She said she understood what I was saying: the tilts don't do anything by themselves; all you have to do is use the tilt when standing up to deliberately move the hip and spine so you don't arch when standing. She tried it then and there. The usual pressure in her lower back was gone. She let her back sag into an arch again and the pressure returned. She said that she previously thought it was her "big behind" that pressed on her back, but now she knew that it was the tilt to her hip and how much she arched her lower back that determined the pressure on her lower back. She smiled and said she knew how to not have any more pain.

Many magazines picture models standing and exercising with their back arched so that the hip sticks out in back and the chest sticks out in front (Figure 2-26). This posture is a major contributor to back pain. It is not attractive. It is weak posture since it does not use abdominal muscles. It is unhealthy for the lower back and shows a lack of understanding of how to use core muscles to control torso posture. It is common to think it is necessary to stick the behind out when squatting or lunging, however this more than is needed, and does not use core muscles effectively. The magazine may state to keep the back straight, or to keep a "neutral spine" but the photos often show arched posture.

How to Stop Lower Lordotic Back Pain when Lifting Things Overhead

Many people arch their back when reaching overhead. That allows their upper-body weight plus the weight of things they are lifting to press down on their lower back. They

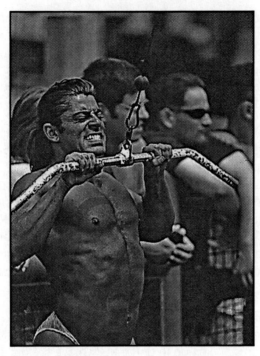

Figure 2-26. Having strong abs does not automatically prevent the arching that loads the low back.

do this dozens of times daily for things as innocuous as putting things on shelves, pulling off shirts, even combing and washing hair. Imagine the damage that accumulates from thousands of repetitions day after day. Try this:

- Stand up and reach overhead. See if you allow your ribs to lift up and your back to arch (Figure 2-27, left).
- Fix this bad posture by straightening your body, as if starting to do a crunch, to take the exaggerated curve out of your low back, but don't curl your body or neck forward (Figure 2-27, right).
- Reach up again, holding this new healthy posture. You'll feel abdominal and back muscles working to hold your body weight. You may also feel your shoulders getting more reach.

Transfer this straightening skill to your daily life for carrying gear, putting bags up on racks, heavy packages on counters, and whenever you lift and reach. Your gear could be a built-in abdominal exercise to maintain healthy position against an anterior load. When picking up a chair or a child, or any load, don't lean back to counter the weight, use your abdominal muscles. When you are washing your hair in the shower, notice if you are arching your back, allowing your weight to rest on your lower back. Fix this bad posture by using your abs to move your spine. If you use your abs in this way for daily positioning, you should notice a large reduction in your back pain.

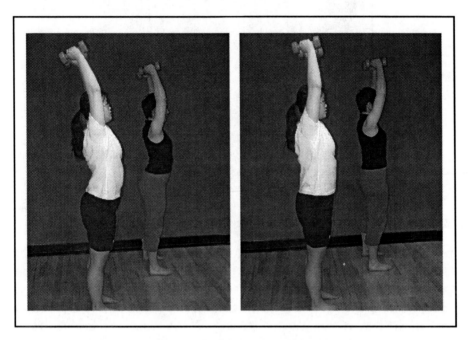

Figure 2-27. To prevent arching when reaching and lifting overhead (left), use abdominal muscles to pull ribs down to hips to deliberately reduce the arch (right), not by tightening, but moving your spine and hip.

How to Stop Lordotic Back Pain while Wearing Backpacks

Heavy bags and backpacks don't make you arch your back or have bad posture. Not using your abdominal muscles to counter the pull and allowing your back to arch is the problem. Use your abdominal muscles to prevent arching and maintain good posture against a posterior load. Your bags could be a built-in abdominal exercise.

- Stand up wearing a backpack. If you notice yourself arching or leaning back (Figure 2-28, left), straighten your body as if starting to do a crunch, but don't curl forward, round your shoulders, or crane your neck forward. Just straighten your body against the pull of the load and maintain your posture (Figure 2-28, right).

- If you find that you stick your behind out to "hike up" the bag, tuck your behind under, enough to straighten out. Don't tuck so much that you lean back or stick your hips forward.

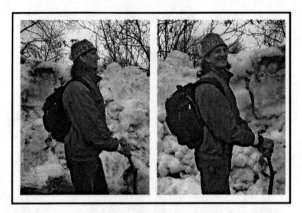

Figure 2-28. It is not the backpack that makes you arch your back (left). Use your torso muscles to tuck the hip and reduce the arch (right).

How to Stop Lordotic Back Pain when Carrying Things in Front

Many people lean back or arch their back to "balance" an anterior load like a chair or a baby. Arching your back shifts the weight of the load plus the weight of your upper body onto your lower back. Many people have heard the false statement that being pregnant makes your posture change and arch. This statement is not true. It is preventable by just using muscles to stand without arching. Of all times to prevent this arching, pregnancy is it. The section on carrying loads shows more examples later in this chapter.

- Stand up and pick up a chair or any load in front of you.
- If you notice yourself arching or leaning back, straighten your body as if starting to do a crunch, but don't curl forward, round your shoulders, or crane your neck forward. Just straighten your body against the pull of the load and maintain your posture.
- You will feel your abdominal muscles working to hold you straight. Your bags and babies could be a built-in abdominal muscle exercise.

How to Stop Lordotic Back Pain when Swimming

The same principles of using your abs when standing up apply to swimming. Many people allow their back to sag into an exaggerated arch, making them look like they are face down in a hammock (Figure 2-29). The fulcrum of the kick becomes their lower-back joints instead of the muscles of the abs and hip, which is why many people are mistakenly told that swimming is good for you except for the front crawl which "makes you arch your back." It is not swimming that makes you arch. It is you allowing it. Use your abs to straighten your posture. Your body will be streamline, your kick will be powerful, and your back will stop hurting from the pressure of "creasing" the lower back by arching.

Vivian didn't have lordosis. She sometimes suffered back pain after using her computer. She enrolled in my class at the university called "No More Back Pain." During the class, I show examples of painful body ergonomics during real life activities from cooking, to sewing, to exercising, to lifting the baby, combing hair, and the many exercises involving legs where people arch their back to move their leg instead of using leg muscles. Vivian had started practicing martial arts the year before. Her lower back never hurt before that. She came back to class the next week and said that she realized she had been doing back kicks by arching her back instead of using muscles to control back posture. She tried the hip-tilt repositioning we learned in class. Instead of flinging her leg backward by arching her back, she kept her hip tucked and used abdominal muscles to hold her spine from arching backward. Her back didn't hurt and she got better exercise from the kick—and a stronger kick.

When Vivian mentioned this, Tom (another student in class) added that he had just applied the same principle to swimming. His last doctor told him to swim to help his back pain. But the back pain continued year after year. So did his shoulder pain. From class, he discovered that when he swam, he was allowing his body to arch in the water, as if he were lying facedown in a hammock. He said it was simple for him to straighten his body using his abdominal muscles. The pain stopped. With the back no longer arched, the shoulder no longer had to overreach, which helped reduce the shoulder pain. With the improved streamline position in the water, he found he was suddenly swimming faster.

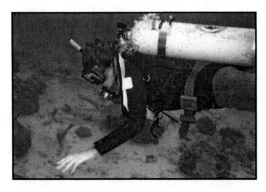

Figure 2-29. For swimming and scuba, use abs to prevent your lower back from sagging into an arch. Tip hip to straighten out for faster streamlined swimming and no pressure in the lower back.

Exercises to Strengthen Abdominal Muscles at the Same Time as Retrain Positioning

Instead of curling forward for crunches, some exercises follow that work your abs and back at the same time, plus train you how to hold your back in healthy position when you stand up. These exercises are good for everyone—especially for those with osteoporosis of the upper back or disc herniation. For these people, bending forward increases the pressures that further their injuries. These exercises teach you how to strengthen core muscles without forward bending.

Isometric Abs

A major purpose of your abdominal muscles is to hold your back in position when you are standing. This positioning does not happen automatically. That important concept is often missed. Many people allow their lower back to sway or arch, whether they have strong muscles or not. They may do "exercises" for the abs and their back pain by lying on the floor or standing against the wall and pressing the lower back (pelvic tilt) to reduce the curve. But that does not change your positioning the rest of the time, and so it does not stop the back pain. You are supposed to use the tilt voluntarily when standing to keep your back in position. By preventing arching you prevent the cause of the pain. This exercise strengthens abdominal and back muscles at the same time and, more importantly, retrains how to hold your back without overarching the rest of the day.

- Lie face up with your arms overhead on floor and your biceps by your ears.
- Press your lower back toward the floor to reduce the arch (Figure 2-30). You will feel abdominal muscles working to prevent your back from arching.

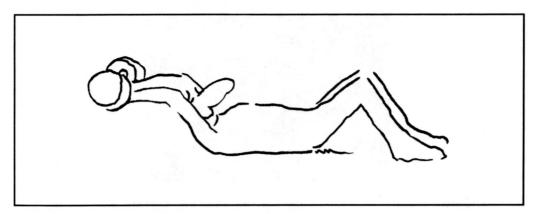

Figure 2-30. Isometric abs exercise with knees bent. Keep your ribs pressed down. Don't let the weight pull your lower back into an arch. You will feel your abdominal muscles working to control spine posture from being yanked upward into an arch.

- Hold hand weights an inch above the floor, without arching your back.

- Keep your lower back against the floor by using ab muscles to straighten your spine.

- Notice that you don't need to tighten your abs to do this. Just use your abdominal muscles, like any other muscles, to move your spine into position.

- When you straighten your spine positioning, the pivot point of lifting the hand weights shifts off the lower back and on to the core muscles. Two more pivot points that are strained with the arched position are the shoulder and elbow. Instead of arching back to lift the weight, you should also feel the weight shift from the shoulder and elbow to the abdominal muscles. Don't let the weights pull your shoulder or elbow joints. Use your muscles.

- Transfer this knowledge of how to use your abs to control the posture of your back when standing, and prevent overarching.

- As you get better at using abs to keep spine from arching, straighten your legs (Figure 2-31) and repeat without letting your back arch under the weight of the hand weights.

- Transfer this knowledge so that you can practice how to keep your spine in healthy position when standing without bending knees.

Some people say you must bend your knees to "protect your back" from arching. But it is your own abdominal muscles that are supposed to hold your back in position. If the way to "protect your back" is to keep your knees bent, how could you stand up and go about your life? It is not the knees that control back posture, but your torso muscles. Use the exercises in this section to strengthen your abs at the same time as retraining standing posture.

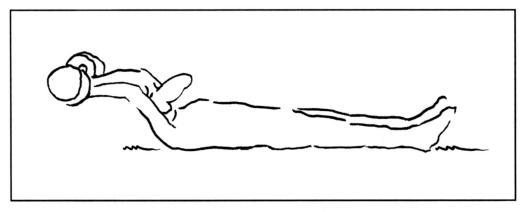

Figure 2-31. Isometric abs with legs straight. Keeping knees bent is not what "protects" the back; it is using muscles to position the spine. This exercise teaches how to prevent overarching when standing. Keep your ribs pressed down. Don't let the hand weight overhead pull your lower back into an arch.

If you habitually stand with your back arched, your back may tighten to the point where you can't straighten it to control your posture because you're stuck in arched posture. You need to stretch and retrain positioning habits. Use this exercise with legs straight to retrain how to reduce the arch by using abdominal muscles when you are standing.

Hold a Push-Up Position

Holding a push-up position can reduce back pain when used to retrain the abdominal and back muscles how to hold the spine and hip in position without sagging under your body weight. Many people do push-ups and allow their lower back to arch (Figure 2-32). Arching hammocks your body weight on the lower back and does not give the intended exercise for the muscles. If you don't control your spine position, doing push-ups can add more back pain.

Tuck your hip to straighten your back (Figure 2-33). You will immediately feel your abs working, and the pressure in your lower back will disappear. The purpose of this

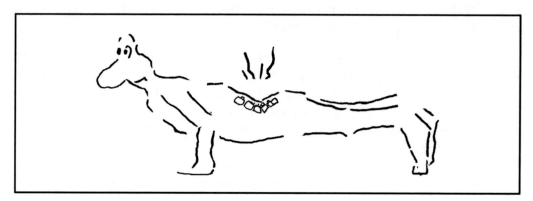

Figure 2-32. Don't let your body weight sag your lower back into an arch.

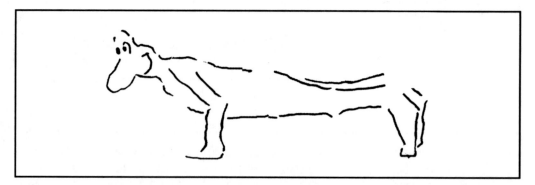

Figure 2-33. Train your muscles how to hold your back in healthy position, and then transfer this straightening to standing and reaching up.

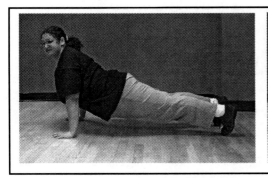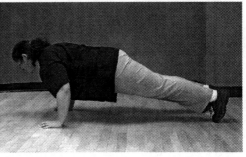

Figure 2-34. Push-ups are often done in ways that do not work the core and strain the back (left). Keep the hip tucked under (right), as if "starting a crunch" to make your back a straight line. You will strengthen at the same time as retrain how reduce arching when standing.

exercise is to train your abs at the same time you relearn how to hold your back from arching when you are standing up. Stay on hands and toes, not on knees. If you can't even hold up your own body weight, you are too weak for normal healthy life.

Keep your back straight, not letting it sag into an arch like a hammock. Don't drop your head. Use a mirror, if available, to see yourself and learn what healthy position feels like. Use this new, healthy position all the time, particularly when you stand and reach overhead.

Learn to Move Legs without Arching the Lower Back

A common but ineffective exercise is to stand on hands and knees and lift one leg in back. Often people arch their back to lift their leg (Figure 2-35). This movement does not work the leg or hip muscles, and reinforces faulty movement patterns. Many people arch their back to move their legs to walk and move instead of powering the movement from the leg and hip muscles.

Tuck your hip (Figure 2-36). You will have to use leg and hip muscles to lift your leg instead of arching your back and pivoting from your spine. Use chest muscles to lift your head; don't bend your neck at a sharp angle. Use this same abdominal technique when standing and lifting your leg in back.

Arm and Leg Lift for Strengthening

The hands-and-knees position gives little exercise and does not train how to hold body weight up against gravity. Instead of spending time on ineffective exercises, get off your knees. Hold a push-up position (Figure 2-37). It will strengthen arms and upper body. Use abdominal muscles to tuck under your hips or you will get no core exercise.

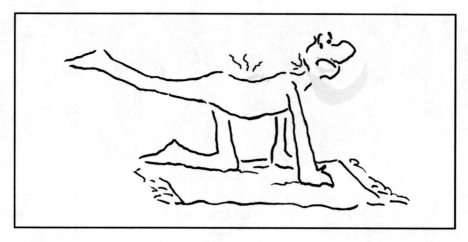

Figure 2-35. It is common to see people exercising by arching their back to lift their leg.

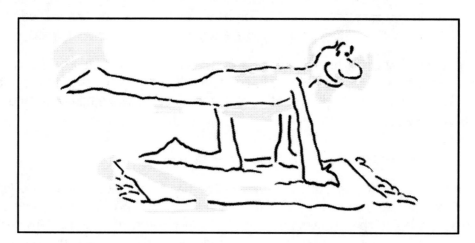

Figure 2-36. Don't arch your back to lift your leg. Instead, tuck your hip under, using your abdominal muscles and lift your leg with your leg muscles. You will feel a big difference.

- Hold a good push-up position with no arching.
- Lift one leg without letting your spine sag.
- When you can hold a push-up position without arching or sagging, lift one arm straight out in front of you.
- Lift one arm and the opposite leg at the same time to straight position in front and back.
- Don't drop your head. Use your muscles to hold you as straight as if you were standing up.

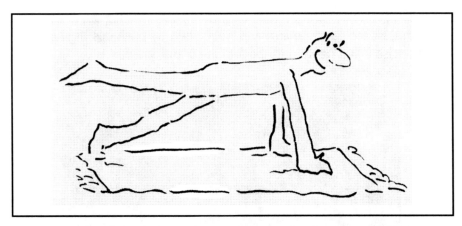

Figure 2-37. Use abdominal muscles to prevent your spine from sagging into an arch under gravity. Holding yourself up will give body and abdominal exercise while retraining how to stand without letting your lower back sag into an arch under gravity.

Oblique Abdominal Exercise

Another fun exercise trains your oblique abdominal muscles to hold your posture against changes in load (Figure 2-38). Hold a push-up position and turn to the side on one arm. Hold your body straight, using oblique abs to prevent sagging in the middle. When you can do this, lift the top leg so that you are standing on one arm and the side of your bottom foot.

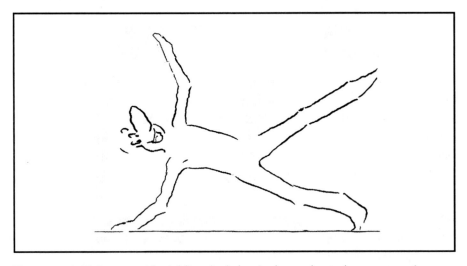

Figure 2-38. Train your side (oblique) abdominal muscles to keep your spine from sagging under loads. Use this side plank to train straight posture for carrying things without sagging.

For a challenge, hold a straight push-up position with one leg out to the side. When you can do this, lift the opposite arm and hold. Then try push-ups as shown in Figure 2-39. This exercise is not needed for back-pain control, just for fun.

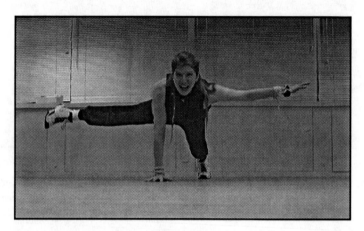

Figure 2-39. Hold a flat "plank" (push-up) position. Hold one leg out to the side. Lift the opposite arm. You will feel abdominal muscles working hard to hold your body in straight position against your body weight.

How Does Using Abs Translate to Standing Up?

You need to exercise your back the way you use it in real life—standing and stabilizing your spine against sagging under gravity and loads (Figure 2-40). This doesn't happen automatically—just by strengthening. It happens with holding your spine in whatever position you need.

Exercises to Transfer Use of Abdominal Muscles to Standing up

- Tie the middle of a long, rubber tube around a doorknob, post, railing, friend, or other device. Hold both ends in front of you. Stand far enough back to create tension on the band. Pull both arms straight down to your sides without leaning back or arching. Hold. Repeat. If you consciously hold your spine in healthy position while doing this, you strengthen and retrain torso-stabilizing muscles.
- With both arms straight, lift both arms overhead without arching your back or leaning back, to retrain how to lift loads with good posture. Repeat. Keep breathing.
- Turn your back to the band. Raise your hands overhead and repeat the above exercise without letting the tension on the band pull you backward into an arch. Don't lean forward against the pull. Hold a straight and healthy position (Figure 2-41).
- Turn to the side and use the same concepts to customize your own exercises to strengthen your back while holding steady for movements you commonly do.

Simulate tennis, kayaking, boxing, throwing, pitching, swinging a racquet, swimming, even combing your hair or writing on a blackboard. The idea is to retrain good postural mechanics during motion. Learn to use core muscles to power overhead activity to prevent back pain (and shoulder trouble, too).

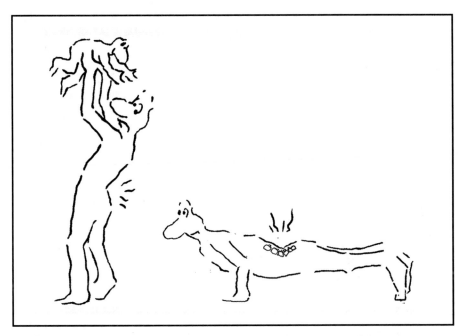

Figure 2-40. Arching pressures the lower back, both standing and exercising on the floor. Pushups done with an arched back does not work your "core" muscles. Practice your push-up position with tucked posture and transfer the idea of using abs during exercise to standing posture.

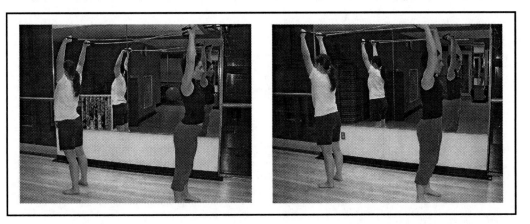

Figure 2-41. Practice good positioning when exercising overhead motions. Don't let the low back arch against the load (left). Use muscles to work against loads that pull your back and shoulder into an arch (right).

Why Not Put a Pillow under the Knees?

Many people are told that when sleeping on their back they must keep a pillow under their knees. The rationale is that lying on the back with legs straight will make the back arch and create lordosis that pressures the back (Figure 2-42). The pillow lets the tight hip tilt back down and reduce the arch. However, this does not solve the problem. Using the pillow to keep knees and hip bent perpetuates the problem. When the front of your hip is so tight that you can't stand and lie flat without your back being pulled into too much arch, you need to stretch your hip to stop that problem, not keep your hip bent.

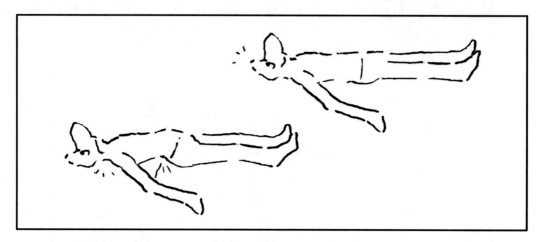

Figure 2-42. Lower-back pain when lying on your back often comes from hips being so tight that you can't straighten your legs without craning your back (left). A pillow under the knees perpetuates the tight hip. To fix the cause, stretch the hip using lunges and other stretches so that you can lie flatter (right), stopping the pain.

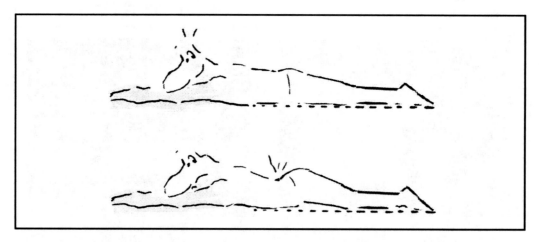

Figure 2-43. Lower-back pain when trying to lie face down often comes from tightness in the front of the hip (bottom). Stretching the front of the hip with the lunge allows you to stretch out flat without back strain (top). If you can't lie flat, then you can't stand up straight, either.

It is also common to hear that you should not sleep on your stomach because that makes your back arch, which is often the same issue. When the front of the hip is too tight to straighten, your back arches when you lie face down (Figure 2-43). Again, it is a matter of stretching the front of the hip so that you can lie flat. Use the lunge and other anterior hip stretches described in Chapter 4 (Figures 4-5 through 4-13). Remember that you also need to stand up without a bent hip and an arched lower back. If you can't lie flat with only a normal lower back curve and your legs straight, you can't stand straight either. No wonder so many people have pain.

What's Wrong with Conventional Abdominal Exercises?

Why not just do abdominal exercises to prevent all the problems? Even though conventional forward-bending exercises activate your abdominal muscles, they don't train how to use abdominal muscles in daily life. Forward-bending exercises round you forward. In real life, you need to use your abs to voluntarily prevent you from arching backward.

It's practically universal to see a gym full of people doing crunches, then stand up and walk away with their back arched and no use of abs, or knowledge that you are supposed to use abs standing up. Simply strengthening a muscle will not transfer the positioning you need for healthy sports and recreation, or back-pain control. Crunches and conventional forward-bending core exercises promote bad posture. The last thing the average person needs, after a day hurting their back by bending and rounding forward, is more of the same. Crunches make a person, who likely spends much of their day already hunched over a work area, practice that hunched posture which may be mechanically promoting the back and neck pain they think they are working their abs to prevent.

Upper and Lower Abs

Anatomically, each of your abdominal muscles are the same muscle throughout, not different at the top and bottom, like the upper and lower gastrointestinal tract. But the upper and lower ends of your abdominal muscles pull differently depending how you use them. All of your muscles do this. One example is bench pressing and push-ups. They are the same move, but in the bench press, your body is still and your arms and hands move. In the push-up, the hands are fixed but your body moves. Forces on your joints are different and stresses on your muscles change. The squat and the leg press are also mirror images. In the squat, your "end segments" (feet) are fixed and your body moves up and down. In the leg press, you sit in one place and your feet are the moving segment. Forces on the knees, cartilage, and muscles are different in each.

When you let your upper body arch or lean back, the upper muscle fibers need to contract more to pull the upper body forward to restore straight position. There is pull throughout the abdominal muscles to straighten up, but more in the moving upper areas. When you move your lower segment out, such as sticking your hips out in back, you need to activate more lower-abdominal muscles by tucking your hips under. Restoring healthy position is free upper- and lower-abdominal muscle exercise throughout the day.

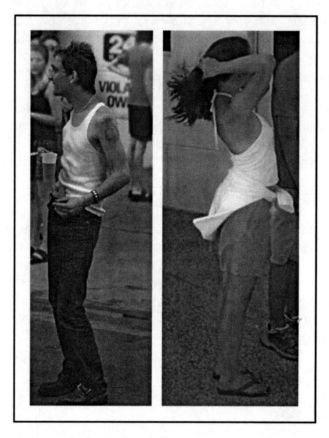

Figure 2-44. On the left is hip forward and upper body leaning back. On the right, the hip is out in back (the upper body is also leaning). Both bad postures arch the low back and create lower-back pain.

It's Not Arching by Itself That Is Bad

Arching your back, by itself, is not the main issue. The problem is the loading of the lower back from letting your lower back fold under your upper-body weight. This loading can occur standing up, when doing exercise such as holding a push-up position and letting the lower back hang like a hammock under your body weight, even doing a headstand or handstand and letting the weight of your legs hinge and fold your back sharply.

In cases where you want to extend the back for stretching, you can get a nice stretch by lying face down and lifting the upper body from the floor. This arches the back but does not load it under body weight. Lying face down and lifting arms, extending the back is an important back exercise. It strengthens the back muscles by contracting them and counters the excessive forward rounding of the back that many people do during most of their day, but it is not loading the lower back under body weight.

In cases where you need to extend the back for sports and reaching, use abdominal muscles to hold your upper-body weight up as you lean or extend backward. In this way, you can extend back without your weight pressing down onto your lower back. This extension is often confused for lordotic arching, and some people think they must never arch their back. Proper back extension is one of the most important exercises for back health and is covered in the previous back-pain section.

Spondylolisthesis

Andrew had played football in high school. Now that he was older, he wanted to stay active, but back pain slowly made him stop favorite activities. His doctors told him he had a condition that was probably genetic, permanent, and disabling. The doctor showed him his x-rays. The vertebrae in his lower back seemed to not line up one over the next. Andrew's doctor told him to never do any activity that arched his back because he had a condition called spondylolisthesis, or "spondy." Andrew gave up gymnastics. He gave up tennis and anything else that might arch his back. His pain increased and he got increasingly out of shape. When he came to me, he was miserable. "I used to be fit. Now I'm a wimp."

Spondylolisthesis is when one backbone slips forward on the next, adding to back arching. This slippage is not a necessarily a surgical situation or an unchangeable disorder. It isn't completely known why vertebrae slip in some people. In some cases it is a trauma from letting body weight continually press the vertebrae until they move. It is more common in people who do sports that forcibly bend the back too much both forward and back. Sometimes the places where the vertebrae attach to each other can fracture under repetitive stress. Andrew didn't have to give up sports or arching; he needed to learn how to use his abdominal muscles to prevent upper-body weight from falling on his lower-back vertebrae while he moved—especially when he extended his back. Sometimes what looks like a "spondy" is not always a true "spondy," just an exaggerated arched posture. Even with spondylolisthesis, it is even more reason not to allow your back to arch more this way. Arching and pushing the vertebrae out of place only enhanced the forces that create spondylolisthesis.

Stenosis

Stenosis means narrowing of a passageway. When you have spinal stenosis, the narrowing can be in the canal of your spinal cord or the small openings in each vertebra where the nerves go out to your arms and legs. People with spinal stenosis often find that they hurt less with bending forward and more with bending back. One of the reasons seems to be the same arching that causes the pain from lordosis. The arched posture makes less room for the spine and nerves. In stenosis, the fit is already tight, so it is easy to pinch or pressure things. Stenosis is all the more reason not to allow your back to overarch without muscular control. Use all the same principles of holding healthy position with abdominal muscles to stop the pain. Many of my stenosis patients report feeling much better with the exercises in this chapter and, more importantly, with the concepts of repositioning while standing, so that they can stand and walk around and have an active life without pain.

Both stenosis and lordosis can, interestingly, cause or worsen a pinched nerve. Arching can bring the vertebrae closer together in back, enough to press the nerves that exit the back of the spine and go down the leg, resulting in pain that can be confused for disc pain and wrongly treated for it. Imagine a person who has normal wear in their discs that doesn't cause pain, but which decreases the amount of space between the vertebrae just enough for a bad arched posture to pinch the nerve. Their x-ray shows decreased disc space and some disc degeneration. They have pain. They get surgery for pretty much normal discs. The pain continues and no one knows why. Sometimes they tell me, "You don't understand. I had to have the surgery. The pain was unbearable." You can stop the pain without surgery. Keep discs healthy with the principles in the disc section of this chapter and avoid the arched posture that is a hidden course of so much pain. Stop the source and stop the pain.

What Else to Check?

Several medicines have the side effects of causing back pain and muscle aches. These include cholesterol-lowering medicine, some prescription allergy medicines, stomach-acid inhibitors, erectile enhancing drugs, anti-anxiety medicines, prescription anti-depressants, prescription acne medicines, medicines for irritable bowel, constipation, and Crohn's disease, the calcium-channel-blocker drug verapamil, the antibiotics erythromycin and clarithromycin, and others. It used to be thought that pain only came with overdose, but it is now known that body aches and back pain is are common side effects of these drugs. Doing a few stretches does not stop this pain. It is better to solve the cause of the problems than to take drugs that cause other problems.

It is important to rule out non-orthopedic causes of lower-back pain, like diseases of the esophagus, pancreas, prostate, and genitourinary system, an aorta (big heart artery) that is ready to dissect (tear open), cancer, infection, thyroid problems, and kidney and gall stones, being a few. Smoking is directly toxic to bone cells and discs. A burning ache around the side of the body or hip may seem like ongoing back pain before the characteristic rash comes out to show it is shingles. Vitamin D deficiency is a hidden contributor to pain syndromes. Get outside for fun activity every day, making sure not to overexpose yourself to skin cancers either. It's a balance. Your doctor has a hard job making sure of where pain is coming from. If it is not something medical, then you have the easy job of just changing simple ergonomic habits.

Several foods are thought to be inflammation promoting—such as dairy, meat, sugar, and white flour. Foods with anti-inflammatory properties are leafy green vegetables, flaxseed, cherries, blueberries, and spices like ginger and turmeric.

Most back pain from poor positioning is not an inflammatory problem, which is why many people taking over the counter and prescription anti-inflammatory drugs don't get the expected relief. Others with conditions like rheumatoid arthritis get more relief from changing food habits to anti-inflammatory ones and getting more sunshine. It is not a bad idea for everyone else to reduce the inflammation processes in the body that modern life seems to promote to excess.

What to Do Every Day to Stop Lower-Back Pain from Lordotic Overarching

- The pain-prevention technique of using abdominal muscles to prevent overarching is one of the simplest of all pain preventions. Don't sag your lower back into an arch. If you let your hips stick out in back, tuck your hip back under you using lower abdominal muscles. If you lean the upper body backward and let the hip jut forward, pull the upper body forward and the hip back using upper abdominal muscles.

- Hold a push-up position with your hip tucked under to keep your back in a straight line, not arched. If you can't hold a straight position without sagging, your core muscles are so weak and untrained that it is no wonder that you sag when walking around all day.

- Isometric ab exercise (Figure 2-31). Lie face up. Arms straight by your ears an inch or two above the surface holding hand weights. Don't let your back arch or your ribs lift. Use abdominal muscles to prevent arching and to hold your posture against the load of the hand weights. This exercise simulates how to use abs to hold posture during the way—by moving spine into position, not by tightening.

- When you pull your chin in, reach overhead, or look upward. Don't do it by arching your lower back. The postural change needs to come from your upper body, not by creating another strain on another part.

- Retrain your exercise habits and mindset away from conventional exercises that curl the body forward to exercise the abdominal muscles and core. Use functional exercises that use muscles while exercising back hip in the straight position you need for healthy, natural function, like the isometric ab exercise (Figure 2-21) and holding a push-up without arching (Figures 2-33 and 2-37).

- Watch other people, especially in the gym when doing exercises. When you see them arching, it is easy to see the pressure they put on the lower back. It will remind you not to do the same.

When to Notice Overarching in Your Lower Back

- The most common times to arch the lower back are when standing and when lifting arms overhead. The most overlooked times are when looking overhead, hugging, washing your hair in the shower, drinking, and taking photos.
- When you lie flat on your back without a pillow under your head or knees, does your back arch, your ribs lift up, or your chin jut upward? If you are too tight to lie flat without these positional strains, you are too tight to stand up straight without lower-back pain.

How to Get Natural Lower-Back and Abdominal Strengthening during Daily Activity

- Instead of letting your back arch, use ab muscles to tuck the hip if it is stuck out in back, or pull the upper body to a straight position if you lean back with the hip forward. You will get free, all-day, built-in exercise for your entire core and lower-back muscles.

Alice was a medical resident. At age thirty-four, she had already suffered with back pain for nearly twenty-five years. She had been told it was because of slight scoliosis and lordosis. Various doctors she worked with and went to as a patient described it as "a pronounced curvature but nothing can help this condition because it is within the normal limits of back curvature." She spent much time reading many medical books on back pain which all repeated the common assertion: "This is the price that we pay for being bipedal (walking on two legs)." She thought it was normal to have back pain and that it was a mystery issue.

As a medical student, Alice had learned that as long as you rule out conditions such as sciatica, spondylolisthesis, disc herniation, and so forth, back pain was the product of how the spine is shaped or is psychosomatic (originating in the mind). Dr. Alice told me she was hoping that she would have the scary physical conditions because then there would be a cause and a cure (surgery) for her unrelenting pain. But she had "back pain, not otherwise specified." She said, "You can imagine my dismay that I could not be 'cured' from surgery."

Alice went to expensive, private yoga classes, which briefly helped but the pain always recurred. She did all the back and abdominal exercises in every medical book. She saw an orthopedic surgeon and a PMR doctor (physical medicine and rehabilitation). Her x-rays were "perfectly normal." She wanted to get an MRI of her spine hoping it would show disc herniation so that she could get the much wanted surgery and be "done" with back pain. The physicians she saw recommended bed rest, NSAIDs (non-steroidal anti-inflammatories), and ice.

Alice studied books about the importance of good posture in back pain. To her dismay, the "good" posture was difficult and uncomfortable. When she came to my back-pain workshop, she told me she hoped we would just learn some exercises so that she could go back to the usual "comfortable" bad posture. She just wanted some exercises, "because it's something you can do for 30 minutes, and have the back pain go away, at least briefly." In class, I showed her how easy it was to change the lordotic position that was causing such unrelenting pain for so long. She told me she was "greatly surprised and shocked" that the pectoral stretch (Figure 1-9) and trapezius stretch (Figure 1-10) made good posture "strangely comfortable." Because her upper body was tight, she had previously been arching her back to keep her upper body upright. She was more surprised to find that going back to her old lordotic position was uncomfortable and made her hurt. She could tell where her pain had been coming from along, and why some of her exercises and yoga had added to it. She had been doing them in the lordotic position that everyone told her was normal. She realized why the pain went away briefly after exercise then returned when she went back to daily life with lordotic positioning. Back pain was no longer mysterious, and in fact, made a lot of common sense to her. She knew that she didn't have to memorize rules and could apply the principles to yoga classes, step machines, weight training, and everything else she liked to do. She felt empowered.

Alice wrote me a few months later, "After a mere four-hour 'No More Back Pain' workshop, I was surprised to find that the whole class knows much more than a lot of PT and orthopedic physicians in terms of diagnosis, evaluation and treatment for 'back pain, not otherwise specified.' We thus received a greater than $1,000,000 education, for medical school and loss of income during orthopedic residency training. I can also go home and teach all my friends and family suffering from back pain. This is a great example of the 'see one, do one, teach one' model of medical education."

No More Lower-Back Pain from Hyperlordosis

Fixing lower-back pain from lordosis (also called hyperlordosis and swayback) can be simple. The cure is not facet injections (shots in the joints of your vertebrae) or just strengthening your muscles. The key is to address the cause. Stop the arched lordotic position that drops upper-body weight on your facet joints and soft tissue.

Some of this is information may be different from what you may have heard. The old stuff wasn't working as well as it could. New strategies were needed. Discard the outdated notion of "tightening" your abdominal muscles, or any muscles to use them, or the old "press navel to spine." You cannot breathe in or function that way, and walking around with "tight" muscles is a factor in headaches and stress- and strain-related muscle pain. Instead, use your muscles to hold your spine in healthy position, easily, no matter what you are doing or carrying. Use abdominal muscles to simply to keep the upper body from swaying back, the lower back from arching, and the hip from tilting forward and sticking out in back, when standing, reaching, and carrying, and doing all you want to do.

A patient sent me a card around Christmas time that she noticed the Christmas dolls in the store: "This year it struck me that one of the pilgrims was standing in a contorted fashion; pelvis thrust forward, back arched, and neck bent forward. It hurt me just to look at him. Now picture me trying to reshape the posture on the dolls!" When I get letters like this, I know that patients know what it means to live a healthy lifestyle, not just do a bunch of exercises.

Preventing Back Pain from Long Sitting

Sitting for long periods can get uncomfortable, whether at the desk, on a flight, when driving, or using a wheelchair. Most lists of instructions for sitting without hurting your back tell you to sit in exact ways at exact angles. This approach is not needed. Instead, it is better to understand the concepts of how and why strain and injury occur when sitting. Then you can sit in healthy ways that are comfortable, easy, and healthy.

Why Is Slouching Bad?

Sitting with a rounded back does several things to cause injury and pain. Rounding forward (slouching) when sitting holds the muscles in a longer-than-normal position, which weakens them. It also slowly degenerates your discs, the cushions between your backbones (vertebrae), and pushes the discs outward to the back—which is how discs herniate, also called a slipped disc (Figure 2-14). A slipped disc can bulge outward enough to press on nearby nerves, sending pain down your leg. One kind of pain down the leg is called sciatica and is easy to prevent.

When Do People Round Their Back?

Many people could sit up straight and rest against the chair back, but they let their back

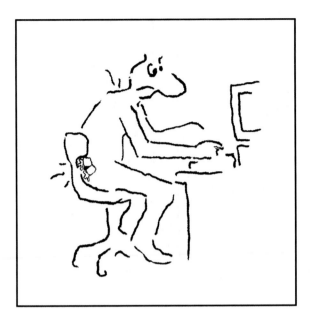

Figure 2-45. Rounding your back pressures the discs in your lower back. Over years, the discs can be pushed outward (herniate), especially the lowest ones that bear the most weight when you sit and bend badly.

round. They round their back all day at work, then round to "relax" (Figure 2-46). No wonder their back hurts.

A problem is that many kinds of seats have a round (concave) back. It is common to sit in these round chairs and allow your back to round to fit the round chair back (Figure 2-47).

Worse, many people not only round into the chair back but round further by hunching forward of the chair or putting a pillow behind their head which only rounds the upper body further (Figure 2-48).

Another common way to make your back hurt when sitting is to sit toward the middle of the chair, and create a "hammock" out of your spine, sagging between the buttock and the upper back. Your body weight presses down on your lower-back discs (Figure 2-49).

Simple Back-Pain Prevention When Sitting

Instead of sitting forward in your chair, move your hip against the back of the seat, and lean back in comfort. If the chair back is rounded, put a small cushion in the space between your lower back and the seat back to preserve the small, normal inward curve, instead of assuming the curved posture of the chair (Figure 2-50). Use this for all sitting, from wheelchair to jet.

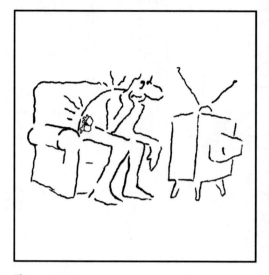

Figure 2-46

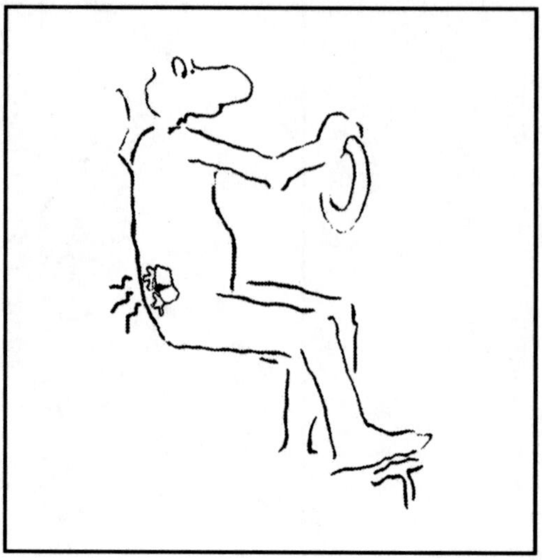

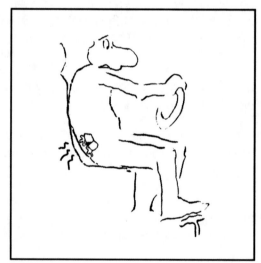

Figure 2-47

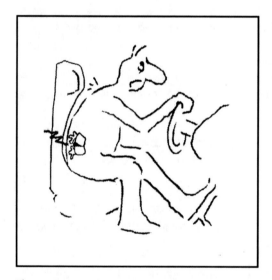

Figure 2-48

Figure 2-49

Making a Lumbar Roll

To feel the right size for a lumbar roll, sit back in a chair and nestle your forearm behind you in the natural lumbar space between your lower back and the chair. Lightly press your upper back against the chair so that the lower back does not press your arm, but rests lightly. It should feel comfortable. Your forearm is usually about the right size for a lumbar roll.

Many things can work for a lumbar roll. Rolls are commercially available—including inflatable ones that pack flat. When traveling, you can use many common soft items. Try a small folded towel, shirt, hat, or gloves. Fold your jacket, just enough to be the size that is comfortable.

Commercial lumbar rolls are sometimes large, solid forms. If it is too large, it will be uncomfortable. Others are a roll of foam. You can make your own from foam, or cut a commercial roll lengthwise (Figure 2-51). Then you will have two, one for home and one for the car. Put the cut side to the seat and the rounded side toward your back.

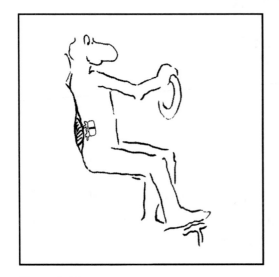

Figure 2-50

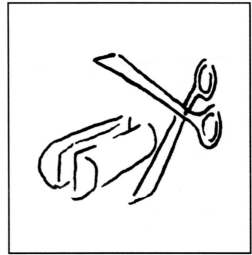

Figure 2-51

Using the Lumbar Roll: Lean Back, Not Forward

Don't use a lumbar roll that feels too large. It will be uncomfortable. If you feel like it is sticking you in the back check to make sure you aren't rounding against it, or that it isn't too large, or extending too high or low on your back. Lift your upper back against the chair instead of pressing against the roll. Don't force into an unnaturally straight or arched posture. Keep head up, not tilted or craned forward. Rounding against the lumbar roll is as uncomfortable and useless as rounding without one (Figure 2-52).

Sitting When Driving

- Move your hip to the back of the seat.
- Move your seat in closer. Then you won't have to round forward to reach the steering wheel.
- Tilt the seat slightly backward.

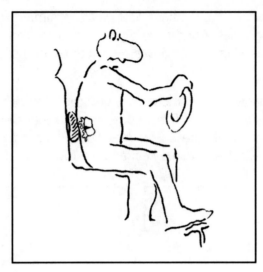

Figure 2-52

- Sit up and lean back against the seat, instead of craning and rounding.
- Use a soft lumbar roll (Figure 2-51). Don't round against the roll, or press your lower back into it. Lean back and press the upper back against the seat.
- A bonus to moving the car seat forward is that by sitting back instead of reaching forward, your chest and face are farther from the airbag, said to be safer.

Sitting at Your Desk

- Move the seat in and sit closer to the desk so you can sit up instead of hunching forward (Figure 2-53).
- Put the computer monitor up on a book, block, or shelf.
- Use an external keyboard for laptops so that you can raise the laptop as if it were a monitor.
- Depending on your height, lower your seat so you don't reach down for the desk.
- If there is a chair back, sit with your hip against the back of the chair. Use a soft lumbar roll (Figure 2-51). Don't round against the roll, or press your lower back into it. Lean back and press the upper back against the chair, not the lower back.

Sitting on Buses and Flights

Commercial airline, bus, and train seats are often rounded, encouraging prolonged, forced rounding. If the seat is very curved, you may need two pillows, one for the small inward curve of your lower back, and the second above that one for your upper back, in the space still left by the rounded seat (Figure 2-54).

Flights sometimes have a video message encouraging in-seat stretching. Often the advice is forward bending, which is the last thing you need after sitting bent forward for so long. Instead, stretch your back and shoulders backward, not forward. Pull your chin in while leaning back. Breathe.

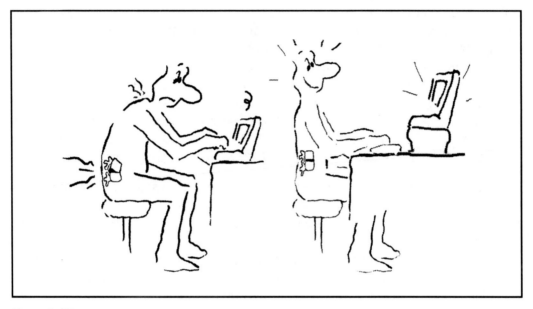

Figure 2-53

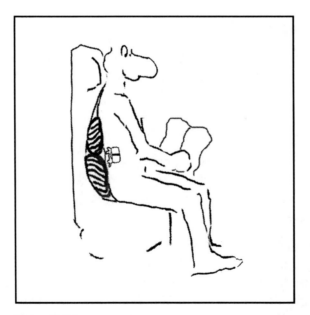

Figure 2-54

Sitting for Exercising

People exercise in hopes of better health, yet often exercise in unhealthy ways. A common way to increase back pain is to lift weights sitting down and leaning forward, supposedly to "target" muscles in the back of the shoulder or back. You know it is unhealthy on lower-back discs to bend over to pick up a package. Bending over to pick up a gym weight is not magically healthy. Pressure on the lower-back discs is higher during sitting than standing. Pressure is even higher when sitting bent forward. Adding lifting weights adds more damaging force. It is not necessary to hurt your discs to "target" a muscle. Instead, exercise your back muscles with extension exercise (Figures 2-11 and 2-12) rows, and push-ups, and other core training exercises without forward bending (Figures 2-30 through 2-39). If you like rows, hold a flat, straight push-up position without arching (Figure 2-33) and lift a hand weight from the floor up to your side. Instead of sitting, stand to lift weights. It's more exercise and better balance training.

Another common injury from sitting exercise occurs when sitting rounded on weight machines (Figure 2-18). After years of unhealthy sitting, rounding against a leg press or other resistance can be too much for the discs. They break down, swell, and press on nerves that go down the leg, sending pain down the hip and leg. The problem is not the amount of weight you lift, or that you are exercising; it is your positioning. Check to see if you sit with a rounded lower back. Change to straighter healthy position. Don't let your hip and lower back round when you bend your knees toward your body to lower the weight. Instead of pushing your lower back against the seat or pad, lift your upper body to sit straight, and push your upper back against the seat.

Sitting for Relaxing

Instead of sitting rounded in soft chairs and couches, use a pillow or other cushiony object to pad the space between the normal inward curve of your lower back and the chair (Figure 2-55).

Don't Forget to Get Up

No matter how well you sit, sitting is sedentary, and time spent bending at the hip. The front hip muscles shorten from sitting. Short, tight hip muscles add to achy hips and backs. Get up from your desk, and out of the car often and straighten the hip from the bent position (Figure 2-56).

Use the pectoral (chest) stretch and the trapezius stretch often to help straighten the upper body (Figures 1-9 and 1-10). To stretch after long sitting, household chores, or exercise, lie face down and prop on elbows (Figure 2-57) or stretch backward over something (Figures 1-11, 3-10, and 4-10). Don't pinch or crane your back or neck. Gently stretch the entire spine and hip the other way. If backward stretching brings on lower-back pain from the arched position, see the lordosis section in this chapter.

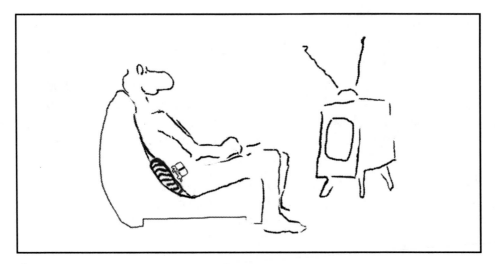

Figure 2-55

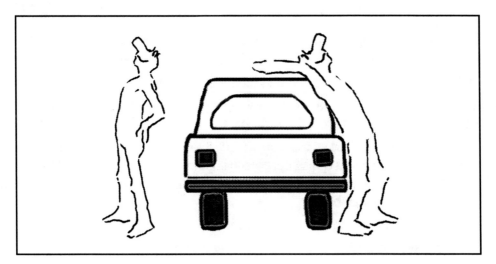

Figure 2-56

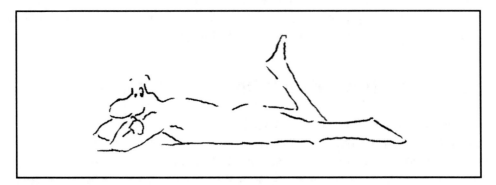

Figure 2-57

No Strange Rules

It is common to hear that you must sit with elbows, knees, or hips at 90-degree angles, hold thighs parallel to the floor, or other strange, strict rules about positioning arms or legs. Don't worry about angles. Get the concepts and then you will know how to make whatever you are doing healthy. Don't sit frozen in place. Movement is important for joint health. Joints don't have high blood flow. Joints move nutrition in and waste out by physical movement. Move freely in your chair instead of sitting still for hours. Moving regularly through a wide range of motion is important.

Sit in healthy position whether the chair has straight back, a round back, or no back. Keep it simple. Sit preserving the small inward curve of your back without exaggerating it. You will prevent injury and be able to get up after long sitting with straight, happy position and no pain.

What to Do Every Day to Stop Pain from Long Sitting

- Watch how other people sit. When you see how bad it looks to sit in unhealthy ways. You will be better able to see and correct it in yourself.
- Notice unhealthy posture featured in fitness and health magazines.
- Move your desk and car seat closer to sit up, not rounded forward. Press your upper back, not lower back, against the chair back.
- If the chair back is curved so that you would sit with a rounded back, pad the space with a lumbar roll so you can sit up, preserving the normal, small, inward lower-back curve. A rolled up shirt or small towel will do. Don't round against the lumbar roll. Sit up and lean slightly back.
- Raise your computer monitor if it is too low.
- Move the keyboard off the "below desk" tray and back up on the desk.
- Raise your television higher. Stop sitting hunched and forward to watch.
- Don't slouch because you think it is natural to let your weight sag. Many things happen naturally if you let them, like drooling and wetting your pants. Sitting right is just healthy, comfortable, natural control of your body.

No More Back Pain when Lifting and Carrying

Healthy lifting is more than "lift with your knees," although few people do even that much. What is often missed in back-pain prevention is how to carry things. More achy backs can be found at the end of the day from poor carrying technique than from bending wrong to lift your packages in the first place. This principle holds for anything you carry, not just packages—whether carrying the baby or groceries, a pet, lifting luggage to overhead racks, lifting weights in the gym, and even the weight of your own body.

Back Pain from Leaning Back when Carrying Things in Front

A common bad habit is to lean backward when carrying something in front of you, like a package, a chair, or a baby (Figure 2-58). Leaning back makes things easier to carry because you don't support the load with your muscles. Instead, you lean back to shift the load onto your lower back, which means your lower-back joints bear the load instead of your muscles. You lose free exercise and pressure and strain your lower back. To prevent this problem and get good exercise at the same time, try the following:

• Stand up and hold any load in front of you, like a backpack, baby, or chair.

• If you notice yourself arching or leaning back, straighten your body to an upright position by curling forward enough to take the excess arch from your lower back. Don't curl forward so much that you round your shoulders. Just straighten your body against the pull of the load. You will feel your abdominal muscles working.

• Maintain upright posture against any anterior load. Your bags, groceries, and babies could be a built-in abdominal muscle exercise.

You may have heard the false statements that being pregnant makes your posture change and arch and that it is the pregnancy that makes your back hurt. Pregnancy is

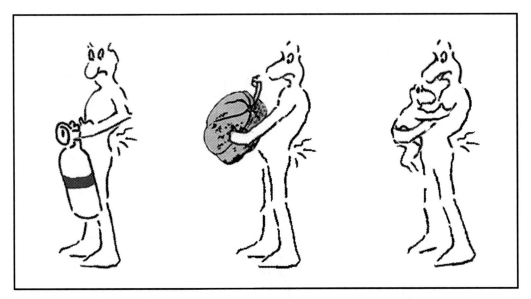

Figure 2-58. When carrying, don't arch your back, lean back, or push your hip forward. Instead, tilt your hip under you to reduce the arch in your low back and straighten your posture against the load.

a case of leaning back to carry a load. The pain is preventable by not leaning back to counter the weight in front. Use your abdominal muscles to straighten your posture so you can stand without arching backward. Of all times to prevent arching, pregnancy is certainly one.

A surprising way to help your back is to strengthen your arms. When your arms are weak, it's more tempting to rest a carried weight on your hip and lean back, letting your lower back take the brunt. Even if you have strong arms, don't lean back. It's not strengthening the muscles, but using your knowledge to position your muscles that will fix your back pain.

Back Pain from Leaning Back when Lifting Overhead

When reaching overhead to stretch, reach a shelf, take a picture, take off your shirt, or lift things overhead, see if you arch your back (Figure 2-59). Arching shifts weight to your lower back. Instead, tuck your hips under you to reduce the arch of your lower back, then reach up again without leaning back. You may be surprised at the difference. You will have to stretch your chest and shoulders more, but that is good, and will save your back.

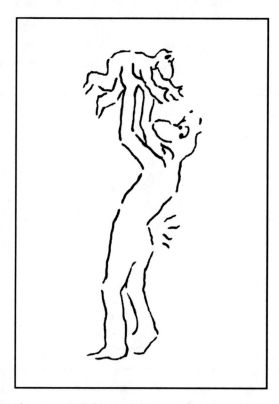

Figure 2-59. It is common to arch or lean back
when reaching and lifting. Don't lean back.

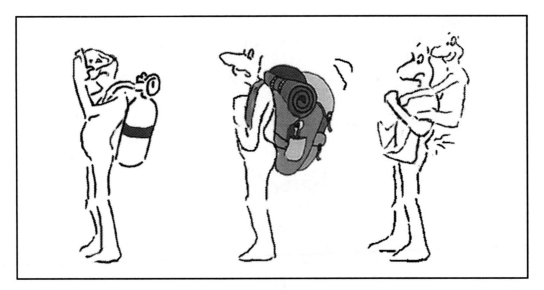

Figure 2-60. A common source of back pain is letting your back arch when carrying posterior loads. Don't let your back arch. Reduce the arch and hold your torso upright. Your pack becomes a free core-muscle workout.

Back Pain from Leaning Back when Carrying Things on Your Back

Heavy bags and backpacks don't make you arch your back or have bad posture. Not using your abdominal muscles to counter the pull, and allowing your back to arch is the problem (Figure 2-60).

- Stand up wearing a backpack or other load on your back. Notice if you arch or lean back. Straighten your body by beginning to curl your torso, as if "doing a crunch" but don't learn forward, round your shoulders, or crane your neck. You will feel abdominal muscles working to do this. Your bags could be a built-in abdominal-muscle exercise.

- Don't stick your behind out to hold the bag. Keep your hip tucked in enough to straighten your body.

- Don't tuck so much that you lean back or stick your hips forward.

Some people let the load pull their upper body backward and their hip forward (Figure 2-61). Instead, pull your upper body forward and your hip back to straighten yourself.

Back Pain from Leaning Forward when Carrying Posterior Loads

With posterior loads like knapsacks, it's common to lean or round forward to counter the weight (Figure 2-62), instead of holding the weight using muscular effort. Leaning forward is easier because you don't have to support the load with your muscles. Leaning forward shifts the weight of the load to your spine. That means your spine does the work instead of your muscles. You lose free exercise, get a round-shouldered posture, and strain your back. Instead, use your back muscles to pull back to straighter position. It's a free workout and you won't be sore after a day of carrying.

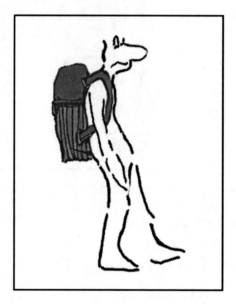

Figure 2-61. Letting the upper body slouch backward pressures the lower back. Pull your upper body up and forward to straighten out.

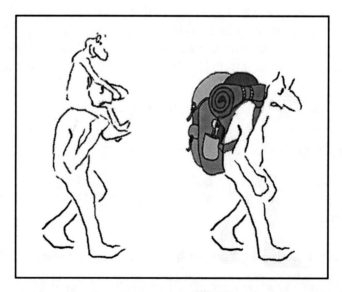

Figure 2-62. A common source of back pain is rounding forward when carrying loads on your back. Instead, use your muscles to keep body upright and chin in.

With extreme weights, it is normal to bend under the weight. It is not healthy, but it is sometimes the only way, for example, rescuing a heavy person or getting a truck out of a ditch. Strengthen your muscles and learn good positioning so you can minimize injury during situations when the weight is just too heavy. For most carrying, prevent rounding forward, and get good exercise at the same time. Stand straight without leaning backward or forward. You will feel your muscles working.

What to Do Every Day for Healthy Carrying Habits

- Watch other people when they carry things.

- When you notice yourself leaning your upper body backward when carrying a load in front or back, pull yourself forward until you are straight, as if starting a crunch. Come to straight position, without curling forward.

- When you notice yourself arching backward or sticking your hips out in back when carrying a load in front or back, pull your hip forward with a tucking motion until you are straight, as if starting a crunch, but without curling forward.

- When you notice yourself rounding forward when carrying a load, lift the upper body up and back until straight. Don't arch your back to do this; use your upper-back muscles.

Good Carrying Habits for All the Time

Is it natural to slouch under your own body weight and the weight of things you carry? It is as natural as wetting your pants, but you learn to "hold it" even when you don't feel like it. Good body positioning is the same. Learn to hold it.

Use your muscles to hold your body in healthy positions when standing and carrying and you'll get natural exercise without going to a gym, and save your back for all the things, big and small, that you lift and carry.

No More Back Pain

The majority of back pain, even pain from arthritis, curvatures, structures not being where they should, and bad discs, are results of unhealthy standing, sitting, carrying, and bending, that mechanically abrade, strain, degenerate, and push things out of place. Stop the cause of the injury and you can prevent and stop the pain that results. Rethink your exercise program so that you don't do unhealthy things in the name of fitness. Moving in healthy ways for daily life gives free, built-in exercise to become strong and mobile. How is your back positioning right now reading this? You can quickly heal from back pain without pills or surgery, and regain your life, better than before.

3

No More Shoulder Pain

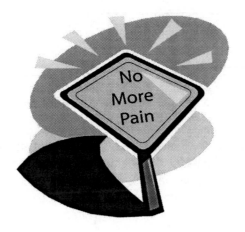

- Mystery Shoulder Pain
- Round Shoulders
- Grinding Shoulder
- Scapular Winging
- Separated Shoulder
- Rotator Cuff

This chapter covers major contributors to shoulder pain that are often missed and simple things that can stop even long-time problems. Most shoulder pain is the result of small, daily habits that slowly injure the shoulder over time. Using the techniques in this chapter, you can understand and relieve most of them yourself. Even if you don't have shoulder pain, the principles can show you how to have healthier, more mobile, and stronger shoulders.

Injury from Forward Head and Round Shoulders

Robert was a top photographer in Philadelphia. Over time, he started losing use in one arm. He saw the big-name doctors in Philadelphia and New York. Each told him it was a serious long-term injury—probably job-related. He must give up his work and learn to use the other arm more for daily life.

I made my house call to his commercial studio. Equipment, props, and papers covered the walls, floors, tables, ceilings, and hung in the air. Prize-winning photos lined beautiful shelves he had carved himself. Products piled on tables waiting to be photographed. He gestured to his work with one arm; the other hung strangely forward. As he talked, the arm would sometimes move weakly and then stop. His face was pained.

He worked long hours craning his head and neck forward over lenses, lights, and work orders. He didn't know that letting your head and neck hang forward (a posture called a "forward head") is a common cause of neck and shoulder pain. Combined with rounding the shoulders, it interferes with normal movement of the shoulder. Robert kept his neck and shoulders tilted so tightly forward that the weight of his head and round shoulders slouching on his spine was like a bowling ball pressing the nerves that supplied his arm. Photography was not the problem. The trouble was the forward head and rounded upper-back positioning.

Robert liked to work while listening to music and craned forward to put a cassette in the player. The tape slipped out of his hand. He said his arm often had problems when he raised it while leaning forward. He pushed his neurological tests to me over the table where he sat hanging his head and going over his fears for his arm and career. The discs in his neck were fine, but conduction tests of how the nerve signal could pass through his shoulder to his arms showed blockage of the nerves that moved the arm, and some damage to the nerves that let him feel, called sensory nerves, which was why he hurt and could not move well.

I explained how the forward head is a factor in shoulder pain. He yanked his head back, hoping the arm would revive. He winced in pain. I told him the good news was that he didn't have to wrench his head back. Tightness and pressure was the problem in the first place. You didn't want to add to it yanking and straining to stand straight.

I showed him the pectoral stretch (Figure 3-3) and the trapezius stretch (Figure 3-4) to restore muscle length so that that he wouldn't have to struggle to hold his head and neck straight. I had him stand with his back against the wall to feel where straight positioning of his head and shoulders would be. Although he rounded forward from habit and years of tightening into a familiar position, he relaxed against the wall and let himself straighten out. I gently pulled each arm downward by the hand to make some room in his hunched-up shoulder sockets. He said he could feel the pain subside in the arm with each stretch. I had him lie flat on the floor to try to relax with his head, neck, and shoulder in a straight position. He slowly waved his newly-working arm to me.

He worked on the concepts and practiced repositioning exercises for a few weeks, along with strengthening exercises for the arm that had shrunk from lack of use (Figures 2-31, 2-33, 2-37, and 2-38). On follow-up six months later, his arm was fine. He insisted to thank me by taking my picture. He said he would "capture the real me." I thought, "Who could do that?" But he did, and that photo is the author photo for this book.

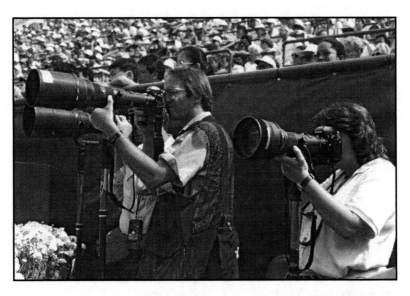

Figure 3-1. Curving the upper back and neck forward can interfere with raising the arm, sometimes producing shoulder pain. You don't need to round your back to take a photograph—even with a heavy camera.

When you slouch with round shoulders and a forward head, the bony ledge of your shoulder rounds forward. Every time you raise your arm, the top of your upper-arm bone jams against the shoulder bone, squeezing the soft tissue between them. What is between? The four muscles and their tendons that make up your rotator cuff. It is called a cuff because these muscles wrap around the top of your upper arm like a sleeve cuff so that they can rotate your arm around in the socket. Rounding your shoulder forward can hurt the rotator cuff over years of raising your arm during daily activities, such as brushing your teeth, shampooing your hair, pulling a shirt off overhead, and putting away groceries and clothes in overhead closets. The injury adds up over time. Rotator cuff pain may be in the front or back of the shoulder, and often in the middle of the arm at the bottom of the deltoid shoulder muscle.

Other things that can be squeezed between the arm and shoulder bone when your head and shoulders rotate forward are the nerves that go from your neck down your arm. When the nerves are squeezed, it is called impingement. Impingement sends pain down the nerve. If you are told you have shoulder impingement, don't think of it as the diagnosis of the problem. It is the result of something else—often the neck and shoulder posture. Fix the cause and you will stop the pain. This approach is better than just getting shots or taking medicine. A small percentage of the population has a shoulder bone, called the acromium, which is more hooked than usual. Surgery is often recommended to shave the hook so that it does not abrade the rotator cuff. Good positioning becomes even more important for people with an acromial hook, and can be enough to prevent injury and the need for surgery.

To feel for yourself how your neck and shoulder need room to work together, let your head jut forward and round your shoulders in bad posture. Slowly raise one arm overhead and notice how you can't raise it completely without feeling like something is in the way. Now stand straight with your shoulders back and your chin in and raise your arm again. This healthy position lets you raise your arm without it pressing against the shoulder, crushing the nerves and soft tissue in between. For many people this change in pasture habit is all they need to restore healthy, pain-free movement and give their shoulder a chance to heal.

Danelle worked bent over a cash register. She sat on a high stool. Her knees didn't quite fit anywhere at her station, so she bent forward to work the register. She sat heavily slouched, shoulders rounded, with her head and neck forward. She was large, so her chair was far back from the counter. Each time she leaned in and lifted her hand to the register she winced in pain. Sometimes her arm would drop. "My doctor said I have a rotor."

"A rotator cuff?" I asked.

"Yeah, something like that. The doctor said it's repetitive strain and I have to use the other hand more." If Danelle used her other arm in the same unhealthy, rounded position, it was more likely that she would get new pain than fix the old. Some simple changes were needed for her to fit in her station. It was more important for Danelle to sit differently in her workstation and not to round and slouch forward when she lifted either arm.

Do You Have a Forward Head and Round Shoulder?

It is so common for people to let their head tilt forward in a "forward head" that many people think it is normal posture. A forward head is the equivalent of a bowling ball hanging forward on your neck and shoulder all the time, pressuring, and getting in the way of raising your arm normally. No wonder it hurts. How do you know if you have a forward head and rounded shoulder?

- Stand with your back against a wall, with heels, hip, and upper back against the wall.
- Does the back of your head touch the wall without arching your back or lifting your chin?

If it is uncomfortable to bring your head against the wall to stand straight, it is likely that the front muscles of your chest are tight. Chest muscles shorten from standing round-shouldered. A cycle continues of shortening so that you are too tight to stand straight, and standing rounded which further tightens and malpositions the shoulder. For many people, this habit is the mysterious cause of long-term shoulder pain, numbness, and tingling in the top of the shoulder, and sometimes pain that goes down the arm.

Two Stretches to Relieve Forward Head and Round Shoulders

Two main stretches restore normal resting length to your shoulder and the front of your chest so that you can stand in a healthy and straight position without pressuring your neck and the top of your shoulder. These same stretches are described in Chapter 1. To recap:

Pectoral stretch

The goal is to stretch the chest muscles, not the shoulder joint (Figure 3-2).

- Face a wall with one elbow bent about ninety degrees out to the side. Place the inside of your arm against the wall (Figure 3-2, left).
- Turn your feet and body away from the wall (Figure 3-2, center), letting your arm be braced back by the wall so that it stretches. Keep breathing. Pull until it is comfortable, not tense (Figure 3-2, right).

- The stretch should feel good in the front muscles of the chest and underarm
- Don't jut your neck forward or arch your back
- Keep your shoulder down and relaxed.
- Hold for a few seconds and change sides.

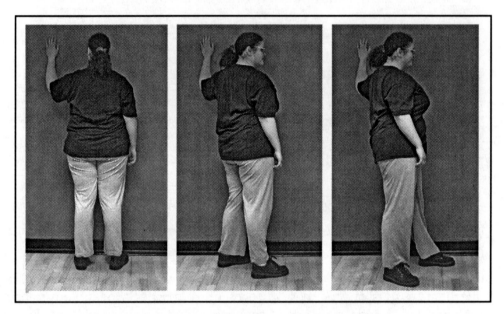

Figure 3-2. Pectoral stretch

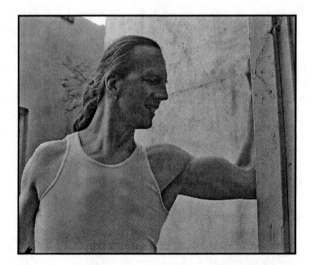

Figure 3-3. Front view of the pectoral stretch. Brace the inside of your elbow against a wall and turn your whole body away from the elbow. Feel the stretch in the muscles of the front of the chest—not in the shoulder joint.

Trapezius stretch

The trapezius stretch restores length to the muscles at the top of the shoulder that often ache from the forward head, or from holding the shoulder hunched or tight (Figure 3-4).

- Put one hand over the opposite back pocket.
- Tilt your head and body down toward that hand. Slide the other hand down the side of your leg to your knee.
- Don't lean forward or round your shoulders.

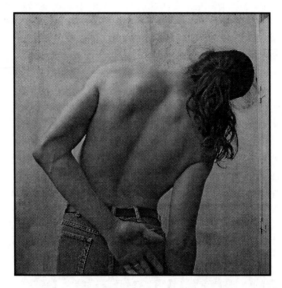

Figure 3-4. Trapezius stretch. Put your hand over the opposite back pocket. Tilt your head and body to stretch the top of the shoulder.

Pierre had pain across both shoulders. He explained to me that he had good posture and was "very attuned to his body because he taught Alexander Technique." I asked how long he had the pain and he said it was just a general part of his life. The Alexander Technique is variously described as a way to become conscious of habits and movements so that you can become able to learn new things ranging from posture to other endeavors. He said that part of the technique was using muscles efficiently with the minimum effort and letting weight rest on the skeleton. It seemed that he was doing exactly that. He was letting his head and shoulders round forward. The weight of his head hanging on the skeleton of his neck was creating ongoing pain in his shoulders.

The rounded shoulders were interfering with overhead movement of his arm. Both his thumbs faced each other because his arms rotated inward from his rounded shoulders. This "crab" position is a classic sign of upper-body tightness (Figure 1-8). I asked Pierre to stand with his back against the wall, with heels, hip, upper back, and head touching. He could not bring his head to the wall without straining and pulling his lower back into an exaggerated arch.

Pierre was doubtful when I explained that the wall stand was straight posture. "But it's so uncomfortable. Straining and tightening is bad," he said. I explained to Pierre why that was exactly his problem. His "comfortable" rounded position was what made him too tight to stand straight. He said that he thought that "blockages" caused his pain. I showed him the pectoral stretch (Figure 3-3) and the trapezius stretch (Figure 3-4). Right after doing both stretches, he was able to stand with the back of his head against the wall without straining. When he looked down at his thumbs, they now faced straight ahead, no longer turned inward. His straighter shoulders no longer rotated his arm bones inward, but held them in healthy position. Pierre said, "They say that the Alexander Technique is supposed to discover unconscious habits so we stop interfering with the body's innate movement, but slouching as a comfortable habit was innate to me. It was just making things worse." I reminded Pierre not to just let his weight hang on his skeleton, but to use his muscles so that he didn't simply slouch to whatever position his body fell into—comfortable or not. By restoring muscle length to the chest muscles, and holding it there, he wouldn't get tight in the first place.

Shoulder Pain from the Tight Hip

Although not obvious at first glance, another hidden cause of shoulder pain occurs when you reach upward and the hip is too tight to straighten. The shoulder has overrotated when raising the arm (Figure 3-5). This problem is not uncommon.

The front of your hip often gets tight enough that you stand with the hip bent at the crease where the leg meets the body. It may sound like a tight hip contributing to shoulder pain wouldn't happen often. Some sports-medicine professionals state that a tight hip only affects the shoulder in "overhead athletes," such as baseball pitchers. However, reaching overhead is something almost everyone does many times a day. You reach in the gym for weightlifting and exercise class, during recreational activities like tennis, basketball, dancing, cheering, swimming, and football, and ordinary activities all day like reaching shelves, cleaning the house, combing and washing hair, and getting dressed. A tight and habitually bent hip is common because most people spend most of their days and nights with their hip bent. They sit much of the day, sleep with knees

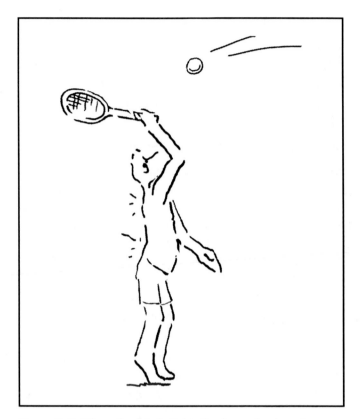

Figure 3-5. When the hip is tight, the lower back and shoulder overrotate when reaching up. A tight hip can hurt the shoulder dozens of times a day in ordinary, overhead activity, at work, and during exercise.

bent, and then exercise by mostly bending forward and bending at the hip. Most people even do stretches for the hip with their hip still bent instead of straightening it.

A bent hip is so common that it looks normal to many people. They think they are supposed to stand with the hip bent, the back arched, and the hips stuck out in back. This bad posture is not healthy or good looking. It is unhealthy posture that contributes to aches and pains. The repeated strain on your shoulder just from daily activity with a bent hip can produce shoulder pain that is hard to rehab if you don't stretch the tight hip that creates the problem. To stop the cycle of tight anterior hip, bent hip posture, and shoulder strain, stretch the front of the hip. One effective and easy stretch that you don't have to get on the floor to do is standing in the lunge position (Figure 3-6).

- The key to stretching the front of the hip is tucking the hip under the body so that it is straight—not stuck out in back (Figure 3-6, left). To tuck the hip, start to do an "abdominal crunch" standing up, but don't lean forward. Reduce the overly large arch in the lower back that comes from not standing with the hip tucked under enough. You will feel the abdominal muscles working and the front of the hip stretch in the back leg. Don't lean your upper body backward. Stand straight. Use this hip tuck when doing throwing activities, to get power to the arm from the core muscles.

- Keep a wide stance with the back foot straight not turned out. Don't lean forward (Figure 3-6, right).

- Feel the stretch in the front of the hip of the back leg.

- To increase the stretch in the front of the hip of the back leg, bend both knees and lower straight toward—but not touching—the floor. Raise and lower straight up and down. Start with five or six and see how you feel. Use a mirror where you can, to see what straight position is. Work up to at least 10 to 20 "dips." Use this lunge for leg exercise instead of "walking lunges." Many people step forward or back, leaning their front knee inward and forward with each step. Keep feet in place when raising and lowering to practice healthy placement. Then apply it to walking lunges, not letting the front knee come forward or sway inward.

- Increase the exercise by holding hand weights. Each time you rise, lift the weights up. Use a variety of lifts: biceps curls, overhead lifts, and out to the side with thumbs facing upward. The combination of lunge and lift strengthens body and arms together in functional ways, simulating lifting daily objects. When you put the weights back down, don't bend over wrong. Use the lunge you just practiced.

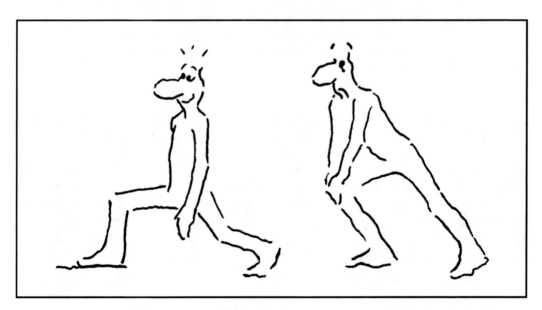

Figure 3-6. Standing lunge. Keep your hip tucked under and your back upright, without hands on your knees (left). Feel the stretch in the hip that is stretched back. If you lean forward or stick your hips out in back (right), you won't get the hip stretch, but can throw body weight on the lower back and front knee joints.

Look at your belt or waistband to see if it tips down in front and up in back. Unlevel, tipped position may indicate that you are standing with your hip bent forward. The hip may be bent from tightness, or just a bad habit. If the unhealthy hip position is the reason for pain, but is not recognized or fixed, the shoulder injury continues and the lower back may hurt along with it. When the tight hip is corrected with stretches and good body mechanics, the source of the damage to shoulder and back can stop. The hipbone really is connected to the shoulder bone.

Tight Shoulder

We live part of each year in Asia. We visited friends in northern Thailand in their traditional house. The grandmother is a slender, straight-backed, silver-haired Thai lady in her 80s. Over the years, every morning on our way to school, we would greet her in the customary respectful greeting called the "Wai" of raising arms with hands pressed together, saying "Good morning, Mama," as she moved unfalteringly for daily chores. She returned the Wai with sure hands.

One year we arrived in the rainy season and found Mama sitting under a yarn blanket, unmoving and pale. She tried to return the Wai but could not raise her arm. She sat, still and defeated. I was stricken. I asked the daughter what happened. Mama had broken her shoulder two months earlier. I asked if she could move it but it was too painful. Each day we greeted her in the morning, but there was no return Wai—or much other movement. She sat under her blanket and dozed in the afternoons. I worried that this was the last year we would see Mama.

It turned out that it was not the shoulder, but the upper arm that had broken. The shoulder was not injured from the fracture. It was stuck from disuse. I launched into lectures about the dangers of lack of movement and how keeping it still was injuring it more every day. They nodded politely. I explained how joints don't have high circulation. Not much blood passes through to bring food and oxygen in—or wastes out. The way joints move things in and out is through movement. The simple hydraulic pumping of moving the joint squished nutrients in and wastes out. Movement was crucial. Without it, debris and increasingly hard scarring would fill the capsule, slowly freezing it. They nodded politely.

One morning I sat with her, massaging her hands and arms. I told them that in the United States, one of the favorite exercises of my senior-age patients was called "Punch the doctor." I made a punching motion in the air. Punch the doctor! I punched the other arm. Her medical care had been good, but she still smiled. Throughout her life she had done martial arts and, until breaking her arm, had practiced every day. I asked her about her martial arts. As she described it, her eyes livened and her head lifted. She did some experimental punches. At first her shoulder was uncooperative, but she kept moving. I told her that my seniors also liked "Kick the doctor." I gave them that exercise to get their blood circulating instead of pooling in their legs when they sit too long. Often, after sitting or lying down too long, blood pressure falls when trying to stand. For some people this becomes a negative cycle of not moving, and being too weak to stand without getting dizzy. The way to stop this problem is not to prevent standing, but to get blood pumping before standing so that enough blood pumps to the head when rising. One easy way to do that is squeezing the fists and pumping the legs. Punch the doctor! Kick the doctor! She rose unsteadily out of her big chair. Her daughter sitting at the desk looked up. Mama started showing us her full martial-arts routine: punch, punch, step, step, kick, crouch down, stand up, punch (Figure 3-7). The daughter's eyes were happy. The next morning we greeted Mama. She raised her arms just enough to return the Wai.

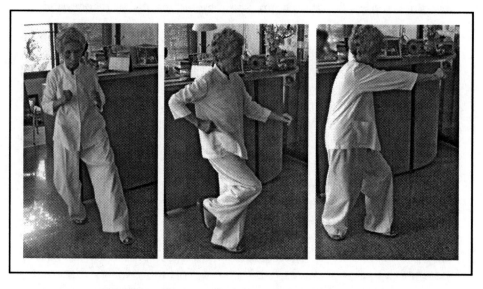

Figure 3-7. Movement every day at all ages is essential to continuing health and mobility.

Good Shoulder Stretches

Some say that those with shoulder pain should not do overhead stretches or exercise. It is true that many people hunch their shoulder or raise their arms with tight shoulders and a forward head, worsening their situation. The goal is to retrain overhead activity so that it is healthy again. You need to reach up for a normal life on a daily basis—to wash, dress, put away groceries, and other activities. It is important not to create pressure and injury to the shoulder while doing them. The goal of relearning movement is to retrain healthy movement to restore function.

Pectoral and Trapezius Stretches

- Two stretches to start every day for your shoulder are the pectoral stretch (Figure 3-3) and trapezius (top of the shoulder) stretch (Figure 3-4).

- Do both stretches first thing in the morning and throughout the day to restore healthy muscle length, and to remind you to keep shoulders from rounding.

Standard Shoulder Stretch

- Stand up and reach your arms overhead (Figure 3-8). Keep your shoulders down. Don't hunch the shoulders when raising the arm. Bend your elbows so your hands can reach your back, as if to scratch between your shoulder blades. If your back arches (Figure 3-8, left), you will reduce the shoulder stretch.

- Flex your trunk forward to straighten your torso, as if to start doing a "crunch" (Figure 3-8, right). Keep your elbows lifted to the ceiling. Feel the stretch move to your shoulder and triceps. Don't drop your head forward since that motion only reinforces the forward head habit.

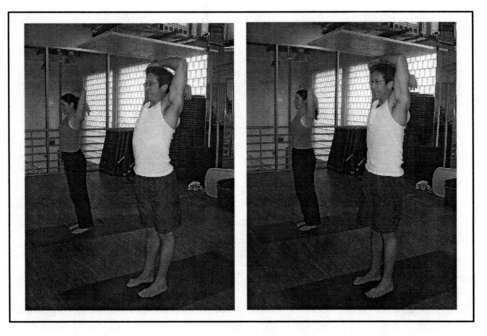

Figure 3-8. If you arch your back, you lose the stretch in your shoulder (left). Tuck hip to reduce the arch, keep head up not forward. Let the stretch come from the shoulder (right).

Shoulder Posture Stretch

- Either sitting or standing, put your hands on hips. See if you let your shoulders come forward.

- Pull shoulders back without arching your back or sticking your chin out. Keep your upper body lifted up without increasing the arch in your back. The stretch comes from the upper body.

- Pull shoulders back with your bands touching behind your back.

- Use this technique to restore and remember straight upper body posture. Use the new position all day, not just as a stretch. Use the stretch throughout the day to remind yourself.

Wall Shoulder Stretch

- Stand with your back against a wall and reach your hands up to touch the wall overhead. Keep your shoulders down. Don't hunch the shoulders when raising the arm. Can you reach up without arching your back?

- Push your lower back toward the wall to reduce the arch. A small arch remains, but not a large one.

- Keep shoulders down and relaxed.

Lying Shoulder Stretch

- Lie on your back on the floor or bed.

- Reach arms back, elbows by your ears, touching hands to the floor or bed. Can you do this without arching your back or hurting your shoulder?

- Keep hips tucked under and your shoulders down and relaxed.

Bed or Ball Stretch

- A fun stretch is to lie back over a ball, bed, or other raised surface, and let your upper back and arms drape over the edge (Figure 3-10). Make sure the stretch comes from your upper back and shoulder, not by arching your lower back. Don't hunch the shoulders.

Good Shoulder Flexibility Helps More than Your Shoulders

A tight shoulder can cause more than shoulder pain. Just as a forward head and tight hip are hidden causes of shoulder pain, a tight shoulder is one hidden cause of lower-back pain. When the shoulder is too tight to reach overhead normally, a person will

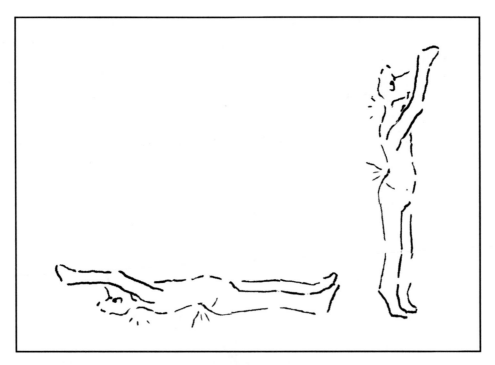

Figure 3-9. Many people arch their back instead of stretching their shoulder. When you lie on your back with arms overhead, your arms should be able to reach your ears without making your back or neck crane back (left). If you are too tight to do this, then you are too tight to reach overhead without pinching and craning your lower back and neck (right).

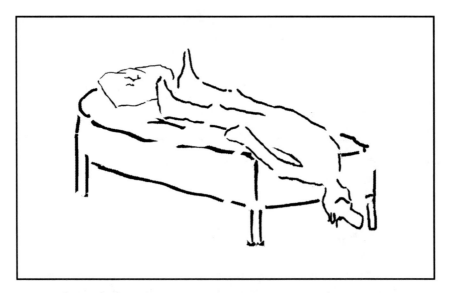

Figure 3-10. Bed stretch for the upper back and shoulders

often arch the lower back instead. Try it yourself now. Stand up and stretch both arms high up overhead. Did you lean back or raise your ribs to do it? Many people arch their back rather than get the rotation and stretch from the shoulders. That is why many people have tight shoulders even though they "do stretches." They never got the stretch. To relearn lower-back positioning to prevent the kind of arching that pinches the lower back, see the lordosis section in Chapter 2.

The contribution of shoulder mobility to saving the lower back is one reason that American football receivers wear smaller shoulder pads than other players. Bulky pads, just like a tight shoulder, get in the way of reaching up to catch a pass.

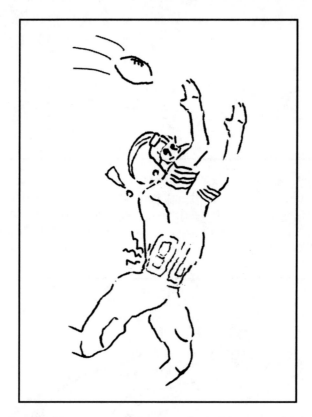

Figure 3-11. When the shoulders are too tight to reach straight upward, it is common to yank and overarch the lower back to raise the arms, making "mystery" lower-back pain.

Functionally Tight Shoulder

When the shoulder is tight, it can hurt during normal movement. Sometimes tightness is not from lack of flexibility. Often normal shoulder flexibility is present, but the person tightens the shoulder to move it. They will pass a flexibility test in a doctor's office or gym, but get continuing shoulder pain from tightening when they move. This tightness is not structural tightness, but functional tightness.

Sheila came to me explaining that she was getting shoulder pain after exercise class. It would have been easy to assume it was something in the class, but I asked her when she felt it after class. She told me when she was driving home. It was her left arm. If it had been her right arm, I would have asked her if she often reached over the front seat for a shoulder bag or a child in the back seat. A common source of right-sided shoulder pain is reaching without using torso muscles, just levering the weight of what you want to reach onto the shoulder joint (described in further detail, later in this chapter). But it was her left shoulder. She said it didn't always happen. She didn't rest it on the door when driving. She said it didn't hurt right then so was difficult to describe.

Her shoulder flexibility was good. I told her that hard-to-describe pain was common from tightening in poor positioning, and was a good indication that it wasn't something torn or so wrong that it would hurt in a memorable way. I clasped my hands in front of her making my arms as much like a steering wheel as I could.

"Drive!" I said. She put her hands on my simulated steering wheel. I held my arms still to give resistance. "Turn right!" I said. She raised her left shoulder and pulled it forward in the effort.

"That's the pain!" she said. Shelia had healthy flexibility in her shoulder. Moving her shoulder wasn't causing pain; it was how she was using her shoulder when she moved. I showed Sheila a scapular mobilizing exercise to train her how to relax her shoulders for activities involving her hands, like driving, preparing dinner, and using the computer.

How to Fix Shoulder Pain from a Functionally Tight Shoulder

- See if you raise your shoulder when moving your arm.
- See if you tighten or raise your shoulders to turn your head to look over your shoulder when driving.
- Keep shoulders down and back, easily. Don't tighten shoulders to force "good" posture.

I have found, after seeing hundreds of patients and students, that they can move their shoulders into healthy position as long as they are not also doing something with their hands. Then, their shoulders suddenly get "stuck" in a rounded forward position. All their shoulder exercises didn't help them in real life. It is important to practice functional exercises.

Scapular Mobilizing Exercise

- Stand at arms length facing a wall. Round your shoulders forward, as if trying to touch them together in front. Then pull them back, as if trying to touch them together in back, pinching shoulders blades together. Repeat several times easily and loosely.

- Put both arms straight out in front of you, reaching for the wall, without touching it. Do the same forward-and-back movement for the shoulders. Keep elbows straight. Your hands will move toward and away from the wall.

- Now put both bands flat on the wall with elbows straight. Move your shoulders forward and back just as before, without bending your elbows or neck. Your shoulders and body should move forward and back.

- Let the movement forward and back come from your shoulders, without bending elbows. This movement is how to mobilize your shoulders to relax them and put them in healthy position when your hands are fixed on a task

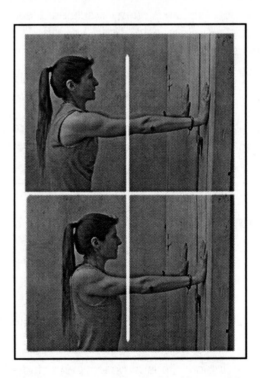

Figure 3-12. Scapular mobilization exercise to keep shoulders mobile when your hands are fixed, such as when driving or typing.

Your shoulders may be surprisingly "stuck" at first, and not move when touching the wall. This lack of movement is an example of needing to practice function when you stretch or do an exercise. When you're driving, you may hold your shoulders forward and tensely, and not be able to move them to healthier position. Don't practice this exercise while the car is in motion. Learn it at home first. Then when you find yourself driving with head and neck craned forward, you can make an easy, safe adjustment to bring them back. Make sure not to raise and hunch your shoulders to look over your shoulder when making turns, changing lanes, entering on-ramps, and checking for oncoming traffic.

Allen was a personal trainer, proud of the muscles bulging from the top of his shoulders. They were strangely out of proportion to the rest of his body. He said his neck and shoulders hurt and he wondered if it was from how he watched television or slept. I asked him to show me how he pointed at something, combed his hair, and brushed his teeth. Each time me moved his arms, his shoulders hunched, bunched, and tightened. He showed me his biceps, and hunched his shoulders when he flexed to "make a muscle." He raised his arms to touch his hair, and his shoulders bunched up. The straining and tensing was hurting his neck and shoulder, and making his muscles into tight, unstretching little rocks. I showed him how holding his shoulders in this unnaturally high and tightened position all the time was causing his problems. I assured him he could still have muscles, without the muscles causing him pain.

It is simple to use your body in a healthy manner when you move. Don't tighten to move. If your shoulders are truly tight, not just from how you use them, use the several stretches and exercises in this chapter to restore normal resting length to the muscles. Then use your healthy range of movement for all daily activity. Don't artificially tighten your neck and shoulder when you move.

Shoulder Pain from Bad Stretches

It seems easy enough that if the shoulder can hurt from being tight, then the answer is just to stretch. A problem comes from doing stretches that add to the reasons it hurt in the first place.

It is common to stand, sit, and move with rounded shoulders. Adding to that, a stretch that many people do is to round their shoulders by pulling their arm over the front of their body (Figure 3-13). This stretch promotes the same round shoulders with which you started.

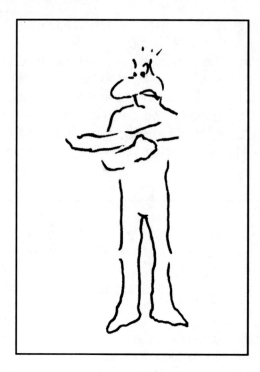

Figure 3-13. You don't need to stretch the back of your shoulders because they are usually already overstretched from rounding them all day. This stretch promotes round shoulders.

Two more stretches that worsen shoulder problems involve pulling your arms up behind you (Figure 3-14). These do not stretch the chest, but often jut the shoulder forward. Pulling the arms back further jams the arm bone forward into the front of the shoulder joint where it is weakest. Bending forward while doing this stretch pressures the discs of the lower back. Instead, do the pectoral stretch (Figure 3-3).

Another stretch that isn't useful for most people is to put your arm against a wall to pull the arm back by forcing the shoulder capsule forward. Some injuries (for example, adhesive capsulitis), where the joint is stuck, a professional in physical rehabilitation can use this technique to mobilize the shoulder capsule. For general stretching and shoulder health, use the pectoral stretch (Figure 3-3).

Forced stretching past a certain range can destabilize the shoulder joint until it doesn't seat well—increasing wear and tear. Unstable shoulder capsules may allow your shoulder joint to slip out of place from forces that healthier joint capsules tolerate. An inflexible shoulder joint is often confused for an unstable joint. The difference is that a flexible joint can still be held in healthy position while an unstable joint has been injured so that it does not seat properly.

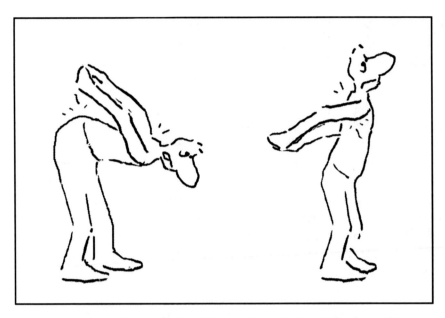

Figure 3-14. These common shoulder stretches don't stretch the muscles effectively but can destabilize the shoulder joint.

Shoulder Pain from Bad Exercises

A common weightlifting and aerobic-class move is raising the arms repeatedly to the side with the thumbs pointing downward. Turning thumb-down rotates the upper-arm bone, called the humerus, so that the bump at the top comes directly under the bone forming the top of your shoulder. This movement can squash (impinge) the soft tissue and rotator cuff tendons. This squashing doesn't only happen in the gym, but when you brush your teeth or reach into cabinets. This problem is similar to the shoulder injury you can get with a forward head. Both repeatedly squash structures like the rotator cuff between them. It can also squash the cushiony sac called a bursa. The purpose of the soft, squishy bursa is to reduce friction where the moving parts rub. If you repeatedly squash them, it can inflame the bursa—which is called bursitis. Imagine the double damage by both rotating thumbs down and letting your neck slouch forward. Keep thumbs facing up when exercising and reaching. You can still exercise the back of your shoulder just by holding your shoulders back in good posture.

Neck and shoulder pain is not uncommon for swimmers. The good news is that swimming itself is rarely the problem, just poor stroke mechanics. Many swimmers do not roll their body to the side, as needed for good swimming form. They keep body level and yank their arms out of the water and crane their neck to breathe. Or they hunch their shoulder to turn their head. Poor stroke mechanics combined with extreme distance work can result in neck and back pain from twisting movements or overarching vertebral segments. This bad habit is easy to fix by rolling to lift the arm, not craning the shoulder. With a good body roll, the arm comes high out of the water in easy position without strain, with a faster stroke. A good workshop in "stroke mechanics" can help you feel and practice the proper positioning.

Another problem for swimmers is the shoulder stretches they do, most importantly, raising clasped hands up behind them. Swimmers routinely do this for a greater range of motion, which can improve swimming speed. The price can be shoulder instability and susceptibility to long-term injury. Ironically, when pain develops, they are often told, "It must be the repetitive strain of swimming, so stop swimming. Just stretch for now." It was not necessarily the swimming, but the stretching. They continue to stretch wrong, which was the cause of the pain, but no longer have the muscle-building activity of swimming. Strong shoulder muscles help to counteract the instability that poor stretching technique can produce. The unstable shoulder joint continues to rub, clank, and hurt.

Grinding Noises from the Shoulder

"My shoulder crackles!" Elaine wiggled her shoulders forward and back. She was happy to make crackling noises from her shoulder for me to hear. I told her the noise was coming from where her shoulder blade rests on her back, over her ribs. She had been trying to keep in shape and had been lifting little hand weights. She strengthened the muscles at the top of her shoulder a little but didn't work the lower muscles. Together with her slightly rounded shoulder position, it tipped the shoulder blade. The top of the shoulder blade, or scapula, was tight on the ribs but the bottom pulled away. It made noise as it moved over the back of the rib. The scapula is supposed to glide over the ribs as you move your arm and shoulder. Instead it was grinding where it tilted.

I showed Elaine exercises for the lower-shoulder muscles, like low rows pulling back elbows, but also showed her how to hold her shoulders back in healthier position all the time so that she didn't round the upper back and tip the scapula. She was surprised. She had deliberately been pulling her shoulders forward when doing "pull-backs" given to her by her trainer because she could get more "umpf" as she put it, to pull back and because she thought it was "sort of dance-y" to learn forward. On six-month follow-up, Elaine said that she had been keeping her shoulders straight and not rounded forward when exercising and for daily life. She could crackle her shoulder if she "wanted to" by holding the shoulder forward, but otherwise the noise was gone and the top of her neck, which often ached from the poor shoulder position also no longer hurt.

Restabilize the Scapula to Prevent Grinding

- Hold shoulders back all the time. Don't arch your back or strain to do so. "Hold shoulders back" doesn't mean to hold them in back of you, arching and straining. It means to bring them back from a forward position to straight.

- Don't round the upper back, which tips the scapula up at the bottom.

- Do "low rows." Pull a cable weight or band that is secured in front of you, to your waist. Pull elbows and shoulders back together.

- Do very low rows. Pull a band or cable weight with straight arms at the sides of your legs. Pull from your sides to behind you. Pull arms and shoulders back together.

Winged Scapula

An interesting thing you can do to your shoulder is to let the shoulder blade, or scapula, stick out at the bottom like a "wing" (Figure 3-15).

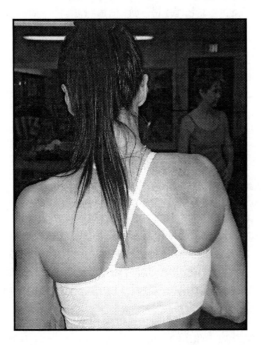

Figure 3-15. "Winged" scapula shows a weakness of the serratus muscles and poor use of scapular muscles. Don't let the bottom of your shoulder blades "wing' out. Keep the upper shoulders back, stretch your chest with the pectoral stretch, and use muscles around the lower areas of the scapula to hold the scapula in place

Trina came to me because her doctor thought she might have a nerve injury. Her scapula stuck out at the bottom. Instead of lying flat on the back of her ribs, the scapula looked more like a wing. Sometimes winging happens when the serratus, one of the muscles that holds the bottom of the scapula in place, isn't working right. The serratus starts on the front of your ribs and goes around your side to the edge of your shoulder blade. The nerve that serves the serratus is called the long thoracic nerve. Trina's doctor worried that she might have a long thoracic nerve injury.

Trina was an aerobics and yoga instructor, and personal trainer. She had been teaching and doing all the usual upper-body exercises—like biceps and chest curls, overhead press, bench press, and deltoid raises. She stretched by bringing each arm in front of her. Her upper scapula was tight on her ribs, and the low end stuck out. She thought that meant she was "cut" and lean enough to see her bones. But a winged scapula is a warning of poor muscle use or weakness. You sometimes see this on young children before they develop their chest and back muscles. It looks like you can hang them up on the back of a chair by their shoulder blades (but don't do that).

The strengthening exercises Trina had been given, like rows and incline press, hadn't worked to reduce the winging. Nothing was wrong with the nerve to her serratus, and it wasn't that she didn't strengthen the serratus; she just wasn't using the muscle.

Retrain Scapular Winging

Several exercises are common for winged scapula, and are often given to strengthen the area, without reminding that the purpose is to retrain you how to stop rounding your shoulder forward all the rest of the day—not just when doing the exercise. Plenty of muscular people have muscles but don't use them for healthy positioning. Use the muscle to keep the scapula from winging. To retrain scapular winging, try the following:

- Use the pectoral stretch (Figure 3-3) and the trapezius stretch (Figure 3-4) to restore ability to stand without rounding your shoulders. Then use this ability during all the things you do.

- Scapula mobilization exercise (Figure 3-12). Start by rounding shoulders forward and back. Try this again with arms out in front, elbows straight. Try this movement again with hands against the wall and elbows straight, so that it is the shoulders that move back and forth—not the elbows bending—that lets you move. When you bring shoulder back, don't round your shoulders to do it. Bring the top of the shoulder back without arching your back, while you move the bottom of your scapula back in. Use this exercise to discover what pulling shoulders back in good position is, so you can use it the rest of the day.

- Take the scapular mobilization further as a combination serratus exercise and positional retraining. With the ability to do the scapular mobilizer above, sit on hands and knees. Keep elbows straight. Sink down letting your shoulder blades pinch together in back. Don't let them wing. Then round up, pushing your chest far from the floor. When you have the idea of how to control shoulder positioning, do this same mobilizer in a push-up position. Sink shoulders down pinching your shoulder blades together in back. Then round upward. Keep your body straight; don't dip your hip down. Keep elbows straight (not locked) but not moving. All motion comes from your shoulders.

You can "wing" your scapula by putting your hand behind your back and letting your elbow hang a little forward which tips the scapula. Some people can "wing" just by pressing the extended hands against a wall. Control this by pulling your shoulders down and back into good position.

Straining the Shoulder Joints Instead of Using Torso Muscles

When throwing and reaching overhead, your torso and legs should power most of the movement. Some people just swing their arm, pivoting at the shoulder and arching their back. Shoulder and back pain can develop. When swinging a tennis racquet, for example, you can overload your shoulder when you let the arm be pushed back by the weight of the racquet and the recoil of the ball. Instead, you want the pivot point to be your hip and abdominal muscles. Instead of arching your back and letting your arm hinge back at the shoulder, push off your feet and legs and bring your hip under you using abdominal muscles. It doesn't mean to tighten the abdominal muscles, but to use them. The abdominal muscles also curl the spine forward. The upper body follows, pulled by the musculature of the body, not just the joints of the shoulder. In that way, your leg, abdominal and hip muscles power the move.

Your shoulder has four interesting joints. One is at the front of the shoulder between the collarbone (clavicle) and the bony ledge of the shoulder called the acromion. The acromion swings around from the shoulder blade in back to meet the clavicle in front at the acromio-clavicular (AC) joint. You can feel and often see the bump at the joint. The joint at the other end of the clavicle where it meets the chest bone (sternum) is the sterno-clavicular (SC) joint. Inside your shoulder, the knob of the upper-arm bone (the head of the humerus) fits into the shoulder socket called the glenoid at the side of the scapula—which is the gleno-humeral (GH) joint. On your back, between your scapula and ribs, the mobile scapulo-thoracic (ST) joint lets the shoulder blade glide and move over your ribs as you move your arm.

A common shoulder-joint injury comes from letting body weight—or the weight of a swung object like a racquet, or the weight of an overhead object or barbell—lever the front of the shoulder backward, instead of keeping the weight on the upper-body and torso muscles. For example, when bench pressing, you can lower the barbell keeping the weight and pressure on the chest and torso muscles, or let the shoulder come forward so that the weight is levered onto the two front shoulder joints. As the arm continues backward, the acromial-clavicular joint, or AC, can be pulled slightly apart. Similar shoulder separations can happen at the sterno-clavicular (SC) joint. Someone who falls from a bicycle onto an outstretched arm and bends their shoulder back can gets this same kind of "prying open" or A-C separation injury. The same happens when letting the shoulder come forward as the arm comes back to swing a tennis or racquetball racquet.

The common recommendation to prevent AC and SC separation when weightlifting is to limit the range by stopping the weight before your chest. A barrel-chested, short-armed person can lower the weight a short distance and touch their thick chest without moving the arm far back. Their elbows will be in line with their body, but they may still be levering the weight with the front of their shoulder. A slender, long-armed person may find that they have to stop with the weight many inches above their chest at this same joint angle. Another way to limit joint injury without limiting the range of the exercise is to use chest muscles more, instead of letting the shoulder joint become the lever point. Then even a person with long arms and a narrow chest can lower the weight all the way and not pry the joint open. Use this principle of using anterior muscles for swinging in racquet sports and overhead throwing. Practice the hip tuck using the lunge (Figure 3-6) to learn how to move the pivot point to the abdominal and core muscles and off the shoulder joint. You can also apply this the same way to prevent injury to the elbow, by keeping the pivot point of the effort on the muscles of the legs and trunk, instead of letting it pivot back at the elbow.

Good Shoulder Exercises

I went to physical therapy for my own shoulder injuries. I had been in an accident with many injuries. Spinal-cord damage in my broken neck and back left me unable to walk for a long time. Doctors, physical therapist, friends, and family called me an unreasonable baby for wanting to walk again and not accepting that I would not. In some of the less-serious injuries, I tore the rotator cuffs in both arms, stripped the cartilage called the labrum that holds the head of the humerus in the shoulder socket, and crushed both shoulder sockets.

When the examining doctors pulled my hand, a large hollow, called a sulcus, formed at the shoulder where the bone pulled out easily. Medical students crowded the exam room to try it. Pull, pull, pull. Ow, ow, ow. I went to physical therapy. I wanted to learn new good information for my own patients, and thought I'd get better from their care.

In PT, I was told there was no fixing such injuries without surgery. At that time, I wasn't able to lift either arm without pain, or even with pain. I couldn't touch my own head. My hair looked funny. When I held food in one hand, all I could do was wiggle my lips at it with my neck forward like a horse, but couldn't get close enough to eat it. They gave me the standard instructions: "No reaching overhead. No lifting anything over a few pounds. No putting any weight on my arms." I was dismayed since they said those rules were not just for the week, but for a long time—probably always. This approach ruled out most of my life. They said surgery was the only way to fix the cartilage tears. I asked about the surgery. It turned out that after a healing period of months, where I would not be allowed to move the shoulder for any reason, I must still not do any of the things on the list of "shoulder no's" or the surgery would fail.

"What's the point of the surgery?" I asked.

"Just to stop the pain." They said I could try PT, but I would be back for surgery. Then, I would need more PT to loosen the surgically tightened shoulder enough to be able to raise my arm again.

They gave me stretchy bands, the usual shoulder exercise, to pull outward and inward with my elbows near my sides. This exercise was for my torn rotator cuffs. An interesting thing going on at the same time was that, because of having broken my neck, some of the nerves to my hands didn't transmit signals. I couldn't hold even a light band without it pulling out of my hand. This problem was still better than the previous months I had spent without being able to move my arms and legs—especially when I had an itch. I had worked hard to get movement back in my hands and finally developed enough grip strength to be able to pull on my own pants. "Armed" with three working fingers, I went to PT to faithfully pull the bands.

The rotator cuff muscles of the shoulder are often neglected in fitness programs. These four muscles go around your shoulder like a cuff, and rotate and stabilize your arm and shoulder. It is common for people to work their deltoids, chest, and back—but not the rotator cuff. It is not uncommon to create a situation where the arm bone can get too pulled up in the socket by the stronger shoulder muscles, and not pulled back to place by the neglected rotator-cuff muscles. This situation can allow the top of your upper-arm bone to push and grind against your shoulder capsule. Good rotator-cuff exercises can offset this problem, and also help rotator cuffs injured by trauma.

I was shown how to practice pulling stretchy bands out to the side with my elbows in. I called this my "flasher exercise" because the only motion in real life to use was a flasher opening his trench coat. It wasn't even useful for opening a door.

The bands come in different colors according to how hard they are to pull. I worked daily and was able to do my "flasher exercise" better each day. I worked until I could do the most difficult color, but would still tear my shoulder out all over again just trying to brush my teeth or dress myself. One day after PT, I stopped in their ladies' room and reached back for the light. My shoulder dislocated there in the bathroom. The front of the upper-arm bone bulged through the skin at the front of the shoulder. My arm was stuck behind me like a tail. I chased my arm around in the dark with my other hand, like a dog chasing his tail, trying to reach it to reduce the dislocation.

It is commonly thought that shoulder pain is caused by weak shoulder muscles, therefore strengthening will prevent and rehabilitate injury. But just strengthening my rotator cuffs wasn't fixing anything. I still didn't have function for daily life. I changed how I exercised my rotator cuffs to the way these muscles need to work in real life. At first it was difficult and I had to go back to the easiest color. I was barely able to reach my face at first, but I kept at it. Around that time, they told me I was pretty much finished with what they could do to fix me. I think that translated to mean that my insurance was almost out. Before I left, I showed them how I changed the physical therapy so that I was getting better. When holding the stretchy bands, instead of opening and closing like a flasher, I showed them how I pulled against the band in motions that simulated brushing my hair and pulling off a shirt, and cleaning the house. These were things that previously had been too painful, and required moving the shoulder in ways it previously wouldn't go.

I showed them how I was starting push-ups. The therapist said to stop because that would push the loose arm bone into the damaged socket. I showed them how I trained my muscles to hold the bone in line instead of pressing into the joint. Then I could use my arm in normal ways that they said would not be possible without hurting it.

Push-ups, done properly, can be good for the shoulder (Figure 2-33). Traditionally this approach was not done. The old thinking was that the shoulder joint is already pressured and inflamed so that you do not want to push the arm bone into the joint further with any weight bearing or weight lifting. The key here is to relearn movement. Don't push the arm bone into the joint; use muscles to hold the socket in healthy position. When you can hold healthy shoulder positioning for the push-up, lift one leg (Figure 2-37), and turn to one side, raising one arm, supporting weight on one hand

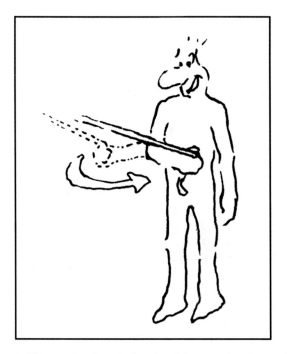

Figure 3-16. When using bands for shoulder exercise, keep chin in and shoulders back. Pull the bands while practicing movements of normal activities—like combing hair, brushing teeth, and fastening clothing items that have zippers or hooks in back. Practice arm actions of your regular sports.

and one foot (Figure 2-38). When you lift packages, don't let the package pull your arm bone, use your muscles to keep shoulder positioning.

What Else to Check

Sometimes muscle or joint aches are caused by common medicines with pain as side effects: statin drugs to lower cholesterol, some prescription allergy medicine, some prescription medicines to prevent stomach acid, the calcium-channel-blocker drug, verapamil, the antibiotics erythromycin and clarithromycin, and some prescription anti-anxiety and antidepressant medicines, and others. Check with your doctor to make sure that pain isn't a sign of medical conditions like heart disease that sends pain up into the shoulder, problems in blood supply that injure or kill the bone, fractures, infections, esophageal problems, heartburn, lack of blood supply that injures the shoulder joint, joint destruction from taking steroids, infections, tumors, fractures, or conditions of the thyroid, breast, or lymph system and other things that need immediate attention. While you treat these with your doctor, you can use the exercises and principles to improve health, keep moving, and reduce pain. The healthy positioning and exercises can make a difference to reducing pain and problems from most causes.

What to Do Every Day to Stop Shoulder Pain

- First thing in the morning do the pectoral (chest) stretch (Figure 3-3) and the trapezius (side and top of neck) stretch (Figure 3-4). Do these several times throughout the day.

- Several times a day, check your upper-body positioning using the wall stand. Touch heels, hip, upper back, and back of head against the wall. If not comfortable, do the two stretches above. If you can't stand straight without discomfort, you can't stand in healthy positioning. See Chapter 1 for full explanations.

- Pull your shoulders back with your chin in, without forcing. It is not necessary to make the area tighter through straining. When you pull your chin in, don't do it by arching your back. The postural change needs to come from your upper body—not by creating another strain on another part. Keep shoulder muscles relaxed and down to pull chin in.

- Check periodically to make sure you can pull your shoulders back with your hands on your hips. If your shoulders come forward when you put your hands on your hips, your shoulders are too tight. Stand up straight with chin in, when doing this stretch. Repeat with your bands touching behind your back.

- When you stand to stretch arms overhead, don't arch your back to do it. Instead, keep your hip tucked under and feel that the stretch comes from your upper chest and shoulder (Figure 3-8). Make sure not to hunch or tighten the shoulders when stretching or reaching.

- Lie on your back with arms comfortably overhead without increasing the arch in your lower back. If needed, start by bending elbows to the side, as if in a stick-up. As you progress, lift arms higher. Can you lift both the same? Keep shoulders down and relaxed. If you can't lie on your back comfortably without lower back pain, see the lordosis section (Figure 2-42).

- Upper-body (upper-back) extension (Figures 1-15 and 1-15a). Extension strengthens the back muscles while unloading the discs that are pushed outward by forward bending. Lie facedown. Lift upper body, gently lower. Try three to five to start. See how you feel, then increase. Work up to at least 10 to 20 at a time.

- Do lunges to stretch the front of the hip and learn how to use core muscles to control torso position (Figure 3-6). Stand with both feet facing straight and slide one foot far back. Keep the back foot straight, not turned out. Tuck the hip under the body so that the behind does not stick out, to feel the stretch in the front of the hip.

- Scapular mobilization exercise (Figure 3-12). Slowly wiggle shoulders forward and back. Repeat holding arms out in front. Then repeat with hands fixed on the wall to simulate ability to relax and reposition shoulder with hands on steering wheel, computer keyboard, or other task. Round shoulders forward, which pushes your back backward, then pull shoulders back and "pinch" shoulder blades together in back, which brings your chest toward the wall. The shoulder moves several inches forward and back. Don't bend elbows or your neck; just move the shoulders.

- When using bands for rotator-cuff exercise, simulate movement of normal activities (Figure 3-16). Pay attention to keeping the hip in position to train healthy use of the whole body when using the shoulder.

- Check your desk. Move computer up and chair in. Keep the keyboard on the desk. These help prevent sitting round shouldered (see Chapter 2).

- Use your muscles—not joints—to hold you up. It's free exercise.

- Get more active. Learn the principles and apply them, instead of memorizing rules and buying expensive ergonomic chairs and beds.

Retrain Shoulder Positioning Under Load

- When lifting weights overhead, keep chin tucked in, and lift upper body upward. Get the stretch from the shoulder instead of arching the lower back and craning the neck.

- Start with just holding a push-up position (Figure 2-33). Don't let your body weight press into the joint capsule. Hold your weight up on your muscles, not squashing the joint. Keep hip tucked under to keep back in a straight line—not arched. If you are debilitated, start by pressing against a wall, without arching your back. Keep head up and chin in gently. Then try a lower position—for example, arms on a stable bench, chair, or bed. Work up to holding a push-up position on the floor.

- Holding a straight push-up position, "walk" your hands and feet sideways, using good shock absorption to strengthen the shoulder while moving, without jarring it. Don't let your body weight press your arm into the shoulder capsule.

- Work up to push-ups, then doing push-ups with the feet raised on a bench, bed, chair, or the wall.

- Scapular mobilization exercise in a push-up position. Hold a straight push-up position with straight—not locked—elbows. Let shoulders sink downward, bringing shoulder blades together, and then round shoulders up, bringing the chest far away from the floor. Repeat so that the shoulders move up and down against the weight of your body.

- Isometric ab exercise (Figure 2-31). Lie face up. Arms straight by your ears an inch or two above the surface holding hand weights. Don't let your back arch or your ribs lift. Use abdominal muscles to prevent arching and to hold your posture against the load of the hand weights. Use your abdominal muscles to control the load; don't let your arm be levered back at the shoulder

- When using bands to train overhead positions and throwing motions, strengthen in functional manner for your whole body while training good shoulder use and position (Figure 2-41).

- Watch other people's upper-back positioning when standing, sitting, driving, eating, and reaching. Seeing other people hunch and round their shoulders reminds you not to injure your own shoulders doing the same. Notice if they sit on stationary bicycles hunched forward, rounding their shoulders, and hunch and round shoulders when lifting arms and weights. These activities are supposed to be for your health. Don't do unhealthy things.

What to Avoid

- Don't reach up with your shoulders or upper back rounded forward.

- Check for exercises that add to shoulder pain (Figures 3-13 and 3-14).

- Don't do things that increase pain. Stretch to where it feels good and releases the tightness—not to where it pinches or strains.

- An often-missed source of shoulder pain is being in a sling for treatment of arm or shoulder injury. The sling is often positioned in the very rounded position that makes the shoulder ache. Check positioning and avoid rounding.

- Don't just "do exercises." Make healthy motion and positioning part of your enjoyable life.

When to Notice Shoulders

- Common times to check if you hunch shoulders forward or upward is when reaching overhead, brushing teeth, preparing food, walking, bicycling, and sitting. Say to yourself, "Relax shoulders down."

- When you lie flat on your back with both arms overhead by your ears, does your back arch? If your shoulders are too tight to raise by your ears without straining the back into an arch, you are too tight to reach up overhead without the same thing happening.

How to Get Natural Shoulder Stretch and Exercise from Daily Activity

- Don't stick your chin forward to pull your shoulders back. Stand and move all the time without letting the shoulders round forward and you will exercise the posterior muscles and prevent shoulder tightness.

- Whenever your reach overhead, each without arching your back. Move from the shoulders. Keep chin in, not forward.

- Whenever your reach overhead for anything, drop shoulders down before reaching up.

- Keep shoulders from rounding forward. Holding them gently in position gives free exercise for the posterior muscles. "Holding your shoulders back" doesn't mean to hold them in back of you. It means to bring them back from a forward position to straight.

No More Shoulder Pain

It was a common idea that shoulder pain is caused by weak shoulder muscles, therefore strengthening will prevent and rehabilitate injury. It is important to strengthen, but of the many causes of shoulder pain—how you position and use your shoulder, and what the rest of your body is doing when you move your shoulder—are the most common and most correctable.

The forward head and the tight hip are two contributors to shoulder pain that aren't immediately obvious, but once stopped, can relieve years of shoulder problems that seemed resistant to standard shoulder exercises and therapies. Several other contributors of shoulder pain are also easy to identify and fix on your own.

Understand the cause of shoulder pain instead of doing a bunch of exercises without knowing what they do and why, then going back to injurious positioning in daily life. Do the purpose of the exercises—not the exercises alone. Shoulder pain can be a helpful warning of tight, unhealthy ways of moving. Fix the cause and you can fix the pain, plus gain a healthier, stronger life at the same time. How is your shoulder positioning right now reading this? Not everything is caused by positioning, but you can reduce a lot of problems. Keep it simple. Learn the concepts of what makes good stretches and exercises so that you move in healthy ways for all the things you do.

4

No More Hip Pain

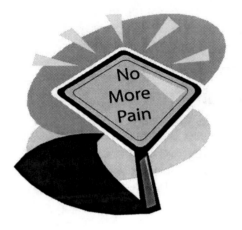

- Hip Pain
- Tightness
- Arthritis
- Avoiding Hip Replacement

A diagnosis of hip arthritis is often thought of as a life sentence of pain and disability that only hip surgery can change. Reducing activity because of pain adds to weakness, disability, and more pain. The good news is that even though no cure for arthritis is currently available, you can do much to stop pain and restore ability. In many cases, the majority of the pain is not from the arthritic changes seen on x-ray. Strained, tight, pressured muscles make the hip ache—just like anywhere else.

The hip has several bones and joints. Some people think of the bony prominence on each side where you can carry a package. Others pat the front of their leg when they want to describe their pain, or only think about the joint at the top of the leg that is replaced when it wears out. The hip is the entire pelvis with three big matching bones on each side, joints that attach the hip to your legs and back, and many muscles on all sides that move the torso and legs. This chapter covers hip pain from all of these areas.

Hip Pain from Tight Hip Flexors

Hip pain in the front of the hip is often from tight muscles that yank and pull at the joint. The crease where your leg joins your body should be able to straighten flat so that you can stand up straight. A major thing you can do to stop hip pain is not to stand bent at the hip. That may sound obvious. But many people keep their hip bent most of the day from sitting, stand and walk with the hip still bent, and then exercise by bending forward at the hip.

The result of all this bending is that the hip gets good at staying bent. It tightens until it remains in a bent position (Figure 4-1). Standing bent forward is long known in scientific studies to put large forces on the lower back—more than other standing postures. Standing with the hip tilted from tightness sometimes puts the leg bone in a poor position so that it rubs and wears at the socket. When the hip is too tight to straighten, it does not even let you lie down flat without pain.

Some of your front-hip muscles cross your hip and attach to your leg. They pull the leg to bend it. The bending action is called flexion, so these muscles are "hip flexors" (Figure 4-2).

If your hip is too tight to straighten with standing (Figure 4-3), imagine how limited and strained it will be when walking (Figure 4-4). To walk, your hip needs to stretch past the straight position to extend behind the line of your body.

Stretch the Anterior Hip: Hip Extension

Several stretches for the front of the hip are often done in ways that keeps the hip bent, rather than straightening. Many people spend time stretching, but don't get results because they are not stretching in ways that provide the intended stretch. Many people

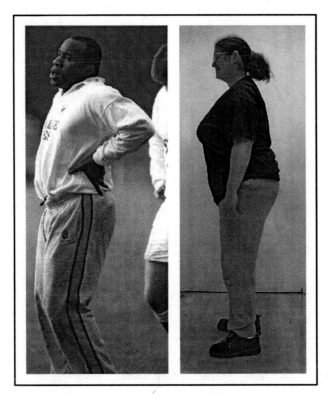

Figure 4-1. When the front of the hip is tight, it often stays bent when standing. People with a tight front hip may either arch their back to keep their head up (left) or stay bent forward (right). Both postures can strain the hip, lower back, and sometimes the knees.

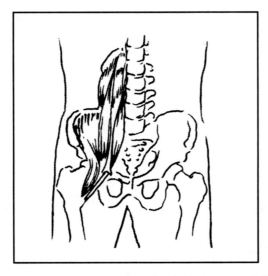

Figure 4-2. Muscles that bend your leg at the hip are called hip flexors. Hip flexors need to stretch and lengthen to prevent pain in the hip and pelvis, but many people only bend and shorten them.

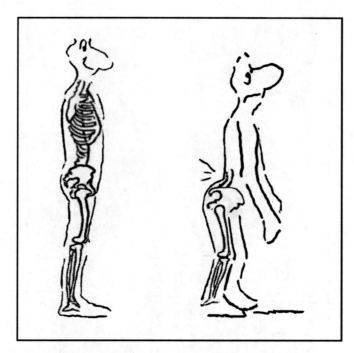

Figure 4-3. Normal hip muscle length lets you stand straight (left). Tight front hip muscles can keep the hip bent when standing (right) straining the back and hip.

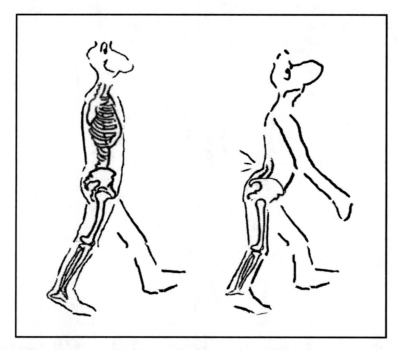

Figure 4-4. In normal walking, the front of the hip must stretch to an angle that is past straight (left). A tight anterior hip stays bent (right) and creates positioning that strains the hip and back.

think they are not flexible. New studies have come out that stretching isn't helping as much as hoped. The reason seems to be that they are doing their stretches in ineffective ways, then not applying the results to how they move.

Lunge

The lunge is a common move to stretch the hip, but is often done in ways that keeps the hip bent—which loses the stretch. Three things make the difference between getting a hip stretch or not:

- Keep the back foot straight. Don't turn the foot outward—even a little. Rotating the leg out turns the front of the hip away from the stretch.
- Keep your weight centered over both legs—not leaning toward the front leg.
- Tuck the hip under you, as if you are "starting an abdominal crunch." This move takes the bend out of the hip of the back leg and reduces an overly large arch from your lower back. You will feel the front of your hip stretch.

You can get a good stretch just by briefly holding the lunge when standing in line or other places. Many people will not stretch with the lunge because they use positioning that hurts their knees. Done properly, good bending can help reduce knee pain and strengthen the muscles that bend the knees. If you feel pressure in your front knee, check that you are not leaning forward. Keep the front knee over the ankle, not tilting forward. If you feel pressure in your back knee, lift upward with your thigh muscles. Make sure you are not letting your weight concentrate downward on the knee.

To add to the lunge stretch, use the moving lunge to stretch and strengthen the hip at the same time.

- Keep both feet in the lunge position. Bend both knees to gently lower toward the ground and back up. Keep your back knee off the floor. Don't kneel use leg muscles to rise and lower. Work up to at least 10 to 20 at a time on each leg.
- Lower straight down. Don't let the front knee slide forward. The key is keeping the knee over the ankle. Use more back-leg muscles and keep your weight centered over both legs.
- If you need your hand on your knee, strengthen and practice balance until you don't need it. Holding your own body weight up using your leg muscles is a bare minimum for normal life.
- Strengthen the hip and legs by holding hand weights as you lunge up and down. To practice functional strengthening, each time you rise from lunging downward, lift the weights overhead, out to the side, and up to the back. When you put the weights down, don't bend over wrong. Use the lunge you just practiced.

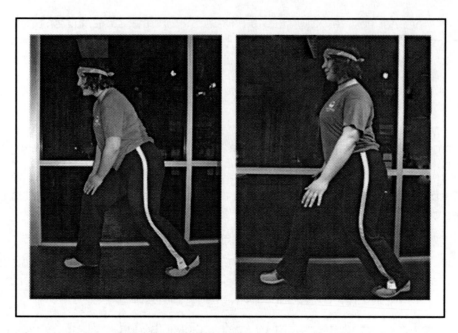

Figure 4-5. Neither of these lunge stretches will stretch the front of the hip. In both cases, the front of the hip is still bent. Note the stripe on the pants.

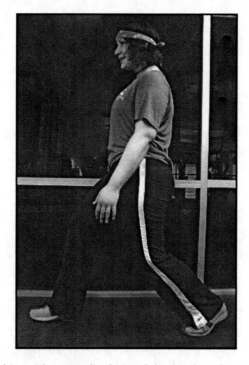

Figure 4-6. By tilting the hip under you, the front of the hip lengthens from the customary bent position. You will feel a nice stretch.

You need to bend for things in normal life many times every day. Bending your knees is normal, good bending for household activities to prevent back pain. Bending this way is built-in healthy movement and stretch. Chapter 5 shows more good ways to be able to use the knees and reduce pain at the same time.

Quadriceps (Thigh) Stretch.

Like the lunge, the quadriceps (or thigh) stretch is often done in ways that does not give the intended stretch. The point of the stretch is to lengthen the front of the hip. For that reason, don't bend the leg forward at the hip or arch your back (Figure 4-7, left). Stretch with the hip tucked and the thigh pulled back (Figure 4-7, right).

- Instead of bending your hip forward to reach your foot, lift up in back to your hand.

- Tuck your hip under you as if starting a "crunch." You will feel a shift in the stretch to the front of the hip and thigh. Tucking the hip also reduces the lower-back arch that pressures the lower back.

- Keep your knee down and toward the back. Some stretching sources say never to pull the knee back because it "makes you arch your back." It doesn't "make you." You control your lower-back arch by using muscles to move your hip. Keep the hip tucked to increase the stretch and to control the lower back so that it doesn't overarch and hurt.

- Push your foot away from your body into your hand instead of pulling your foot toward you.

- Standing on one leg is good for balance, too. If your balance is poor, it is beneficial to improve it—not to make things worse by only holding on to things. Stand near a

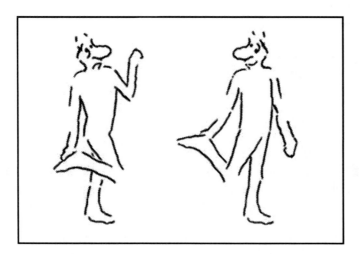

Figure 4-7. Quadriceps stretch. If you bend the hip and arch the back while sticking the hips out in back (left) you lose the stretch. Tuck the hip to move the stretch to the thigh.

wall for safety. Use a finger (if needed) to briefly steady yourself against the wall to get started. Then let go and get a free balance exercise while you help your hip. Keep safety in mind by not subjecting yourself to conditions where you can get hurt.

- Hold for at least a few seconds and switch sides.

Lower Body Extension

Your front-hip muscles must lengthen enough to let your leg extend behind you for normal walking. Use lower-body extensions to train stretch and strength for healthy movement (Figure 4-8). This same extension exercise helps the lower back. Extension strengthens back muscles while unloading the discs that are pushed outward by forward bending.

- Lie facedown, comfortably, with your arms wherever you want them.
- Lift both legs up, keep your knees straight, and then gently lower.
- Don't yank or force; just use muscles to lift.
- Start with one leg (if needed), and then progress to lifting both.
- Progress to at least 10 to 20 lifts up and down.

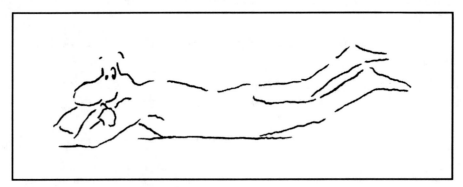

Figure 4-8. Lower-body extension

Stretch over Bed, Pillow, or Ball

It is common for people to keep their hip bent and their back arched all day, then stretch the same way—never straightening, let alone stretching the hip (Figure 4-9). When using a ball, bench, or bed to stretch the hip, make sure you are stretching your hip and not just arching your back (Figure 4-10).

- Move the ball or edge of the bed under the hip—not the lower back (Figure 4-10).
- If you let your back arch, you will feel pressure in your lower back when you do stretch. Instead, tuck your hip to reduce the arch and move the stretch to the hip.

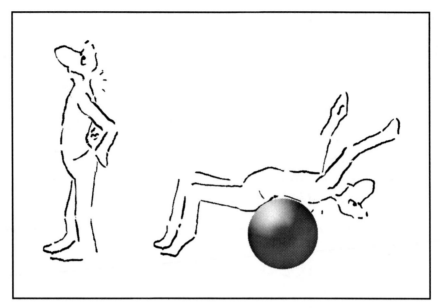

Figure 4-9. Are you really stretching? If you stand with your hip bent all day and then lie over a ball the same way, you are not getting the stretch.

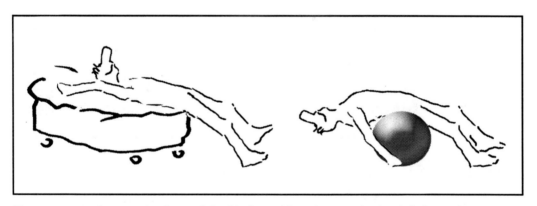

Figure 4-10. Make sure the front of the hip is positioned to get the intended stretch.

Facedown Anterior Hip Stretch

This set of stretches works well and feels good:

- Lie facedown. Draw one knee out to the side. Keep both hips flat down (Figure 4-11). Don't lift or tilt toward the knee.
- Hold for a few seconds. Keep breathing. Relax the muscles. Don't hold them tightly to "stop the pain of the stretch." Don't let the stretch hurt. Go gently and move to a position where it feels good.

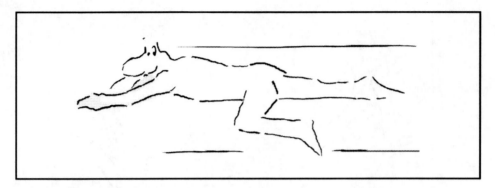

Figure 4-11. Facedown anterior hip stretch, part 1

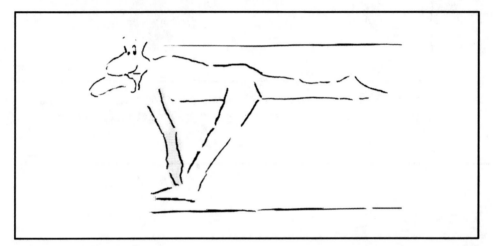

Figure 4-12. Facedown anterior hip stretch, part 2. Keep leg and arm wherever comfortable.

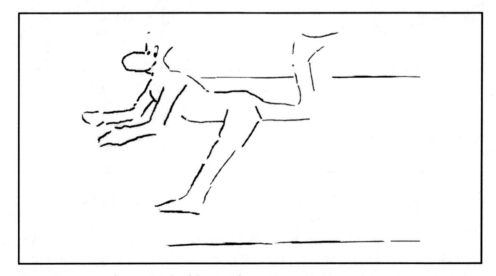

Figure 4-13. Facedown anterior hip stretch, part 3

- Straighten your leg out to the side toward your hand, as close as comfortable (Figure 4-12). Hold for a few seconds

- Gently prop on elbows to increase the stretch. Don't crane your neck or lower back. Hold for a few seconds. Keep breathing. Relax shoulders.

- Next, gently bend the back knee for more stretch (Figure 4-13). Hold for a few seconds.

- Don't force and don't tighten; just stretch pleasantly.

- Stretch the other leg the same way.

Stretch and Strengthen the Anterior Hip

A tight front hip is often weak. Sometimes one side is weaker than the other, putting unequal force across your hip as you move through the day.

Hip Bridge Leg Lift

The hip bridge strengthens the front of the hip while stretching it (Figure 4-14).

- Lie on your back with both knees bent and feet on the surface (bed, bench, or floor).

- Lift one leg out straight, lining up your knees.

- Lift hips and hold for a few seconds. The aim is to use muscles to make the front of the hip straight, not still bent in front.

- Hold the lifted leg at the side of the other leg.

- Try the other side and compare.

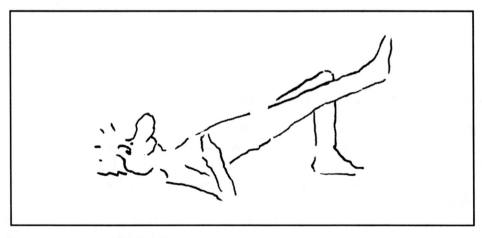

Figure 4-14. Hip bridge leg lift

- Work up to at least 10 "lift and lower" movements on each side.
- If holding the leg out is too much, start with both feet down. Progress to crossing one ankle over opposite knee, then to lifting and holding straight.

Tom was an emergency department physician who asked me for a consult for his hip pain. He was diagnosed with "sacroiliac" pain. Sacroiliac pain is a common, catchall term for pain at the back of the hip where the sacrum— the wide flat plate of lower-back bones—meets the top hipbone, called the ilium. Sacroiliac pain is usually around the sacrum, just above the backside. It used to be that almost any pain in the lower back was called sacroiliac pain—whether it had anything to do with the sacrum and ilium or not. Tom stood with the classic bent-hip position. His belt tilted down in front. The side seam in his pants tilted forward at the hip. His lower back arched enough to fit a football in the inward curve of his lower back. He did his crunches and leg lifts thinking he was "working his core" to help his pain, but all the forward bending was only shortening the front-hip muscles, encouraging his usual way to stand with his hip bent. When he tried to pull his shoulders back to "stand straight," he kept the hip bent and arched his back more. Tom's case was one of classic lower-back pain from lordosis. You can read about this in the Chapter 2. The cause of his lordosis was tight anterior (front) hip muscles that pulled him into a position that pressured his hip where it joined the lower back.

I showed Tom how to tilt his hip under him to straighten his hip and reduce the large arch in his back. The pressure and ache he had for so many years lifted from his back right then. When he let his hip bend and his back arch again, the pain returned. He needed hip-extension stretches to lengthen the front of his hip, so that muscle shortness didn't keep the hip bent when he stood up.

Tight Anterior Hip Prevents Lying Down Comfortably

A big indication of tightness in the front of the hip is lower-back pain when lying on your back or stomach. When trying to lie with the legs out flat, the tight, bent hip pulls the lower back up into an arch—pinching and pressuring it. Many people are told to only sleep with a pillow under their knees. With the knees bent by the pillow, the back can flatten even though the hip is still bent. The pain from the arching stops, but the pillow does not stop the source of the pain, it perpetuates it by keeping the hip bent and tight. A better approach is to stop the cause of this kind of arching, which is the tight front hip. Use the extension stretches (Figures 4-6 through 4-14) to make it possible to lie flat. Sometimes all it takes is a few well-done lunges with the hip tipped under so that it stretches the front (Figure 4-6). Soon it should become not only comfortable, but also enjoyable to straighten out.

Beverly could not lie on her back without pain in the back of her hip. She had gotten many shots and treatments for her pain, and was fitted for orthotics, without success. She was surprised to find that tightness in the front of her hip was the reason for the years of pain. With a few lunges to loosen the area, she was able to lie flat for the first time in several years. I reminded her that the hip would tighten again when she went back to walking around with a bent hip. Over the next weeks, she prevented pain by regularly stretching the hip with the lunge (Figure 4-6), lower-body extensions (Figure 4-8), bed stretch (Figure 4-10), and other hip extension stretches (Figures 4-11 through 4-14). More important, she practiced keeping her hip from bending when standing and used the quadriceps stretch (Figure 4-17) to practice tipping the hip to a stretched position when standing.

Anterior Muscle Tightness Is Not Necessary or Unavoidable

Catherine was a massage therapist with back and hip pain. I arrived for her house-call appointment in her office. The room was overflowing with bolsters, pillows, and blocks of foam in assorted shapes. When I asked her to show me if she could lie face up with her legs straight, she chastised me that such a position "was not natural." She said it was a fact that the anterior (front) muscles of the body had higher natural tension than the muscles of the back. She said that studies showed that lying on your back increases the tension of the muscles in front, stressing them. The flaw in these conclusions is that when you are tight then, yes, muscle tension increases when you try to lie flat. The solution is to stretch the anterior muscles so that you are comfortable lying flat. Then you don't need any pillows. If you don't do these stretches, a cycle of tightening and needing the pillows continues unbroken. Catherine mulled it over in her mind for a moment, looked at the room full of expensive cushions, and said, "Whoops."

Tight Anterior Hip Increases Risk of Hip Strain and Groin Pull

Marta was a Pilates teacher with a sticking pain in the front of her hip. I see many Pilates teachers as patients—mostly for back, neck, and hip pain. They practice a kind of exercise routine that focuses on bending forward to strengthen the core muscles. Many people who exercise mostly do moves that bend the hip—like leg lifts, touching toes, bringing knees to chest, bending over to lift weights, stair machines, and traditional core training that involves bending forward at the back and hip.

Marta's hip was very good at being bent in front. She was surprised that strengthening the muscles didn't prevent the pain. She didn't let her back arch, but the muscles in the front of her hip were so tight that they yanked on the hip bones in front. I asked her to lie flat on her back, which she could do. I asked her to lift one leg up, as if to stretch it. The leg went high in the air. The other leg lifted from the floor a bit along with it. This result is an interesting sign of tightness in the front of the hip—lifting one leg "drags" the other one with it (Figure 4-15). A looser, longer front-hip muscle would allow the leg to flatten to the ground.

We worked on hip-extension stretches and keeping the lower leg flat when stretching the upper leg. The problem of the bottom leg dragging forward happens during all kinds of regular activities—such as taking the stairs, stretching, kicking a ball, raising legs in exercise class and box-aerobics, even just running or walking (Figure 4-16). When the standing leg is yanked forward during a kick or leap, it can sometimes result in a groin pull. The tight anterior hip is a hidden contributor to pulls and strains.

Marta had been taught to keep one knee bent when raising the other leg to "protect" the back. I showed her that her own muscles keep the back in healthy position and bending the knee only results in bending the hip, which lets it stay tight. I showed Marta a system of exercises that I developed to exercise the abdominal and core muscles without forward bending (Figures 2-30 through 2-34, 2-37 through 2-39, 2-47, and others). The training system is called "The Ab Revolution" because it is a change in thinking about using abdominal muscles in the way they need to hold you when you move in real life. Abdominal strength does not automatically hold your spine and hip in position, any more than having a strong arm makes your arm stick up in the air. It is how you hold your spine and hip your muscles. Marta incorporated the hip-extension stretches and the core training without forward bending into her classes. When I checked in with her, she reported that she and her students got a better workout without pain.

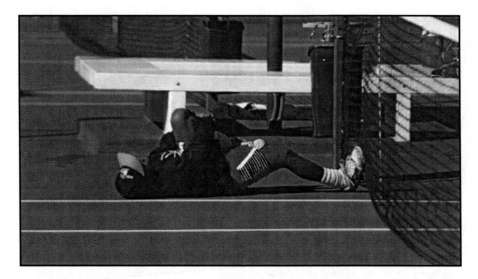

Figure 4-15. If the bottom leg lifts from the ground when lifting the top one, it is frequently because the front of the hip is tight.

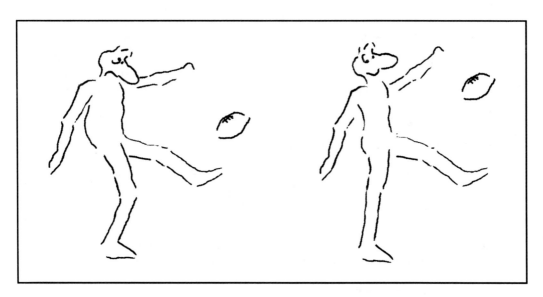

Figure 4-16. When the front of the hip is tight, raising one leg pulls the standing leg forward (left), which may result in a fall or groin pull. Stretch the front of the hip with stretches and during movement by keeping the hip and knee of the standing leg straight (right).

Stop Hip Pain from the Posterior Hip

It used to be thought that if the back of the hip were tight, it would make you stand with a flat low back. The resulting posture would push the hip forward keeping the back tight, and lengthening the front hip muscles. It is now known that the back of the hip can be tight in just about any position, even with the front of the hip bent and the behind stuck out.

Elenya came in with back pain that radiated into one hip. She said her doctor thought her sacral joint was "out of alignment." She went for cranio-sacral therapy, which she liked because it didn't hurt like doing exercise and she didn't have to move.

Elenya said she thought it was a hip condition because "movement of the hip hurts like heck when I do back extensions or try to stretch my hamstrings or any of the muscles along my upper-leg or gluteal area." I touched the back of her hip. It was like a block of stone. It was not in spasm; it was tight. It is often hard to be sure of the difference between muscle spasm and habitual tightness, and then to distinguish that from hip pain from some degenerative process.

A difficult cycle occurs when someone has a simple but severe muscle tightness, which is not uncommon. Trying to move the hip through range of motion pulls on the tight area. It is painful. The person goes to the doctor with a painful hip. The doc moves it and pain results. It is easy to conclude that there is some process at work like arthritis or bursitis. X-rays often show some arthritis, which many people have just from normal wear and tear, but is not what is causing the pain. The person is told to restrict activity because they have arthritis. More tightness results.

Elenya was able to reduce the extreme tightness that was causing her pain with some simple posterior hip stretches (Figures 4-17 through 4-20). We concentrated on her learning to move her legs without tightening the back of her hip. Then she was able to do back extensions lying facedown and lifting legs up behind her without tightening and forcing. She transferred easy motion of her hip to normal ability to extend the joint during walking and exercising.

Laxshmi worked diligently at everything she did. Not being complainer, she didn't come to me until the pain progressed to the point where she could not walk or sit down without pain and a burning, rubbing sensation over her "sit bones." The bottom hipbone is called the ischium. The bumps are the ischial tuberosities, and are located where your hamstrings attach to your hip. When Laxshmi stretched her hamstrings, she did not let discomfort stop her from her task. She pulled so hard that she strained the hamstrings where they start on the ischial tuberosity. The hamstrings are also "fed" or innervated by a portion of the sciatic nerve—adding to the posterior hip pain. Doing gentler stretches for the entire back of the hip helped the area heal.

Stretch the Posterior Hip

Sitting Figure-4 Stretch (Figure 4-17)

- Sit with one ankle crossed over the opposite knee. This position makes your legs look like the numeral 4.
- Hold your shins. Pull chest up. Keep your back straight—not rounded.
- Push the bent knee downward.
- Sitting straight makes the difference in this stretch. If you roll back, you lose the hip stretch—which is helpful to know when sitting in any chair. By slouching, you round your hip and lose the normal stretch. The back of the hip can get tight.
- Try this stretch when sitting at a desk, stretching enough to keep the bent knee under the desk.

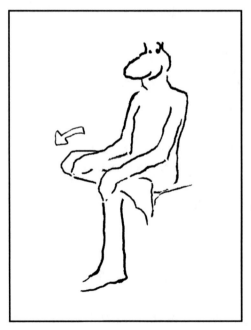

Figure 4-17. Sitting figure-4 stretch

Standing Figure-4 Stretch

- While standing, cross one ankle over the other knee, similar to the sitting figure-4 stretch.
- Bend the standing knee as needed to reach your foot. Vary the bend to vary the stretch.
- Keep your back straight.
- Putting your shoes and socks on and taking them off every day while standing in can be a pleasant way to stretch your hip, with the extra benefit of improving balance to prevent falls.

Lying Figure-4 Stretch (Figures 4-18 and 4-19)

- Lie on your back and bend both knees with feet on the floor.
- Cross one ankle over the opposite knee.
- Push the crossed knee away with your hand to stretch the front of the hip for a few seconds. If you can't reach your hand to your knee, bring the other foot closer.
- Keep head and upper back relaxed and straight.
- Raise your foot from the ground to get a pleasant stretch in back of the hip.
- Hold for a few seconds. Keep breathing.

Lying Figure-4 Twist (Figure 4-20)

- Drop your crossed legs to one side and hold for a few seconds.
- Breathe in, and as you breathe out, move the same crossed legs over and down to the other side and hold briefly.
- Recross your legs the other way and drop to both sides in turn. This movement stretches the hip inward, a stretch that many people need and never get.

Strengthen the Posterior Hip

Lower-Body Extensions

- Extensions (shown in Figure 4-8) are excellent for strengthening the posterior hip, lower back, and upper legs.
- Lie facedown and gently lift legs up without bending knees.
- If lifting both legs is too much exertion, begin with one leg at a time and progress to lifting both legs.

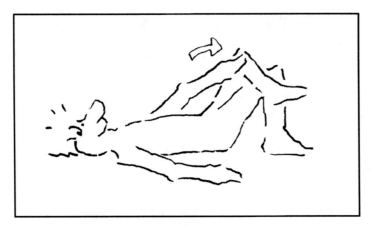

Figure 4-18. Lying figure-4 stretch

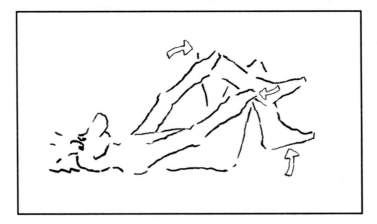

Figure 4-19. Lying figure-4 stretch increases with the bottom foot raised

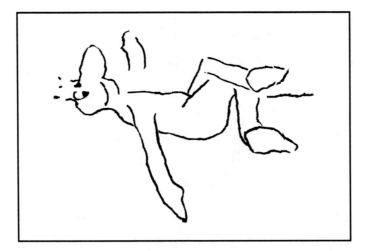

Figure 4-20. Lying figure-4 twist

Hip Pain from the Side of Hip

Bob was a runner. He wanted to run a marathon, but each time he ran more than eight miles, the side of his hip burned. His doctor ruled out fracture, tumor, and hernia. Hernia can cause hip pain, mostly anterior hip pain, but it was good to check. His x-rays showed some arthritis, so he was told to cut down his mileage.

I asked him to run for me. He turned his right foot out. The left leg stayed straight. I asked him to walk a bit. He walked with the right foot turned out. The left leg stayed straight. When we checked, Bob's right hip was tight on the outside. The tightness on one side was pulling his leg that way. The tight structures rubbing the side of his hip were inflaming it. We worked on keeping both feet straight and stretching the side of his hip so that tightness would not rotate his leg outward. The pain subsided and Bob could run as far as his conditioning would take him, instead of being limited by hip pain. A few months later, I stood at the finish line to watch him and other patients do their dream and finish the marathon.

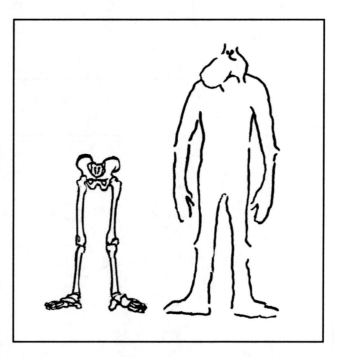

Figure 4-21. Walking with your toe out can tighten the side of the hip. In turn, tightness on the side of the hip encourages toe-out walking. Both can rub and inflame the side of the hip.

One of the causes of side hip pain is a tight iliotibial band, called the IT band for short. It is a long, tough fibrous band. It goes down your side from your ilium bone of your hip, to the side of your lower leg bone, the tibia. The band can hurt from several things. You can get side hip pain if you roll in on your arches (pronation), if the side or back of your hip is tight, sometimes if your quadriceps muscles are tight, if you let your hip tilt to one side a lot, and if you walk with your feet turned out. Turning the feet out usually results from being too tight on the outside of the leg, and too weak on the inside to counter it. If it doesn't feel normal to walk straight, it is better to fix it than allow it.

Sometimes the IT band can be so tight that it snaps over the knobby the top of the leg bone (called the trochanter) at the hip. This condition is called "snapping IT band." A tight or snapping band (and other tight side-hip structures) can press the bursa at the side of the hip making it hurt, also. This condition is called trochanteric bursitis. This kind of bursitis makes a sharp pain.

Stretch the Side of the Hip

Sitting IT-Band Stretch (Figures 4-22 and 4-23)

If your pain is from a tight IT band, bursitis, arthritis, or a combination, the sitting IT-band stretch helps the hip in several ways. Don't do these stretches if you have a hip replacement or if pain increases.

- Sit upright on the floor. Cross your knees until one knee rests on the other (as much as tightness allows).

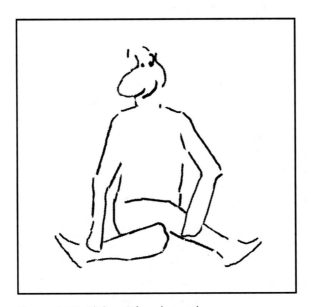

Figure 4-22. Sitting IT-band stretch

- Keep feet forward and away from your body so that the front of both lower legs make a straight line.

- Hold your shins and pull up to feel the stretch in the side of your hip. Hold for a few seconds while breathing in and out.

- Gently bend to each side, breathing in and out (Figure 4-23). Keep your upper body upright without leaning forward. Hold a few seconds on each side.

- Change sides. Cross your legs the other way, pull up to stretch, and then stretch to both sides.

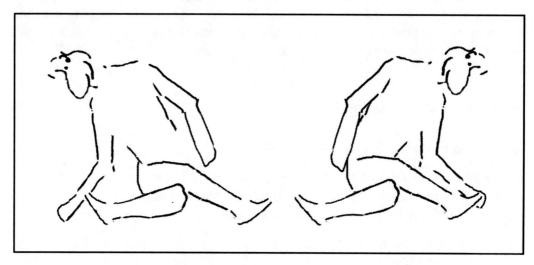

Figure 4-23. Increasing the stretch of the sitting IT-band stretch. Lean to both sides. Cross legs the other way and lean to both sides again.

Mick already had four hip replacements. He was active and wanted to stay that way. After replacing both hips the first time, he wore out the replacements over the next eight years and went for more surgery to replace the replacements. The second replacement is called a revision. Now, several years later, he came to me because he was wearing out the revisions. I asked him what an artificial hip felt like when it was wearing out.

"Arthritis!" he said.

"Wow," I said. "That's a biofidelic [like real life] hip. It even hurts like the real thing." One of the problems with hip-replacement parts is that they wear out faster than the real thing—which is limiting for people who need to be active. I watched Mick walk. He walked hard, with impact. With each step, one side of his hip tipped down. When walking down stairs, he came down hard—with his knee practically straight. This type of movement bangs the joint with each step and adds extra load.

I showed Mick how to walk without sagging his hip to the side, and a trick to not walk so hard. Instead of landing hard with each step, he had to first tighten his leg muscles then place his foot down. This technique is one of many "setting" exercises for the muscles. You don't want to always walk by tightening, but you need to train your muscles to know when they are about to handle a load, instead of jarring your bones with each step. It is similar to a child learning to catch a big ball. When you first throw the ball to them, you knock them over. Then their muscles learn that when they are about to receive an incoming weight, they need to decelerate it. If you have ever picked up something that you thought would be heavy but turned out feather light, you probably lifted it faster and higher than you expected. Your muscles were expecting a certain load and prepared a matching tension. Learning to walk and do all your activities with muscular deceleration is similar. Instead of just dropping your weight down on your legs and hip, your leg and torso muscles engage.

Nicolina had hip pain right in the joint where the leg fits into the hip socket. She felt it when going up the stairs. As I watched her ascend, each time she put her foot on the next step, the hip sagged out to the side under her body weight. Moving this way bangs the joint with each step and adds extra load on the IT band. Learning how to not let her hip shift sideways or drop downward under her body weight stopped her pain when going up stairs and curbs.

The side of Andy's hip ached. Andy was thin. He had purchased a hard bed because he thought it was good for you. But it made his hip ache. He was a side sleeper. Covering the fancy, new, hard bed with inexpensive 'egg crate" foam took care of the hard bed pressing on his bony hip.

Stop Hip Pain on the Inside of the Hip

Kumiko was one of my students in my martial-arts classes. She worked hard in class, learned everything quickly, and also walked, jumped, and kicked with her knees facing each other. Her knees didn't hurt, but her hips did. Unlike many people who let their knee sag inward, stressing the knee, she rotated the entire leg inward. This movement is something she had been taught to do since childhood. Kumiko told me how her grandmother put coins and candies between her knees for her to learn to hold her knees facing inward like a good Japanese girl. I explained to her how the hip can be strained from the habitual position and how important it was to position the legs facing straight ahead. She agreed and nodded. Months passed. Her positioning didn't change. Kumiko was intelligent and I knew she understood me. She was being polite in agreeing with me about something her training would not let her do. Each week we would begin class kneeling on the floor "Japanese style," feet folded under us. One day I asked the class to sit tailor fashion with knees apart.

"Even women?" Kumiko blurted out.

"Yes, even women can sit this way. This is America." I joked. She smiled but wasn't sure she wanted to sit that way in public. She and I decided that she could stretch the inside of the legs at home and practice rotating them outward to try to undo some of the pull of walking turned in for so much of the day. As she became more comfortable, she could try incorporating more into daily life.

Ian played rugby on a tough team. Several players developed groin pain. One was out with stress fractures. In such a tough game it didn't seem surprising. But the reason for the pain was interesting. When they stepped their weight on one leg to kick the ball, they were tipping the hip sharply and dropping their weight where the hipbones join in front, stressing the groin. Simple kicking retraining, along with some inside-leg stretches, stopped the pain.

How to Stretch the Inside of the Hip

Rocket Ship (Figure 4-24)

- Lie face up. Bend each knee to the side, touching the bottom of the feet together. Your knees face away from each other like the fins of an old-fashioned rocket ship. Arms rest anywhere comfortable.
- Add a nice upper-body stretch by raising hands overhead like the nose of a rocket.
- Try rocket ship with the lower legs folded side by side instead of feet touching (Figure 4-25). This movement is often easier on the hip socket and stretches the front hip muscles too.

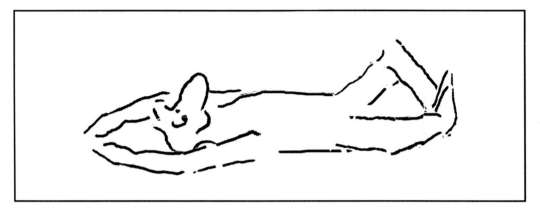

Figure 4-24. Rocket-ship stretch

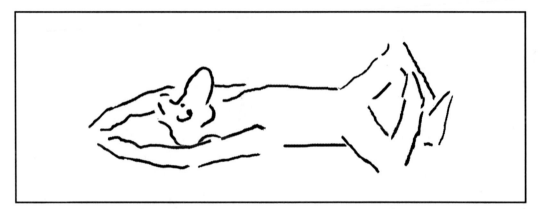

Figure 4-25. Rocket ship with legs folded side-by-side

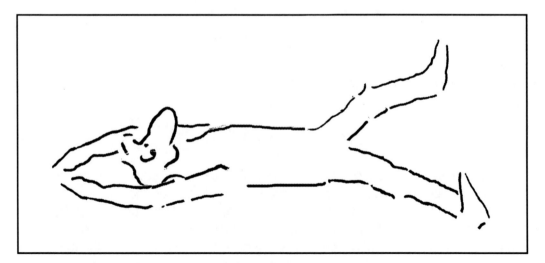

Figure 4-26. Rocket ship, legs apart stretch

Rocket Ship, Legs Apart (Figure 4-26)

- Lie on your back.
- Straighten knees with legs as far apart as comfortable.
- Add a nice upper-body stretch by raising hands overhead.

Legs Up and Apart, Inside-Hip Stretch (Figure 4-27)

- Lie on your back, lifting legs up in the air as far apart as comfortable.
- Keep head and shoulders relaxed and down
- This stretch can also be done relaxing your legs against a wall.
- Add a nice upper-body stretch to this by raising hands overhead.

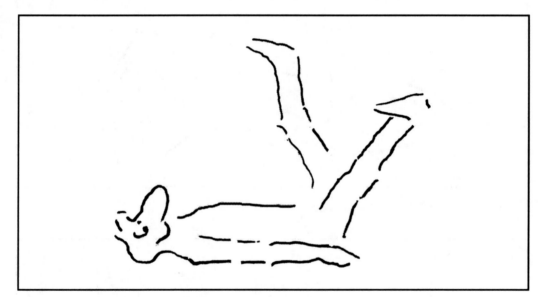

Figure 4-27. Legs up and apart, inside-hip stretch

What Else to Check

Moving, stretching, and exercise often help you feel better—regardless of the source of pain. Still, check with your doctor for medical conditions of the hip like fractures, dislocations, and problems with the blood supply that can kill the bone. Check for things that harm your health that only seem to be hip pain—tumors, conditions of the reproductive system, infections, hernias, and gastrointestinal trouble. Pain at the side of the hip, along with burning or numbness in the front of the leg, can be a nerve injury called meralgia paresthetica. This condition can come from seat-belt injuries, surgery, even tight waistbands in pants that press the nerves. A persistent, burning ache around the side of the body or hip can seem musculo-skeletal before the characteristic rash comes out to show it is shingles. Find and treat these with your doctor. You can still use the exercises, good body mechanics, stretches and principles in this chapter for relief from pain, healthier hips, and healthier exercise.

Many common medications can cause achy muscles and joints. Taking several of these medicines together is common: cholesterol-lowering medicines called statins, some prescription allergy medicines, stomach-acid inhibitors, erectile-enhancing drugs, anti-anxiety medicines, prescription anti-depressants, prescription acne medicines, medicines for irritable bowel, constipation, and Crohn's disease, the calcium-channel-blocker drug, verapamil, the antibiotics erythromycin and clarithromycin, some HIV medications, and others. Try to address and change the original problem in healthy ways, instead of taking more medicines.

What to Do Every Day to Stop Hip Pain

- First thing in the morning, turn facedown while still in bed, to help get the hip in good straight position. If lying facedown is uncomfortable for your lower back, see the lordosis section in Chapter 2.

- Stand without bending your hip forward at the crease where the leg meets the body.

- Stretch your hip to the back with extension stretches (Figures 4-6 through 4-13).

- Strengthen your hip with extension exercise (Figures 4-8 and 4-14).

- Do lunges with your hip tucked to strengthen and stretch the hip at the same time as training a functional way to bend (Figure 4-6). Movement feeds and lubricates the hip joints. Lunges also warm your body, making stretching easier.

- Stretch the back and sides of your hip to reduce pain and dysfunction from a tight hip, as well as tight muscles in the backside that can press on the sciatic nerve—mimicking pain from bad discs (Figure 4-17 through 4-20, and 4-22 through 4-27).

- Walk, move, and exercise, with feet and legs pointing straight ahead—not turned out.

- Practice getting up and down from the floor without hands to increase strength and balance.

- Use the muscles on the side of your hip (called medius muscles) for shock absorption and to keep hips in comfortable level position, not sagging side to side with each step. Keep hips from jarring into tilted position when walking and going up and down stairs.

- Don't let an uneven surface— such as a banked track or side of the road—shift your hip sideways when walking or running. Use your muscles to keep the hip from tilting unevenly, and so that your weight rests on your muscles not the hip joints.

- Cushion your hip joints by using your leg muscles for shock absorption with every step, instead of thumping your body weight down. Walk lightly. See if you can walk across the floor or stairs without making a sound, using a normal gait.

- Try a soft pad if you have a hard bed and like to sleep on your side, so the side of your hip isn't mashed onto a hard surface.

- Wear hip guards for playing hockey and football.

- Don't let your knees sag inward ("knock-knee") when you walk, move, and exercise. Use muscles to hold your leg from sagging. Leaning in on your knees can make the hip hurt and rub at an angle in the joint.

- When you watch a lot of television, instead of sitting in a chair or recliner, lie on the floor or bed and stretch your legs. Lie face up and facedown, and stretch legs in all directions, the way children do when they watch while lying down. It can be fun and gives some natural motion, exercise, and stretch.

- To maintain hipbone density, load the upper leg and hip through weightlifting, by using squats and lunges for all bending, and moving more in daily life. Osteoporosis affects both men and women. Every year, men suffer one-third of all hip fractures, and one-third of these men die within one year.

- Retrain your exercise habits and mindset away from conventional exercises that only bend the hip forward for stretching and strengthening. Instead use lunges (Figure 4-6) to exercise your hip in the straight and extended positions you need for healthy, springy, natural function. For abdominal exercise, use the exercises in Chapter 2 (Figures 2-31 through 2-39) instead of forward rounding.

- Watch other people to see what it looks like when they stand with the front of the hip bent.

What to Avoid

- Avoid standing and moving with the top of the hip tipped forward and the hip bent at the crease where the leg meets the body.

- Avoid the usual exercises—like leg lifts and forward bends—that tighten the front of the hip.

- Avoid letting your hip sink out to the side under your body weight when standing, walking, and going up and down stairs.

- Avoid a sedentary lifestyle. Sedentary older people risk losing bone mass in the hip and other areas, which can lead to osteoporosis. Sedentary young people are setting themselves up for osteoporosis later, which can easily be prevented.

- Avoid fad diets that severely limit calories. You need foods with calcium and the several nutrients needed for calcium to be absorbed and work in the body. Avoid eating high amounts of animal protein, which increases calcium loss. Drugs that decrease bone mass include the anti-convulsant phenytoin (Dilantin), the birth-control shot (Depo Provera), and long-term use of steroid medications for allergy, asthma, some pain syndromes, and some immune conditions. Check with your doctor for interventions without these side effects, or for ways to counter them.

When to Notice Hips

- Frequently overlooked times to notice hips are standing around and on the stairs. See if you keep both hips bent at the crease of the leg so that your behind tips out in back. Check if you let the hip press out to the side. When standing around, do you stand with the hip pushed forward? When exercising, do you keep the front of the hip bent, even when standing up?

- When you stretch the quadriceps, do lunge stretches, or stretch over a ball, make sure the front of your hip actually stretches. Instead of arching your back, tip the hip under you to lengthen the hip muscles. If you don't, you will only arch the back instead of getting the intended stretch in the front of the hip.

- If you can't lie comfortably on your back without a pillow under your knees, the front of your hip is tight. Similarly, if you can't lie flat facedown without lower-back pain, or lie facedown and prop up onto elbows, the front of your hip is probably too tight to stand straight without yanking your back into arched, strained position. Do anterior hip stretches (Figures 4-6 through 4-14).

How to Get Natural Hip Stretch During Daily Activity

- Put on shoes, socks, and pants standing up. For extra balance and hip involvement, retrieve the other shoe or sock from the floor while still standing on one foot in standing figure-4 hip stretch

- Walk with both feet facing straight ahead, not turned in or out. Turning out tightens the outer muscles of the hip.

- When walking, stand straight—not bent forward—to prevent the front of the hip from getting tight.

- When going up stairs, step up with the heel down on the step, standing straight—not bent forward—with the hip stuck out in back. If your feet are too big for the step, keep the heel down at the lowest position off the step without your foot slipping off. When coming down stairs, don't let the hip push out to the side on the leg that steps down.

- For hip stretch, strengthening, and better balance to avoid falls, pick up objects or clothing around the house with your bare foot. Lift and transfer objects to your hand. Practice safely. The object is to build strength and skill to reduce risk of falls and injury, not create uncontrolled situations where you lose your footing.

- For every time you bend for things using a squatting motion, keep both heels down. Don't stick your behind out in back. Tuck the hip slightly, but not so much that you round your back. Use good bending for the many times a day you bend around the house and workplace to strengthen your hip and legs.

No More Hip Pain

People who exercise often concentrate on moves that bend the hip forward, like leg lifts, touching toes, bringing knees to chest, bending over to lift weights, stair machines, and most traditional core training. Tightness of the hip and forward bent daily posture can result that adds to pain and poor function. You may have heard that you must keep the hip bent "to protect the back" when exercising, but it is not true. Your own abdominal and core muscles should position your back. Positioning does not come from bending the knees and hip. Use your own daily life activities to restore healthy movement that strengthens the hip and stops pain.

5

No More Knee Pain

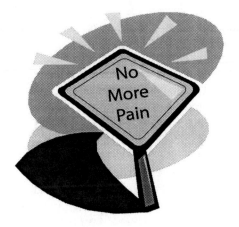

- Knee Cartilage Injury
- Knock-Knees
- Arthritis
- Duck Feet
- Hyperextension Injury
- Twisted Knee
- Bursitis
- Quadriceps and IT-Band Tightness

Knee pain can be uncomfortable and frightening. Luckily, knee pain is usually not difficult to fix yourself. Most people know that bending wrong all the time will make your back sore—even injured. The same is true for knees. Legs have posture and position during standing and movement. After years of bad habits they can begin to ache. A knee injury that may begin suddenly is often just a "last straw" after pressuring and straining over months or years. Of the many things that make knees hurt—from arthritis to being hurt in an accident—you can use the principles given in this chapter to reduce pain and get back to being active and having fun.

Marlyn was 40 years old when she called me as a last resort. Her doctor was talking to her seriously about knee replacement.

I rang her doorbell and she let me in for the house-call appointment. As she walked ahead of me to lead me to her living room, I watched her walk. Because I make house calls, I can see how someone walks and moves on a daily basis.

With each step she took, her feet turned out like a duck's and her arches flattened to the floor. Each kneecap faced a different direction, neither one straight ahead. She bent to pull out a chair for me and I watched as she threw her knees forward and together, with all her body weight forward so that her knee joints—not her thigh muscles—took the pressure of her body weight and the weight of the chair. Her knees wobbled inward as she placed the chair down for me. She clomped into the kitchen to get me a glass of water, walking so heavily that the skin on her face shook with each step. When she returned, I watched her step down the three stairs to the living room, with her knees forward, inward, and with such lack of shock absorption that you could hear each step: "Whump! Whump! Whump!"

Marlyn's doctor had wisely sent her for physical therapy. At PT they gave her strengthening and stretching exercises and recorded each exercise she did with weights and bands.

"Yes, they told me 'Lift right and lose weight,' but they might as well have told me, 'Go to the moon.' It hurts my knees to lift right. How do I even begin?" They gave her arch supports and orthotics. The physical therapists worked hard for her but the knee pain intensified, and her knees began to swell.

They told her to give up running, which was her great love. Now she was almost 45 pounds heavier. She had constant pain and took strong and expensive prescription anti-inflammatory medications several times every day, which upset her stomach. She was on more medicines for the stomach pain but the stomach pain continued. She had gone for weekly hyaluronate injections into both knees to try to improve the joint fluid. Hyaluronate is a compound made to be similar to the natural fluid in the knee joint. She wasn't sure if it helped or not. It had been almost two years like this, and she had "tried everything" except knee replacement. Her doctor told her it was the next and only thing left to try. Calling me was something she didn't expect to work.

Just standing up straight and "good posture" won't cure bad knees, but movement patterns influence pressure on the knees and whether you injure or strengthen them with your daily habits. We started with repositioning knees when bending and going up the stairs. I showed her how to keep her weight back toward the heel and not let knees sway inward. By the end of the first day, she could go up the stairs and could bend to pick up small things from the table with no pain by using the new positioning. She still had to come down the stairs one step at a time. We worked on repositioning her legs and using thigh and hip muscles to decelerate instead of flopping her weight heavily down on the stair below. Soon she could go down stairs without pain and could bend properly to pick up chairs and things from the floor. It was a good cycle of good leg exercise that saved her knees and back, and increased her ability to get more exercise.

At her two-month follow-up, Marlyn laughed to me that she now took the stairs for fun where she used to avoid them to avoid the pain. Her knees had strengthened and her weight had been coming down. At her three-year follow-up, she was still pain-free enough to not yet need knee replacement.

Knee Pain Fix #1: Keep Cartilage Healthy

A common habit that can eventually injure knees is letting body weight fall inward toward the inside of the knees and the arches of your feet. Weight pressing inward pushes your leg inward at the knee. The inward angle is not unavoidable or something you are born to have. Think of watching a beginner on skates. Their ankles and knees often sag inward because they have not yet learned to hold them straight. Learning to hold the ankles and knees straight is just simple repositioning that makes you skate better and stops the knee and ankle pain that comes from letting them sag inward. You can do the same for normal walking.

Letting your weight fall in the inside of your knee joint, instead of holding your weight evenly on your knees using your leg muscles, adds load and wear to the cartilage on the inside of the knee, stresses the anterior cruciate ligament (ACL) in the middle, and overstretches the ligament on the inside of the knee. Ligaments move with your bones but are not supposed to stretch much. They are supposed to keep their same length to hold your bones in line. When an injury overstretches them, they are like an

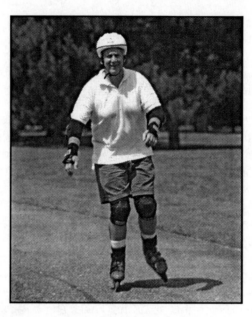

Figure 5-1. Letting ankles and knees sway inward can damage knees. It is not a "condition." It is something you can control using your own muscles to hold your ankles and knees straight.

old elastic waistband that doesn't snap back into normal length. They can't hold the joint together properly anymore. The joint can start to rub and grind at unhealthy angles.

Another problem is twisting. If you plant your foot and turn your body in a different direction, it will twist your knee. This twisting can injure the cushiony knee cartilage, called the meniscus, and also other cartilage. You can also gradually injure your knee by letting your weight fall inward, which makes the leg bones twist in a similar way on a smaller scale, day after day, year after year.

Letting knees sway inward also interferes with normal thigh muscle use and how your kneecap moves when you walk. When you let your weight slump on your knee joints instead of using your thigh muscles, the kneecap can start to move slightly sideways instead of up and down each time you move your knee to walk. This rubs the cartilage on the inside of your kneecap. The friction can eventually break down and wear away the cartilage.

Many people are told to accept knee degeneration as nothing more than aging, with unavoidable pain and disability. They may be told their leg rolls in because they are flat-footed, or have a problem called pronation, which roughly means turning inward, or that they have "knock-knees." But often, the cause is avoidable. Letting your knees roll inward is often easily corrected by using your leg muscles to hold your knee from sagging. It is the same as not letting your shoulders round forward.

Linda's knees touched each other when she stood up with her feet apart. It wasn't that her thighs were that heavy, but that she stood with so much weight on the inside of her knees that they bent inward enough to touch. She let them rest against each other. Her doctor told her that women get knee pain because their hips are wide. I told her that idea used to be commonly thought, but it wasn't the fault of gender. Plenty of men had wider hips than she had. There were at least four studies I knew of that revealed that the higher injury rate was not a gender issue but training error and physical fitness.

It is normal for the upper-leg bone to angle slightly inward as it joins the lower-leg bone. The angle at the knee is called the "Q angle," and allows us to walk upright on two legs in a smooth gait. Animals that normally stay on four legs don't have this Q angle. When a dog or monkey walks on hind legs, they waddle side to side. The Q angle of human legs allows walking upright with a smooth and narrow gait. When bones are dug up, one thing that is looked for is the slightly angled surface at the bottom of the femur, the upper-leg bone. It is one of many markers that tell if it is human.

The Q angle varies slightly from person to person, male and female alike. It also changes during development from the bowlegged baby to the knock-kneed child, to the straighter knees of adulthood.

It used to be commonly believed that nothing could change your Q angle, or stop you from being knock-kneed. But people with a tendency to have a higher angle from letting their weight sag can change to a more normal angle but not letting the knee sag inward.

When Linda stood with both feet facing straight forward, her kneecaps faced inward. It pressured the inside of her knee joint and allowed her kneecaps to rub instead of gliding smoothly. You can voluntarily reduce this problem, too, by holding your leg from sagging—if you have a tendency to sag like Linda did.

Other people keep their kneecaps facing forward but stand with their lower leg and feet pointing outward. This positioning is called tibial torsion because it twists the knee at the tibia. It is another way of standing that can increase Q angle. When someone with tibial torsion tries to just turn their feet parallel, their knees often turn inward. If they keep the whole leg straight, they can reduce the torsion on the knee and the knee pain that comes with it. It is not unchangeable.

We began retraining Linda's knee positioning using lunges, raising and lowering keeping the upper body upright (Figure 3-6). She stood with one leg in front and the other in back. When she first bent her knees to try the first lunge, the front knee swayed inward immediately. I patted the outside of her thigh to show her to use the outside thigh muscles to pull outward to keep her knee right over her foot instead of sagging inward. She repositioned her knee without trouble. We made sure she wasn't just rocking her weight on the outside edge of her feet—which is another poor position. When she bent to pick up her water bottle from the floor, her knee swung inward again.

"I can't believe I did that," Linda laughed, "after I just practiced bending right ten times."

"Lunging and bending without turning your knee in is for all the time," I told her, "not just for ten repetitions."

"Who would think it!" she joked.

We went on to practice shallow squatting (Figure 5-4), helpful for bending for many daily chores. Instead of lunging with one foot in front of the other, in the squat your feet are straight across from each other—useful for picking up a laundry basket, grocery bag, or child. Her knees swayed inward again.

"Healthy knees when you squat, too," I reminded her. She said it felt like the same muscles, so it shouldn't be hard to apply the same idea. I brought her over to a step bench and asked her to step up.

"Oops," she said as she stepped with her knee swaying inward.

"Okay," I told her. "Now step downward and don't let you knee fall inward." She stepped down, and the knee swayed only slightly.

"Oooh, it makes such a difference," Linda said. "I can feel my muscles controlling it and it doesn't hurt when I control it."

Her physical therapist was a mutual friend. "You're wrong," she said. "The valgus knee (inward knee, or knock-knee) is heritable and the bony articulation is fixed (you're born to be that way and can't change the bones)." I told them that I wanted to catch Linda's pronounced inward sag before it deformed her bones so badly that her pain would come from that and not from the bad positioning that was the present cause. For many people, it is just sagging inward that makes the position and the pain. "You're still wrong," she said. "If you change her knee positioning, you'll damage her hip." That used to be commonly thought, too. People would help one problem but cause another when they didn't reposition the whole leg, and instead, just yanked the knee into position. We didn't want to do that with Linda. We made sure her repositioning came from the entire leg in healthy manner. It was more likely that letting the knee sag inward would eventually hurt the hip. It is usually better to hold things straight. I checked in with her every six months or so, for many years. Her legs were beautifully straight. Her thigh muscles newly developed. Taking the stairs no longer hurt. She said it was free exercise.

When the tires on your car are crooked, they will wear out sooner than they should, and won't move on the road in the safest manner (Figure 5-2). The cure for tire wear is neither to stop driving (give up activity) nor to change or rotate the tire (wear orthotics or have surgery). To fix the cause of the tire wear, you straighten the tires so they don't tilt. It can be the same thing to check why your knee is crooked and stop leaning on it in wears that wear it out prematurely.

Many people are given orthotics or told to never walk barefoot, which is often unnecessary. Practice correcting your leg position until you can walk with healthy and straight leg positioning that keeps weight on your leg muscles—not on the cartilage and joints of your knee.

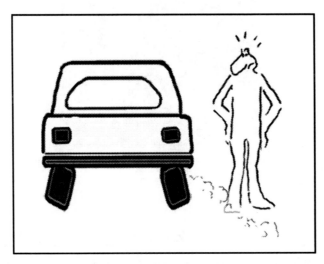

Figure 5-2. Just like tires that tilt inward, knees that tilt inward can wear out too soon.

Prevent Pain from Turned-In Knees

- Look in a mirror and see if your kneecaps face inward or your arches flatten downward under your body weight.
- Learn to hold your leg in healthy position by using your muscles, not letting your weight sway and slump onto your knee joints, making then tilt inward or outward
- Use leg muscles to lift weight off your arches, gently, without rolling too far to the outside of the soles. Like any new habit it may feel strange at first.

- See if your knees are facing straight but your feet turn out. Straighten the whole leg. If you just turn the foot so it points straight ahead, the knees will turn in. Keep feet and knees both facing in the same direction. Similarly, if your kneecaps face straight when your feet turn inward, straighten the whole leg, don't just yank the feet straight.

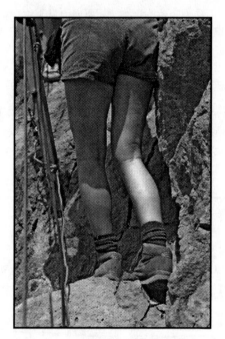

Figure 5-3. Don't let knees turn in as you put weight on them to bend, step up, or down.

Knee Pain Fix #2: Keep Knees from Hurting When Bending and on the Stairs

Satish had knee pain from doing squats and running. His doctor had told him to stop squats and running until the knees quieted down, and to use ice. He said that worked fine. He would stop all his workouts for one to two months and the pain would be gone. It would come back the first week he started running and doing squats again.

His legs were rail thin. I asked him if he would show me how he did squats. He suddenly threw his weight downward, knees quickly sagging inward and forward, up and down, three times before I could stop him. "Okay, I get the idea," I said, "Can you show me how you run, a little more slowly and please don't hurt your knees like that." He ran fairly heavily, bringing his knees far forward each time his feel struck the ground, with weight shifted toward the toes. I asked him if he had pain at the moment. He said he did. He had just started exercising after yet another two-month layoff and was getting discouraged. I showed Satish that when he bent his knees, he was letting the knees come forward, which transmitted his body weight through the knee. Instead, I showed him how to bend by keeping his heels down and knees back, over the ankle (Figure 5-4). I told him this approach is how to bend for everything—even to pick up a towel. He practiced his squatting position and rocked his weight back to the heel, off the toes. He said he could immediately feel the difference in muscle use in the thigh, and that the familiar pressure pretty much disappeared from his knees. On follow-up a year later, his pain had not returned and he was able to run and do squats as he pleased. His legs had also filled out, both from finally using the thigh muscles instead of putting the weight forward on his knee joints, and from being able to exercise without having to stop two months for every month he exercised.

A common contributor to chronic knee pain is bad bending. Many people refuse to "lift with the legs" to save their back because it hurts their knees. The good news is that bending knees properly will not hurt, but help heal and strengthen. Many people around the world habitually bend and rise from the floor many times a day. Their legs remain mobile and strong. A major contributor to knee osteoarthritis is weak thigh muscles. Become more active and your legs will strengthen enough to allow you to do more.

Bending Using a Squat

Most people bend by letting the knees come forward. Instead, keep weight back toward the heel, distributed over the whole foot—not just on the toes (Figure 5-4, right). Many people, who previously could not bend without knee pain, find they can bend without pain with this modification. This technique creates a good cycle of proper bending, which is good for the back and knees, and strengthening so that you can bend more with less pain.

- Keep knees back, over your ankles, not pressing forward.
- Keep knees far enough back when you bend that you can see your toes.
- Don't let your back arch; keep hip slightly tucked.
- Use a mirror to practice healthy knee position.
- If you can't figure how to keep your knee from coming forward, put the front of your knees against a bench or other object to train yourself to keep them from slouching forward.

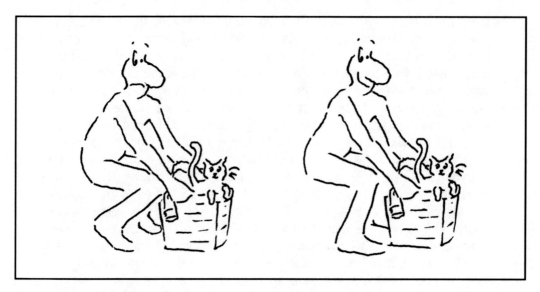

Figure 5-4. Bad bending, with knees forward, puts weight on the knees (left). Good bending with knees back and heels down puts weight on your muscles, and off your knees. It's good exercise and healthy for your back and knees.

Weightlifting Squats

For squats in a gym:

- Stand flat on your whole foot.
- Don't prop up your heels on a block or stand on your toes.
- Lean your weight back to your heels.

Bending with One Foot in Front–The Lunge

- Put one leg in front and one in back. Center your weight on both legs (Figure 5-5).
- Keep the front knee over the ankle, not forward. Keep your weight toward your heel of the front leg, not pressing forward on the front of the foot. Pressing forward transmits body weight to your knee joint, instead of leg muscles.
- Your back heel can come up, but the front heel is down with your weight toward the heel.
- You bend many times a day. Healthy bending is good exercise for your knee and entire body.

Use the standing lunge (Figure 3-6) to practice healthy leg placement and to strengthen the legs. Keep both feet in place, instead of starting with "walking lunges."

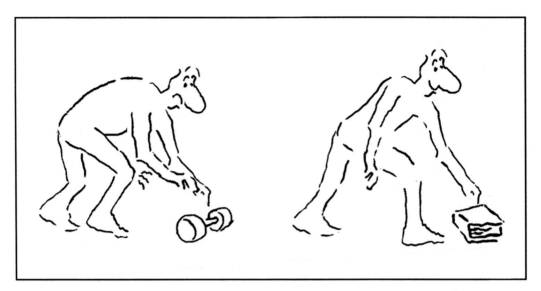

Figure 5-5. When bending with the lunge for all the many dozens of times you bend every day, don't let your front knee come forward (left). Keep front knee back over ankle with weight on heel (right).

Many people step forward or back, leaning their front knee inward and forward with each step, compounding the twisting and pressure on the knee with hand weights. Don't start with walking lunges. Keep feet in place. Raise and lower to practice healthy placement. Then apply the placement learned to walking lunges, not letting the front knee come forward or sway inward. Add to strengthening by holding and lifting hand weights as you rise up and down in the standing or walking lunge. Training knee positioning while lunging is more important to rehabbing knee injury than doing the lunges or lifting the weights. When you put the weights down, don't bend over wrong. Use the lunge you just practiced.

Squatting to Rest

For gardening, resting, doing chores, or stretching, keep heels down and your body weight back. Avoid squatting on the balls of your feet with your heels up (Figure 5-6). That throws your weight forward onto your knee joint and squashes the knee under body weight. Research shows that the meniscus (cushiony knee disc) injuries of professional baseball catchers often comes from chronic squatting with their weight shifted forward on their toes.

• Keep your heels on the floor with body weight back toward your heels. This positioning reduces pressure on the knees and is a great stretch for your Achilles tendon and calf muscle in the back of your lower leg. This sitting posture is customary in much of the world.

- Don't let your feet turn out or let your body weight press inward on your knees or arches.
- Keep knees over your feet, not drooping inward.

My friends in Asia ask why Westerners can't sit on their heels. I explain that they don't practice it. They ask how Westerners sit to eat and wash and do daily tasks. I tell them they sit in chairs and the back of their legs gets too tight to squat. They often think I am kidding that Westerners are so tight that they can't do ordinary life activities. They ask me how Westerners go to the bathroom and I tell them they sit in chairs. They think I am funny.

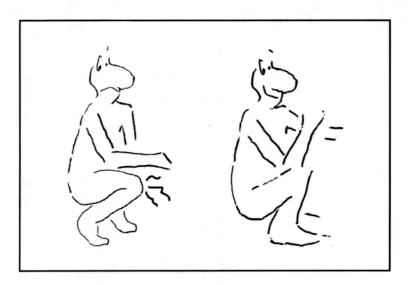

Figure 5-6. Many Westerners are not accustomed to squatting. To sit in a squat, stay on heels (right), not toes (left) to take harmful pressure off the knee and get a nice stretch for the lower back, back of the calf, and Achilles tendon.

Going Up Stairs

Commonly, people step up allowing their knees to sway inward. This movement is injurious to the knee over time.

- Keep knee over your foot, not sagging inward. Use the muscles on the side of your thigh to pull outward so that your knee stays in place without wobbling.
- Keep your arches from rolling inward or flattening.
- Keep your heel down and your weight back toward the heel of the foot that is stepping up. Many people don't step this way because their legs are tight and weak. They throw their weight forward, stepping up onto the toe. Doing so transmits body weight onto the knee joint in a negative cycle of weakness and pain. Keep your

weight back. You will feel the reduction in strain through the knee and free exercise for the muscles.

- Step up with feet parallel, not turning toe-in or toe-out, where stairs are wide enough to allow it.

- Stand more upright. You will be surprised how much you lean forward on the stairs.

- Use these techniques for stair machines in the gym, too.

Going Down Stairs

A move that you do not usually see in step aerobics class is stepping down forward from the front of the bench. It is considered too likely to result in injury, because people so often throw weight forward and let knees sway inward. But stepping down stairs or curbs is part of daily life for most people.

- Don't let knees sag inward. Stepping down with all your weight on this angulated knee grinds the cartilage.

- Keep your arches from rolling inward or flattening as you bend you knee.

- Keep your weight more on the foot on the upper stair. Don't flop heavily down. Keep the heel on the upper leg down as far as comfortable on each step down, without it pushing your knee forward.

- Step lightly down onto the ball of your foot, using thigh muscles to decelerate. You will get more exercise for your legs, more natural Achilles and calf stretch, and less strain on your knees.

- Step down with feet parallel, not turning toe-in or toe-out, where stairs are wide enough to allow it.

Step Aerobic Class

- Step up with your weight back toward the heel of the foot that is stepping up. Sure, it's easier to lean forward on the toe than keeping weight back using thigh and backside muscles, but the point of stepping is to use your muscles.

- Don't let knees sway inward when stepping up or down.

- Step down using leg muscles to decelerate. Don't come down full force under your body weight.

Bending Knees for Rowing

- For rowing machines or a real rowing shell, push back with your whole foot, with weight on your heels, not only your toes.

- It is a better stretch for the back of the lower leg, better thigh and hip exercise, and puts less pressure on the knee.

All Knee Bending

Retrain your bending habits. Good bending strengthens your knees and prevents back pain at the same time. You can become more mobile and strong while reducing pain, by using your muscles instead of throwing your body weight forward on your knee joint.

What about Arthritic Knees?

Straightening your legs again after bending is called "terminal extension" because it is the last few degrees of straightening, and straightening a joint is called extension. Sports medicine professionals discuss that people with knee arthritis should not do the knee bending of lunges or squats. During terminal extension, the tibia (or lower-leg bone) naturally rotates a bit under the femur. This rotation happens because the two sides of your knee are shaped slightly differently. Some say that because of this rotation, which has the funny name "the Screw-Home Mechanism," that any exercise involving terminal extension is too stressful for an arthritic knee. Instead, they only allow straight-leg exercises. These exercises usually are things like sitting on the floor and doing small leg lifts, working up to wearing a leg weight, sitting on the floor and pressing your knee straight, and other small straight-leg exercises.

The problem with this seemingly sensible approach is that the person goes about their day without the good bending that strengthens thighs to prevent arthritis and reduce pain. Good bending keeps the joint moving through a range, which is crucial for joint health and prevents injuring your lower-back discs from bad, straight-legged bending. These people are told to exercise their knees by lying on the floor wearing a five-pound leg weight. But these same people need to walk around carrying their entire body weight to do normal activities, step up curbs, stairs, and bend around the house just to do minimal, normal-life activities.

Practicing small standing lunges (Figure 3-6), retraining front knee position to keep weight back toward the heel has allowed my patients with arthritis to bend for many things that constitute a normal life, without adding load and pain on their knees, and to able to take the stairs again. Don't do huge bends with poor positioning, of course, but see if good positioning allows you better motion with less pain. If pain increases, don't do this. But for many people, the strengthening and movement help create a positive cycle of use and decrease of symptoms. If you need your hand on your knee, strengthen and practice balance until you don't need it. Holding your own body weight up without assistance is a bare minimum for normal life ability.

Bess lived in a third-floor apartment until her 80s. She walked the stairs several times a day. Then she moved to a new place with no stairs. A few months later when visiting a friend, she was surprised to find that she was unable to go up the stairs without discomfort. This injury was not unchangeable. She started practicing standing lunges (Figure 3-6) and remembered to bend well for everything around the house (Figure 5-5). She strengthened her thigh muscles so that she could stay mobile. Movement keeps joints healthy, increases knee strength, and reduces knee pain.

Knee Pain Fix #3: Check for Duck Feet

Walking with feet turned out (Figure 5-7) contributes to knee pain, to tightness of the leg, to hip and heel pain, and predisposes to bunion because you push off each step on the side of the big toe, pushing the toe inward. "Duck-foot" can result from letting weight fall inward, from tight Achilles tendon, tight side of the upper leg (iliotibial band, or IT band), tight bottom of the foot (plantar fascia), even tight big toe (hallux rigidus) that doesn't bend and allow normal foot motion.

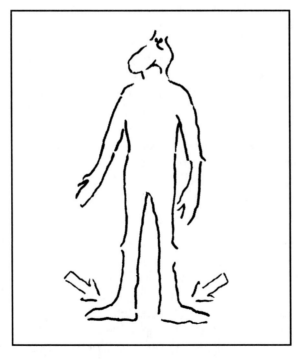

Figure 5-7. Turning out when you walk can pressure the knees.

Sometimes the turned-out position can come from the hip, turning the whole leg outward when the person walks. Sometimes the knee twists to turn out while the upper leg stays facing straight. In both cases, the forces fall inward on the knee and ankle when walking forward.

Danny was a computer "geek" who ran for recreation. He had pain in the front of his knees, around the kneecaps with running, going up or down stairs, and rising from squatting. The pain had started gradually and increased over a few years. Previously it would come and go. Now it hurt more often and more intensely. The pain was cutting down how long or far he could run. The pain would stop with rest, but return with activity. He said he had gained about 10 pounds over the previous year. He had gone for a sports-medicine evaluation that checked his kneecaps and found they were fine, and that since he only ran short recreational distances, overuse was not a problem. He said that it didn't hurt if he ran backward. They had suggested that he run backward from then on.

I asked Danny to run for me. Forward. He pounded around, each foot hitting hard, which is called a "hard-strike phase." As each foot slapped down in a turned-out, duck-footed position, it would roll inward more than normal—looking like his feet were sinking into marshmallows on the insides. It is usual for the foot to strike slightly on the outside of the heel and then roll slightly inward. In this way, you get natural spring and shock absorption. It is this tendency that makes shoes wear slightly more on the outside of the heel, and sometimes leads people to think that they are not walking straight and need a special shoe to prevent that movement. A small (not large) heel-strike on the outside is natural. But Danny turned his foot inward before even hitting the ground. He let his hip follow the arch of the foot sinking downward, so that each hip dropped with each foot strike—like a runway model in expensive sneakers. His knee bowed slightly inward with each foot strike. He turned his right foot outward and the right knee inward far more than he did on the left. His stride length was short, looking like he was too tight to take a normal-length step. When his foot landed, the tight hamstrings made him pull the ankle back more than normal, with his weight farther forward than normal.

Danny had been to physical therapy where they carefully tested the flexibility and strength of all of his muscles. His evaluation was thorough, and reported that he had hip-abductor weakness (hip abductors are the muscles that pull your legs away from each other), tight-hip adductors (the muscles that close your legs), hip rotator tightness (rotators turn your leg inward and outward), hip-flexor tightness (flexors bend the hip at the crease of where the leg meets the body), and hamstring tightness, in the back of the thighs. They gave him a roll of hard foam to roll on the side of his leg to stretch the tight muscles. He said it hurt so he didn't do it often. They gave him an exercise to do 10 times a day—to stand on one foot and bend the knee. He said that made his knee hurt the same way it did when he ran, so he didn't like doing that one, either. He did a similar exercise sitting down with his knee bent over the foam roll, wearing an ankle weight, straightening the knee against the weight. He said they told him that his inner-quadriceps muscle needed strengthening to help keep his kneecap from sliding sideways from the outer quadriceps pulling harder than the inner ones, making the kneecap tilt and rub as he ran. His thigh got stronger, but when he stood up after doing this exercise and walked around, he went back to the same inward rolling on his knee.

Danny showed me his hamstring stretches, sitting bent forward rounding his upper back. He was already round shouldered so he said he liked that one because it felt normal. I showed him to stretch by lying on his back so that his back didn't bend and the stretch had to come from his hamstrings. This feeling was new for him. We worked on knee positioning and Danny found that his pain was relieved by altering mechanics and positioning to healthier foot strike and not letting his knees turn in and his feet turn out. We retrained the "stork" exercise he had been given, to stand on one foot and bend the knee up and down, so that his knee and hip didn't sink inward. He kept weight on his muscles instead of his knee joint. His tightness stayed pretty much the same. At first he didn't believe the pain was relieved from the change in gait. I reminded him that he was originally running backward to stop the pain. Running backward was one way to change the pressure on his knees. Now he had a healthy way to keep the forces on his knee healthy, with the benefit that he could run forward and see where he was going.

Some say that turned-in (or -out) legs are the result of natural difference in hip-joint angles and that fixing bad ankle and knee posture will just cause pain in the hip or other problems. If you only turn feet in without correcting the source of the problem, the rest of the leg turns in with it, making more stress—which is entirely unnecessary. Keep your entire leg position healthy and less pain, not more, will result.

Prevent Pain from Turned-Out Leg Positioning

- Find the source of your turned out foot position. Sometimes it is nothing more than a bad habit.
- If the turned-out position is from a tight hip, tight iliotibial band, or tight foot structures, stretch them and retrain positioning.
- Don't let knees sway inward or arches to roll down.

- Use your muscles to walk with your legs facing straight ahead. Doing so keeps body weight more evenly distributed, and more on your muscles and off the joints of the hip, ankles, foot, and knee.

Knee Pain Fix #4:
Your Own Body's Shock Absorption

Many people walk, run, exercise, jump, and step heavily, letting each foot flop down without muscle use to decelerate. Shock transmits to the joints of your ankle, knee, hip, back and neck, and can strain your calf muscle and Achilles tendon. It is easy to see injury in progress when seeing people stomping, flopping, slamming, and straining knees and Achilles tendons, and calling it exercise.

- When going down steps or a hill, for example, use thigh and hip muscles to step down lightly.
- Instead of just falling onto the lower step, keep weight on the upper leg to lower yourself lightly.
- Add shock absorption from the leg that steps down. Bend the knee as you step down. Don't come down on a straight knee.

Use the same principles for all walking, moving, and running. Use it for exercise classes using a step bench or balance platform. You will get free leg exercise, burn more calories, and reduce shock and wear on the knee.

Knee Pain Fix #5: Don't "Lock Out"
the Knee Joint with Hyperextension

I took a box-aerobics class because I had a coupon for a free week at a local club. Participants swatted at the air like knocking on a door. Most of the participants hung their heads forward in a disc-injuring position that didn't look tough—it looked ninety-years old. If any real boxer put his head so far forward you would be able to knock him out from arm's length. The woman in front of me was bouncing up and down as she swatted the air. Her knees bumped together every time she landed. Her feet were at least ten inches apart yet her knees bashed together, over and over. It was alarming. It worsened during the jump rope section. During the kicking section, she would fling her leg out, her knee slamming straight at the end of each kick. When she stood still to stretch, she threw her behind out in back and straightened her knees so much that they curved slightly backward.

Some people stand and move while "locking" the knee out straight, pressing it backward (Figure 5-8). Hyperextending the knee straightens the joint as far as it normally goes, then forces against the end-range position until the joint gives a little more. The cartilage that protects the ends of the bones gets rubbed instead of seating naturally in position. When you look at a chicken bone, the knobby end is shiny and smooth. This material is the cartilage. Cartilage covers the ends of bones to make them glide smoothly. You don't want to rub this nice surface off. Hyperextending the knee also pulls on the two crossed ligaments that hold the lower-leg bone from shifting forward under the upper-leg bone. Because the ligaments are crossed they are called cruciate ligaments. The one in front is the anterior cruciate ligament (ACL). The one behind it is your posterior cruciate ligament (PCL). Both of these ligaments can be forced to lengthen too much with knee hyperextension. You also have a necessary pad of fat in the knee, no matter how thin you are. This fat pad cushions the knee and can be one of the several structures injured by hyperextension.

When the hyperextended position is a regular habit, it is sometimes called "splay-legs," or "splayed knee," and makes the leg look more crescent-shaped than straight. Many people push their knees into hyperextension when standing and walking. Others "bang" the joint into straight position in exercise classes. This locked-out position is

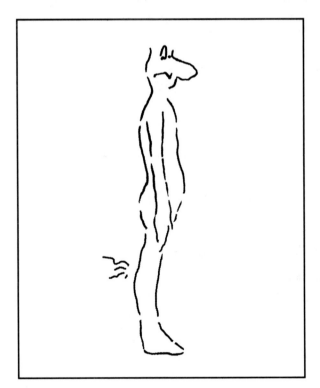

Figure 5-8. "Locking" the knee out straight, or
pushing it back in hyperextension, can hurt the joint.

occasionally taught in yoga and dance classes. Pain is commonly felt after long sitting or upon waking, even when not exercising. To avoid this, stand and move without locking the joint straight.

Wilson was helping move a couch up a flight of stairs. As he stepped up pushing the couch ahead of him, his foot slipped to the stair below. The couch slid down on his knee, pushing it backward. He came to me two days later with a knee so swollen he couldn't raise his pant leg enough to show me. He was amazed he couldn't get an appointment at his doctor's office for another two weeks. I told him that two weeks was a quick appointment for many centers.

When he first tried to tell me what happened, he looked around for words. I said, "Looks like you hyperextended it."

He pointed at me and said, "Yes, like that! How did you know?"

"Because you stand like that on the other knee, too. You push your knees back. Can you bend them both, just a little, to see how that feels?" He said that both knees felt better when he did. He said he liked to keep active. I told him to make sure to move the hurt knee for exercise every day—whether it is walking or dancing or taking the stairs. He said he did martial arts so would use his "katas," or forms, to move through a range each day. He would also use ice afterward, and elevate it. All three of these things help to move out the swelling. We went over how to stand and walk and move on the stairs without "locking out" or pushing back against his joint when he straightened his leg. By his appointment time two weeks later, his injured knee was pretty much healed. The other knee, which had "creaks now and then," had stopped creaking.

Prevent Pain from Hyperextension

- Walk and move without banging the knee joint straight.
- Stand without "locking" the knee straight.
- Stand without pressing the knee backward.
- Bend knees when landing from jumps, or stepping down. Use leg muscles to decelerate and step down lightly. Don't land on a straight or hyperextended knee or let the landing jar the knee.
- Avoid stretches and exercises that push the knee joint backward.

Knee Pain Fix #6: Move without Twisting

Dan was a yoga instructor and proud of his ability to twist his knees sideways in several different poses. He was taught that knee flexibility would prevent injury, but one day he stepped off a curb and his knee nearly slipped out of joint. He said that it had been feeling a bit "raw" before that and tried to stretch away the pain. He had made his knee so unstable by the sideways twisting that it no longer seated properly. It "rattled" and rubbed with each step he took. I showed Dan how the knee joint is shaped to bend and straighten, like a hinge on a door. The shoulder and hip joints swivel, but the knee is not shaped to swivel or twist more than a small amount. When the knee twists, it is like twisting a door sideways on the hinge, or the drumstick from a chicken.

Usually when you think of twisting your knee, it sounds painful. Sometimes people twist their knee deliberately, thinking they are stretching it (Figure 5-9). It is not a good stretch because when you twist your knee sideways, what stretches are the ligaments that hold your knee together. Your knee is a hinge joint, because it swings only two ways like a hinge. Like the hinge of a door, your knee is supposed to open and close but not twist much. That twisting would ruin the hinge. Your door would hang loose and not open and shut properly anymore.

A ligament holds one bone to the next, like the latch that holds a briefcase closed. The job of the ligamentous latch is to hold its position, and not overly stretch or stress. If a ligament becomes overstretched, it is like having a loose "latch" allowing the bones to rub and grind—which hurts and also slowly injures the joint.

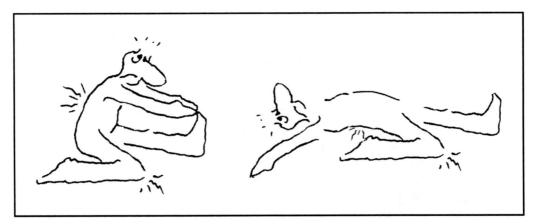

Figure 5-9. Your knee joint is not shaped to bend and twist too much at the same time. That can overstretch the joint and make it loose, so that it rubs and wears out sooner than it should.

Dan's knee joint wobbled slightly when I pulled and pushed it in a series of knee tests that I call "Zissurt Tests." I hold your knee and gently push the joint this way and that, asking, "Does Zihss-urt? Does Zissurt?" We don't want it to hurt; we only want to see what might be making it hurt.

Dan was worried his knee instability would be permanent. I showed him how he could hold knee positioning with his leg muscles. He would have to concentrate at the beginning to do the work that a normally working knee would do on its own. We worked on good lunge positioning with knees not sagging inward. Because he was so used to twisting his knee sideways, the knee easily turned inward, twisting it further. I sympathized with Dan. I had also heard long ago that if you practiced turning a joint into a twisted position, that if you fell down that way, it would not result in a painful twist or tear because it would already be accustomed to bending like that. The problem was that in every day life the knee was not staying in healthy position. Trying to prevent a one-time injury resulted in an on-going injury to his anterior cruciate ligament and the two ligaments on the sides of his knees called the collateral ligaments. Dan checked in with me a month later and said that he had incorporated the properly positioned lunge into his yoga classes instead of the twisting moves, and found he got better knee exercise without the raw feeling.

George was a runner and regularly stretched his thigh muscles, called the quadriceps. He stood on one leg and bent his knee so he could hold the foot behind him. His hip stayed bent in front and he arched his back. I asked him to tuck his hip under, as if he were "starting a crunch" but without bending forward. As he tried it, the front of his hip lengthened for the first time. "Wow, that's a whole different stretch," he said. I told him that when you arch your back you usually aren't stretching your thigh. By removing the arch, the quadriceps muscles of the thigh have to lengthen to reach the foot to the hand. I reminded him not to bend forward at the hip either, since the point was to stretch and lengthen the front of the leg, not bend and shorten it. Keeping his hip tucked under took care of both problems.

George also did a thigh stretch called "the hurdler's stretch." He sat bending one knee behind him. This position can sometimes be all right if you turn your leg out by rotating the hip, but George's hip was too tight to do that so he did the stretch by twisting his knee. That twisting isn't good, but alone didn't seem enough to give him the deep, sharp pain he came to see me about, or the meniscus tears on his MRI scan. A magnetic resonance imaging (MRI) scan is a way of getting a picture of soft tissues and bones without x-rays. I watched him run. I saw that when he turned or changed direction, he would do that by planting his foot on the ground, and then turn his leg and body without also moving his foot. This movement causes a classic twisting injury.

We worked on positioning so that when George changed direction, he pivoted lightly on the ball of his foot. At both the six-month and one-year follow-up, he said he was running with no knee pain. He was pivoting properly to change direction and also stopped doing the hurdler's stretch. I had showed him at the initial visit how a few lunges would give him a better and faster warm up, and stretch his legs at the same time.

Planting the foot and turning at the knee while keeping the knee bent twists the meniscus. Planting the foot and turning at the knee when it is straight can hurt the ligament that crosses side to side through the knee, called the anterior cruciate ligament. It is called the anterior cruciate because it crosses in front of another one going the other direction in back of it, called the posterior cruciate ligament. The anterior cruciate ligament is at its tightest position with your knee straight. It goes lax when you bend your knee. If you change direction suddenly by planting your foot and twisting a straight knee, it can be too much for the cruciate. These injuries can happen suddenly with one big bad twist, or build up gradually over time with small, repetitive, and bad twisting.

Sudden twists also happen in skiing, basketball, or with slips and falls. A sudden twist injury is common with sports spikes. The spikes dig in the ground, holding the foot. If the athlete pivots, the leg turns but the foot is held still by the spikes, which can tear the meniscus or the anterior cruciate. The rotating spike was developed so that you could plant your foot and pivot your body. The spikes dig in but the foot can pivot.

Smaller twists that injure over time can happen with small twists when going down stairs where the stairs turn, when changing direction when walking and running, and when getting in and out of a car, or even a desk chair.

Joni called me about a year after we fixed her Achilles tendonitis. Her Achilles didn't hurt anymore, but her left knee had started hurting. Her x-rays were normal and clean, and testing by her regular doctor showed "nothing wrong" with the knee—except that it hurt too much to exercise. We checked to make sure she hadn't just replaced one injury with another. It wasn't the new, healthy foot repositioning that was hurting her knee. It seemed that something else was going on.

Joni had just started going back to the gym after seven years with an Achilles injury, and didn't want to give up her hard-won ability to exercise again. She was convinced it was something she was doing wrong at the gym. We checked everything she was doing and all looked good. When I looked at how she moved for regular activities at home, we found that the knee pain was probably the way she descended the stairs at home. As she gained energy from weight loss and regular exercise, she developed the habit of jumping down the last two stairs, putting her hand on the banister, and twisting her left leg as she began to walk down the hall. She did this at least 10 times a day. We retrained her to turn her foot and leg together, pivoting lightly on the pad of the front of the foot. Now that she was no longer of twisting her knee everyday, the pain stopped. She promised to use the information for all stepping down—from stairs, to curbs, to getting out of cars, to step class.

Prevent Twisting

- Check to see if you are twisting your knee without knowing it.
- Don't let your knees sag inward. Keep knees over feet.
- Keep knees and feet both facing in the same direction.
- Pivot by turning your whole leg and body. Don't plant your foot and turn leg so that you twist your knee.
- Walk and land lightly.

Knee Pain Fix #7: Tight Iliotibial Band

Your iliotibial band is a fibrous band that attaches from the ilium bone (the side of your hip) to your tibia, or lower-leg bone. Your iliotibial band (IT band) passes over the side of your hip and attaches to the side of the knee. An IT band can be so tight that when the band moves over the side of the hip and knee during normal movement, it rubs and hurts instead of sliding. Tightness can even change the way you walk. A tight band can pull the side of your knee enough to rotate your leg outward, so that you walk "duck-footed" instead of legs facing straight forward. Walking "duck-footed" leads to other pain and problems. Stretching the band will feel good and help your knee, hip, and back. Two easy IT-band stretches follow (Figures 5-10 and 5-11) with more IT stretches in Chapter 4 (Figures 4-20, 4-22, and 4-23). Check with your doctor before trying any of these if you have a hip replacement.

Standing IT Stretch (Figure 5-10)

- Stand sideways at arm's-length from a wall.
- Cross the outside leg in front of other.
- Push hips forward, and then lean the hip toward the wall.

- Experiment with bending forward and back to move the stretch to where you are tightest.
- Hold at least a few seconds, then turn around and switch sides.

Lying IT Stretch

A better IT-band stretch than the standing IT stretch is done lying down (Figure 5-11).

- Lie on your back and move one leg wide out to the side.
- Cross the other leg on top of it. Keep both hips down on the floor. Don't tilt to the side.
- Hold for a few seconds for a comfortable stretch and then switch sides.

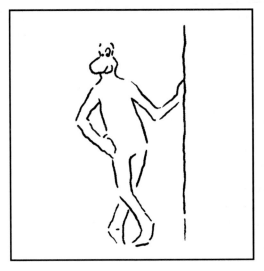

Figure 5-10. Standing iliotibial-band stretch (IT-band stretch)

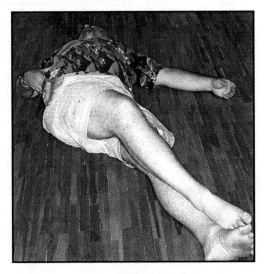

Figure 5-11. Lying iliotibial-band stretch (IT-band stretch)

Knee Pain Fix #8: Tight Quadriceps

Your quadriceps are four muscles in the front of your thigh. The root "quadri" means four. All four muscles come together into a tendon at your knee. Your kneecap sits inside and under this tendon. Sometimes tight thigh muscles can pull on the kneecap when you move in certain ways. When a tighter outer quadriceps muscle pulls on the kneecap, it can pull sideways, instead of gliding up and down in its track, causing kneecap pain. Other people with tightness notice pressure on the kneecap of the back leg when using the lunge.

The most common ways people do a quadriceps stretch usually does not give much stretch. The common way is to stand or lie down and grasp the foot behind you with your hand, with the hip bent forward at the crease, or with the back arched so that movement comes from the lower back instead of lengthening the thigh and hip. Instead, keep hip tucked (Figures 5-12 and 5-13).

Standing Quadriceps Stretch (Figure 5-12)

- Stand and bend knee up behind you to grasp your foot.

- Keep your knee down and behind the line of your body, not in front.

- Tuck your hips under, as if starting a crunch, but without curling forward. Pull foot back and away from your behind. Keep hip tucked. The tuck is to reduce the lower back arch to get the stretch from your leg—not from arching the back. Many people stand with the lower back overarched, which makes the lower back ache and reduces stretch to the hip. The lordosis section in Chapter 2 explains pain from overarching, with effective stretches and exercises.

Lying Quadriceps Stretch (Figure 5-13)

- Lie on your side with both knees bent in front of you, like curling in a ball.

- Keep the bottom leg bent in front of you. Bending the bottom leg reduces the lower-back arch that would lessen the stretch.

- Pull the top leg back, keeping the knee down. Hold your foot in your hand behind your body. Keep a space between your foot and body; don't pull the heel to your behind. Let your shoulder roll back and stretch the upper body too.

- Stretch until your top hip is at least straight, not bent forward at the crease.

Knee Pain Fix #9: Bursitis

A bursa is a small, helpful, fluid-filled cushion for your bones. You have about 160 bursae all over your body. Major ones are under the tendons of big muscles that pass over joints like your shoulder, hip, elbow, and knee. Your knee has three bursae. One is right over the kneecap and is called the prepatellar bursa. This bursa helps protect your kneecap against the pressing and squashing of kneeling. When any bursa gets hurt and inflamed by too much pressure and squashing, this condition is bursitis.

Constantine had bursitis. It was puzzling to everyone he went to see. He wasn't fat—a common contributor to bursitis of the inside lower knee, called pes

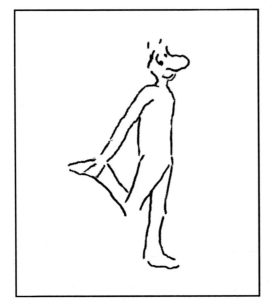 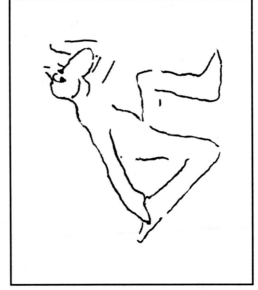

Figure 5-12. Standing Quadriceps Stretch   Figure 5-13. Lying Quadriceps Stretch

anserine bursitis. He didn't do deep knee bends, or swim the breaststroke—two more contributors to anserine bursitis, because the tendons of three muscles heavily used in the breaststroke kick and deep knee bends pass over this bursa.

He didn't do sports with jumping, which can inflame the bursa just under the kneecap, called the infrapatellar bursa. He didn't kneel, or wash floors on his knees, or install carpeting or flooring, or do roofing. He didn't even do any exercises on his knees, which contribute to inflammation of the prepatellar bursa, the largest knee bursa on top of the kneecap. He hadn't fallen, or been kicked, or hit his knee against the dashboard in an automobile accident. He didn't play volleyball and dive on his knees, or wrestle which can rub the front of the knee into the mat. He didn't do gardening. Because his religion was Eastern Orthodox, he didn't kneel in church.

The knee and elbow are two places where bursa can become infected, but it was determined that he did not have an infectious bursitis called septic bursitis. He had no swelling in other joints, so it was felt that this was not a systemic problem.

Sometimes no identifiable reason can be found for bursitis, so he had gone to physical therapy to be treated with rest, ice, and anti-inflammatory medicines. He had gone for massage and heat. He stretched all the muscles around his knees so that tightness wouldn't pressure the bursa. He did lunge exercises to strengthen the knee. He went to the doctor's office to have the swollen bursa drained two times. But it kept coming back.

I make house calls. When Constantine let me into his house, he said, "Here, let me get the door for you, it always stick." He bashed the front of his knee against the heavy door to shut it. After checking all the hard stuff, sometimes it can that easy to see what causes knee pain.

Role of Body Weight in Knee Pain

Some people are told they have knee pain because they are fat. Often it is the case that they stand, bend, and walk with weight poorly distributed on the joint. When we change that, the pain diminishes. I have seen patients, some greatly overweight, who say that retraining gait and stance stopped their knee pain, so that they could go out and walk and exercise for the first time.

Other people who are not overweight, but walk with poor mechanics, poor positioning, or poor shock absorption, can often put more weight on their knee joint than a heavier person who walks in a healthy manner. High body weight can stress the knee, but how you use your body is also important in determining if you have pain and how you can stop it.

Strengthening Exercises Should Transfer to Daily Life

Like weight loss alone, strengthening alone doesn't fix knee pain from poor mechanics. Many muscular people have pain—even thin people get pain. They may do their knee exercises, but strengthening doesn't change leg positioning or unhealthy movement habits. Many people are not strong enough to bend properly, so they bend with weight on their joints, instead of their muscles. The best exercise is to bend properly—heels down, knees bent but positioned over the ankles feet not drooping forward, for all the many dozens of times you bend for things every day. It will strengthen and retrain your knees, save your back, and give you free exercise all day.

Stephanie worked part-time as an usher for the Philadelphia Phillies baseball team at Veterans Stadium. She hyperextended her right knee sliding into first base at the Labor Day softball game. It was the final employee game, and her single scored one of the winning runs for her team. The RBI also left her with pain in her right knee that lasted long after the game ended. Whenever she stood up, the underside of her knee would tense and hurt. It was worse in the morning when she first stood up, and after long sitting—common with hyperextension injuries. She told me that she was able to "walk it off" and continue exercising. She wanted to continuing exercising because she was heavy, but was concerned about further injuring her knee.

After six weeks of pain each time she stood up, Stephanie asked me about it after the yoga class I teach. Her knee was feeling better after class, but when she went back to her normal routine after each class, the pain returned. We looked at where her knee hurt (the underside) and how long it lasted (when she first stood up after sitting for a long time). I told her, "I don't have x-rays of your knee. Hyperextending the knee can press what is called the 'fat pad' that cushions the back of the knee. It often hurts after sitting and if you stand with your knees hyperextended. But even though the pain started when you hyperextended it, pressure seems to be continuing from the way your knees are bending inward. You're falling in on your arches. In class, I always make sure students don't do that."

"Huh?" she said. "I've never had a problem with my arches. And besides, pain is in my knee, not my feet."

We looked at our reflections in the full-length mirror. Stephanie watched me exaggerate her poor standing posture, then straighten my leg and ankle angle. She mimicked the simple shifting of her weight from the inner edges of her feet to distribute it around the sole. It made a difference. She said, "That's ridiculously easy to correct."

Over the next week, she practiced shifting her weight from her arches to the sole of her feet, and not standing with her knee joint pressed backward. Just realizing when she was "doing it again" was more than half the battle. Walking and standing were such routine actions for her, she had never considered how she was standing and walking. She said that once she became aware she was standing and walking poorly, fixing it was "a snap." The more she stood and walked correctly, the less her knee hurt, which encouraged her to continue to practice standing and walking correctly. The pain hadn't come only from the single incident that hyperextended it, but years of pressuring the knee. By the time she returned to class the following Friday, she could stand and walk without pain, even after sitting. She said that exercise had become more than just getting a workout, it was the power of knowledge of how we use our bodies, not just in class, but also in our daily lives.

What Else to Check

Your doctor can check for knee pain from diabetes, fracture, infection, Lyme disease, and problems that are coming from the hip, such as Perthes, a temporary loss of blood supply to the hip mostly seen in children, and slipped capital femoral epiphysis (SCFE), where the growing end (epiphysis) of the thigh bone (femur) slips from hip joint—also more common in children. Sometimes, aches and joint pain are not from injury or disease, but from common medications. Prescription medicines with the side effect of muscle and joint pain include statin drugs for cholesterol, some allergy medicines like Allegra (Fexofenadine), common antidepressants and anti-anxiety medicines, prescription medicine for constipation like Zelnorm (Tegaserod), and prescription acid-prevention medicines called proton pump inhibitors. A cycle may develop of prescriptions for joint pain causing stomach pain, taking stomach medicines that cause more joint and other pain, then more medicines for the depression and anxiety that follow. Instead of taking medicines that cause problems, look for the causes of the problems and solve them so that you don't need the medicines—or so much of them.

What to Do Every Day to Stop Knee Pain

- Keep knees and feet facing straight, not rotated inward or outward.
- Keep knees from sagging or angling inward or outward.
- Keep body weight on the soles, not the arches of your feet.
- When squatting to pick things up, keep knees over ankles, with heels down. Keep your weight back toward your heel. It strengthens knees while preventing knee pain and is the same good bending you need for a healthy back.
- When stepping up stairs or an incline, put your whole foot down, and press through the heel so that your muscles lift you, not your knee joint. Don't step up on your toe. Don't stick your behind out. Hold yourself up straight and use thigh and hip muscles.
- If you feel knee joint pain when bending, check if you are letting your weight press down and forward on your knees. Instead, hold your weight upward using leg muscles. It will take the pain and pressure off the knee.
- When stepping down, step toe first, bend your knee on contact for shock absorption, and step down lightly with your weight held up on the leg on the upper step. Don't step down heavily. Using thigh muscles to decelerate is free leg exercise and keeps shock off the joint.
- Ice injured areas after exercise.
- Walk, move, and exercise lightly, using muscles for shock absorption. Move normally, but see how lightly and quietly you can move.
- Walk and run by rolling heel to toe. Although you will step lightly, don't do it by trying to walk or run on your toes.

- Stay mobile to increase knee strength and reduce knee pain.

- Watch other people. See what it looks like when they walk hard without shock absorption, or let their knees sway inward. People may exercise this way because it is easier than using muscular effort, but it is not healthy.

- Watch your own knee positioning in a mirror. See if you let your knees face toward or away from each other when standing and walking.

What to Avoid

- Don't lock your knees straight or press them backward.

- Don't bang knees straight when rising from a bend or when doing kicking motions.

- Avoid repeatedly hitting your knees whether to close doors or to do exercises that involve repeated kneeling on the floor. Instead of exercising kneeling. Hold up your own body weight using your muscles. For example, hold a full push-up position not on knees (Figures 2-33 and 2-38). Instead of hands and knees leg lifts, do these off the knee (Figure 2-37).

- Don't let knees sway inward. Keep kneecaps facing straight in line with the toes.

When to Notice Knees

- Notice if you let your knees sway or wobble inward when you bend down for things, when you take the stairs, and when bending your knees for exercise moves.

- If you don't have the strength and balance to get up from the floor without using your hands (or even with them), your legs are too weak to support your knees for normal life. Use good bending for all daily activities to strengthen them.

How to Get Natural Knee Strengthening during Daily Activity

- Whenever you bend for anything, bend your knees. Don't bend wrong at the waist. Many people won't bend right to save their back because it hurts their knees. Bending right can help the knees. Bend knees, keeping the knee over the ankle. Keep heels down and your weight over the heel and whole foot, not forward over the toe. This positioning keeps body weight on the leg muscles and off the knee joint, helping prevent knee pain. Imagine getting a natural knee and leg strengthener hundreds of times a day for all the times you bend for normal activities.

- When going up stairs, keep the heel down on the upper leg as you step up. Keep your knee back over the ankle, not letting it rock forward. Stand upright instead of leaning forward. When going down stairs, keep your weight back over your heel on the upper leg, and your knee back, as much as possible, as you step down. Keep your knee over the ankle on the lower leg, without letting it rock forward. Step down lightly using muscles. In short, stand up straight and use your muscles. You will get a natural, healthy strengthener with each step, while stopping the pain that comes from pushing body weight forward through the knee joint.

- Rethink knee exercise as something you do as a part of daily, healthy movement. Many people who exercise and strengthen their knees with leg lifts and knee rehab exercises may still have poor knee positioning that creates injury and pain. Holding up your body weight without letting knees sway inward and being able to get up from the floor are important to health and living an independent life.

No More Knee Pain

In Shakespeare's *King Henry IV*, Lady Percy said, "He had no legs that practised not his gait." Practice good knee positioning during daily activity. Allowing your body weight to sag into your knee instead of using muscles loses the benefit of doing exercise to help knee pain, and slowly wears on the knee joints. As a child you were told, "If you make a funny face, it will stick like that." That means if you keep your knees pressing at unhealthy angles, the bones may eventually deform, tighten, and stick like that.

At least 50 years ago, physical therapies given before surgery were studied to see how they would help a person after surgery. In a surprising number of cases, by surgery time many people didn't need the surgery. The physical intervention was what they needed. Your knee pain may be just the thing your body is telling you to live healthier, with more activity and muscle use. Not all knee pain is caused by—or helped by—positioning. At the same time, it is not necessary to add to knee problems with unhealthy habits. Rethink daily life to see it can be a playground of built-in strengthening and mobility. Keep knees in healthy position during walking, standing, lifting, and moving, for better, healthier exercise, and free knee rehab without going to the gym.

6

No More Ankle and Achilles Pain

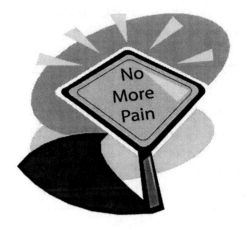

- Sprained Ankles

- Ankle Pain

- Weak Ankles

- Achilles Tendon Pain

M any people sprain or turn their ankle over and over, or have continuing pain or Achilles tendon tightness. Luckily, ankle and Achilles problems are easy to fix with fun practice and use during normal standing and movement. You don't need special or supportive shoes or bracing. This chapter tells why and what to do.

Why Ankle Pain?

Recurring ankle sprains sometimes come from overstretched or torn ligaments at the side of the ankle that allow too much movement. A more important and often overlooked factor in continuing ankle trouble is that weak or injured ankles do not have control of balance, or normal "knowledge" of how your foot is positioned—a knowledge called proprioception. In every place your muscles attach to your bones, little receptors tell you how that part is positioned. Even with your eyes closed, you know if your arm is out to the side or overhead. You know if your foot is facing right or left.

When you slip or lose your balance, your leg and ankle receptors send quick signals to your muscles to rebalance you so that you don't fall. When you injure a joint, it is like getting hit on the head. The receptors get "stupid" and can't remember how to do their job. After a sprain, your ankle receptors aren't good at knowing if your foot is starting to

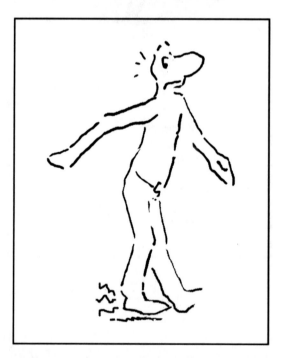

Figure 6-1. The most common way to sprain your ankle is to let your weight shift to the outside so that your foot turns, overstretching the outside of the ankle. This kind of sprain is called "inversion sprain."

roll to the side. The receptors don't send quick signals to your ankle, foot, and leg muscles to steady you. Your weak, slow, overstretched, and "unaware" ankles turn and let you fall before your muscles recognize and correct it.

Nan phoned to tell me that her story was complicated and that she would tell me about it—the next time she phoned. I asked her if she could summarize it at that time, and she said that she wanted to make an appointment to call me back to tell me the full story. I told her that was fine, but if she could tell me in brief, I could tell if I could help her and save us all some time. She tried again to delay. I tried one more time and she almost whispered that the problem was that she sprains her ankles. She wanted me to call her back so that we could talk—all about how her case is unusual and complicated. Against my better judgment, I agreed and phoned her the next day.

At our appointed call, Nan told me she sees several doctors, therapists, and podiatrists. She takes five treatments a week for ultrasound, heat and cold packs, electric stimulation, whirlpool, balms, massage, and acupuncture. I asked her what she was doing to physically strengthen her ankle so that she could use it better. She said that she just told me—heat, cold, ultrasound, massage, and so on. I told her those things will not strengthen or train the balance receptors in the ankle to reduce the chance of losing footing and spraining it again. She asked to see me for an appointment.

At the first visit, I found that Nan kept both ankles tightly taped and wrapped. She walked with a cane, when she walked at all. Each day she drove to work and then took a cab from her parking space. She was so terrified of hurting her ankle again that she didn't attempt physical activity. I asked her to stand on one foot. Anger flashed in her eyes. She said I was endangering her. She said she would not try because she was afraid of falling, even surrounded by a chair, the wall, and me. She would not let me touch her foot. It was easy to see that she was deconditioned from her self-limiting. The deconditioning had become the issue, not the ankle. I told her it was easy to address this kind of thing. You build muscles to support your weight and regain balance by practicing. She told me I was moving too fast for her. She was 32-years old.

Nan had let the ankle, and in fact her entire body, become so deconditioned that without her tape, wrap, heavy shoe, and cane she would tumble over her weak ankles like a puppet. Knowledge of where your parts are positioned and how to move them is called your kinesthetic sense. Nan had no kinesthetics or stabilizing musculature. In fact, she had almost no musculature at all—and she didn't want to do anything but talk about it.

Nan wanted me to know each detail of her MRIs—exactly which ligament was sprained. She gave me a stack of MRI reports and a stack of papers in her own closely-written handwriting—her journal of her years of ankle problems, day-by-day, hour-by-hour. She said in a hushed voice that she had been diagnosed with "sinus tarsi," which meant that she was doomed. Sinus tarsi syndrome is a kind of ankle sprain. She was only doomed by her own thinking.

I told Nan that it was my opinion that there was good news, that this kind of thing can be fairly easily reversed. The majority of her problem was not from the sprain. It was within her own control to fix the problem. She must get moving and restore ankle strength and balance. She had robbed herself—through self-enforced atrophy and disuse—of the strength and balance to make normal gait possible. Several secondary problems occurred from walking bent over, with poor gait, and so on. She needed simple, specific strengthening and retraining of the ankle—and the rest of her body, too. She asked me to conference with her "team." I called them, one by one, that afternoon. I was interested to see what they said. I first phoned her internist who told me he was baffled by "how hard she works and how long she battled this terrible problem." He couldn't understand why she wasn't better when they send her for so much rehab. I explained that she wasn't getting exercise to improve agility, strength, or balance to reverse the problem. He said, "That rehab stuff so often fails. I think it's time for surgery anyway." I told him it failed because she hadn't done it.

I phoned Nan's physical therapist. He told me of his bafflement that, after so many years of physical therapy, she was not better. I asked him what she did for physical therapy. He said she does bands, BAPS board, and water therapy. BAPS stands for Biomechanical Ankle Platform System. It is a small board with a ball attached to the underside so that you can practice standing on a wobbling surface to regain strength and balance. The board moves in all directions, depending how you use your stabilizing muscles. These physical modalities should strengthen and train the balance she needed. But no gains were made. I checked with the aid who administered the modalities. I found that when Nan used the BAPS board, she did it sitting. She never bore her own weight or had to balance. She only used it to make little circles with her ankle. The bands were also used sitting. The water therapy was done floating on a tube, never bearing even her body weight underwater. I told him that she wasn't doing PT, that she was not doing anything functional. I told him that she walked with poor gait, when she walked at all, putting large stress on her ankle. "What a brave lady," he sighed. "She does PT four times a week, year after year. We just don't understand why she doesn't get better."

I went to see Nan for her next appointment ready to educate her with the obvious answer. "This can be so easy," I told her. She told me about her last PT who told her to stretch her quads by pulling her foot behind her. She said that when she held her ankle to do this, she "injured herself badly." On questioning, it turned out that meant it felt uncomfortable. She made a point of telling me the grave risk she faced to do anything physical. I told her bluntly that her risk of everything, including osteoporosis, falls, heart disease, and continuing pain and debility were far greater by not being active.

I told Nan that her extreme self-limiting behavior was not preventing ankle injury. It was continuing it. It was like paying less than the minimum on a credit card, producing more loss than the minimal contribution made. This approach is disastrous in the long term, whether financial or physical. I told her she was deconditioning faster than any of her minimal efforts would help. She was injuring herself more comprehensively than any tumble she could take on a weak ankle. She wept and said that she did not believe she could recover.

What did her several MRI reports say? One showed a herniated disc in her lower back. She was not concerned about that when I mentioned it. The rest of the scans? Sprained ankle, mostly one foot, the other was barely injured. The first sprain occurred when she was 17. They gave her Valium and told her to give up all sports. She used a wheelchair for several years—that someone else pushed for her. She had stayed on Valium ever since.

I asked Nan to hold a three-pound weight. Just to hold it. She was peeved. "It's too heavy. It's too heavy. It hurts!"

"Yes," I told her. "Now think what your body weight is doing to your back and ankles." She could not distinguish muscle injury from any actual use of her muscle.

I gave Nan an exercise to try—a functional strengthener for her whole body. She resisted saying, "That isn't an ankle exercise. I want ankle exercise."

I said, "Here is a basic ankle exercise."

"I can't do that one, I'm afraid I'll fall if I do that." I had her do a balance move. "I can't do that. It hurts my back."

I said "Okay, let's do a back exercise for that."

She said, "That isn't an ankle exercise. I want ankle exercise!"

Nan insisted that she was working hard and doing much. She was seeing four different practitioners two to three times a week each. They did ice, electrical stimulation, ultrasound, acupuncture, massage, cranial sacral therapy, relaxation techniques, and all said, "Gee, we're doing everything. Nothing is helping." But they were not doing the thing she needed—gait retraining and strengthening for her entire body in addition to her ankle. She insisted that was too advanced. She was like a sly child. I told her that she was wasting everyone's time. I fired her as a patient.

How to Stop Ankle Trouble

The most common cause of ongoing ankle pain or recurring ankle sprains is incomplete rehabilitation from the last injury. It is not high-top shoes or Ace bandages or taping that help prevent sprains. The most important thing you can do for healthy ankles and preventing sprains is to improve the strength of your balancing and positioning skills.

Many people who are given exercises after an ankle sprain are told to "spell the alphabet," where they move their foot in the air outlining the letters of the alphabet. This kind of exercise works only on range of motion. Although commonly prescribed, it does not strengthen, or retrain your foot and ankle to balance and adjust foot position when moving to prevent repeat sprains. Spelling in the air can also stretch the side of the ankle, which is not needed and can contribute to the original problem of the ankle being likely to turn.

Prevent Overstretching the Side of the Ankle—Inversion

Ankle flexibility in a forward and backward direction helps walking, bending, and many sports like swimming. Too much motion side to side is not good. Looseness on the outside of your ankles increases chance of ankle sprain because your ankle can bend too far sideways if you stumble. Stretching your muscles is often good for health. But you don't want to stretch your ligaments, which are tough "straps" that attach bones to each other. Ligaments are not supposed to stretch much. You need them to stay constant to hold your bones in place. Ligaments are like old underwear; once they stretch out, they hang loosely. Loose ligaments allow the ends of your bones to rub against each other instead of holding in place. An unstable joint that flops loosely is also predisposed to sprains and dislocations.

Avoid Stretches that Turn Your Ankle to the Inside—Inversion

- The groin stretch, sitting with knees bent and soles of the feet touching (Figure 6-2) can overstretch the side of the ankles if the sides of the feet are left on the floor and the leg bent up at the ankle, rather than kept in line with the lower leg.

- Several yoga poses, if done incorrectly, overstretch the outside of the ankle. Example are crossing the legs in lotus and bending the feet upward at the ankle, and stretching by pulling foot to head and turning the ankle, instead of keeping the ankle straight. Let the stretch come from your hip, which is the idea of these moves, rather than twisting the ankle up sideways.

Strengthen in the Other Direction—Eversion

Make sure that your ankle can bend in the other direction, toward the outside rim of the foot. This movement is called eversion. Eversion is the opposite action from

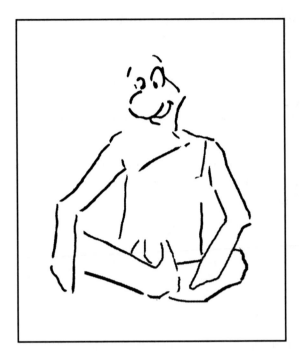

Figure 6-2. Don't let ankles turn up to the side when sitting cross-legged. Keep ankles straight. You'll feel a better stretch from the hip.

the turning motion in ankle sprains called inversion. You want to have strong eversion muscles.

- Press the outside rim of your foot against a wall to start working the muscles. Hold foot position; don't let the pressing turn the ankle inward.
- Play "footsie" by pressing the outside of your ankles against things, the outside of your other crossed ankle, or willing friends.
- Stand on your toes, with weight over your big and second toe, not letting your feet teeter over the little toes.
- Lift your leg up to the side, knee in, and press the outside of your ankle against your hand. Make sure to lift the outside rim of the ankle up against your hand in the "anti-sprain" direction.
- Loop a large band over both feet and practice pulling your ankles outward in the "anti-sprain" direction.
- Practice being able to quickly evert your foot—turning it the way you would need in case of an unexpected moment where your ankle stumbles and turns inward while moving.

Improve Knowledge of Positioning (Proprioception)

Daren came in limping badly, bearing no weight and using a cane. "Oh, I murdered my ankle and tore cartilage in my calf muscle doing aerobics. I don't get it. I warmed up on the treadmill. Look at the calf, all swollen."

"There is no cartilage in your calf muscle," I told him. "Can you tell me what happened?" He explained how he turned his ankle three weeks before. His x-ray showed nothing broken. I asked him, "How is it possible to have such pain three weeks later?"

"Oh," he said. "It doesn't hurt at all."

"No?"

"No."

"Why can't you walk?"

He looked at me surprised. "I thought I was supposed to stay off it."

His doctor, a good general-practice physician, did everything right, then said, "Stay off it and come back in six months if it still hurts." Daren thought it meant to stay off the foot for six months.

I told him "You're not supposed to stay off it six months, even six days." He put his foot back on the floor and walked around. On exam, it seemed that the calf swelling was blood pooling from the inactivity. He had no pain, good range of motion, and the only weakness was from having been off it for the previous three weeks. I taught Daren fun exercises to regain placement and strength to reduce the likelihood of him turning it again in the future. People saw him limping in on a cane and easily walking out shortly later. That was a good day.

Many people use a treadmill or other walking machines for rehab and general fitness, but then sprain their ankle walking on uneven terrain because they are only used to flat, unchanging surfaces. Other people avoid anything except flat, stable surfaces for fear of falling. They have poor ability to adapt to moving or changing surfaces because they don't train their body for it. Their ankles need knowledge of how they are positioned (proprioception) to send the right requests to your muscles to hold you in healthy position.

Proprioception Training

- A simple way to get started strengthening and moving after a painful sprain is to pedal a bicycle or stationary bicycle. It is gentle movement, supporting some weight. It is also useful to ride a real bike when your ankle is too sore to walk everywhere. Ice the ankle after exercising.

- Probably the best exercise after ankle injury combines strengthening with the balance and positioning needed to prevent future sprains. Stand on your toes without allowing your weight to teeter outward over your little toes. Keep your weight over your big and second toe, using leg, foot, and ankle muscles. Rise up on toes. Hold for increasingly long periods. When you can do this, do repetitions, at least 10 at a time, rising up and down, maintaining positioning over the big and second toe.

- Walk on your toes. By not allowing your weight to teeter to the outside of your foot, you retrain ankles to not turn under your body weight.

- Practice walking backward on your toes, with weight on the big and second toes, not only teetering outward on little toes.

- When you can rise to toes and lower while standing on both feet with good positioning, and walk on toes with good positioning, raise and lower on one foot. At first, you may want to hold on to something for balance, and then practice without holding on. This basic skill is how your foot moves in real life when you walk over uneven surfaces, and descend stairs and slopes. You need to retrain it to hold you without turning and wobbling

- Stand on one foot with good positioning. Raise the other leg behind you and hold for increasing time. Keep your back as upright as you can without rounding forward. With the back leg still raised, move it side to side to challenge your balance while maintaining foot position. Practice moving into different poses that you invent while standing on one foot.

- Work up to hopping on each foot softly and safely. Play hopscotch. Hopscotch is a game possibly developed for Roman soldiers to exercise their feet and ankles.

- Safely hop on and off a block of foam, a pillow, or other lightly moving material.

- More ankle exercises while moving follow in this chapter in the section on developing balance.

Joy sprained her ankle hard three weeks before. It made that wet popping noise. Joy was active and had a lot of work to do at the camp where she worked. She was no complainer and wouldn't have asked for herself, so Dr. Tom, the camp doctor, brought her to me. The camp director joined us. Joy was wobbly on that ankle and wondered if something was wrong that would make her sprain it again. I was pleased that she knew this. Her foot below the sprain was swollen and bruised from old blood that drifted down after the initial tear. I knew the camp doc. He was knowledgeable and caring. When Dr. Tom told me he checked the ankle and no fracture or problem was apparent other than the sprain, I knew I could believe him and concentrate on the fix.

Joy showed me the soft, elastic brace she was wearing for the last three weeks. I asked her, "Are you ready to get out of this? By now, the wobbling is more from the brace than the injury. With the brace, your ankle doesn't have to work to hold itself. It gets weaker. It forgets how. It is the opposite of what is needed." The camp director asked if Joy should wear a heavier boot for support. I told them that, as much as it was commonly hoped that a boot would help, it was the same problem as the brace. Without your own ankle muscles working to hold and balance you, the ankle gets weaker, more unstable, and less able stay straight so that you don't sprain it again. In most instances, supportive shoes are no more needed than putting your mouth in a sling to keep it from falling open when you walk around. Thinking you need supportive shoes to brace up uninjured ankles for hiking and walking is a common myth that perpetuates weak ankles. I told them that all over the so-called "Third World," people walk the bumpy paths and hills in bare feet and flip flops, holding their own ankle positioning.

We took off her brace and shoes. Joy stood gingerly on the cold floor. I asked her to stand on the uninjured foot. She balanced without trouble. I asked her to stand on the injured side. She stood unsteadily, waving her arms, with the soft-spoken camp director ready to catch her in a basket and shoot me. Joy was a trooper and said it didn't hurt, just felt so weak and unsteady that it was hard to stand on it. I reassured them that it was from the disuse of the bracing and the past three weeks of decreased use. She quickly started balancing. We tried again. Again balance improved just from practicing it. I gave her the next thing—rising on both feet to toes without letting the feet teeter outward over the little toes, keeping weight on the big and second toe. She quickly saw that the teetering she was learning to prevent was the same that sprained her ankle in the first place. Joy could feel that the muscles she was training would prevent that and improve the balance needed too. Next I had her walk around on her toes, keeping straight ankle positioning, without "teetering." Then I had her stand on one foot and swing the other leg around in all directions to challenge the strength and stability of the ankle. When she stood on both feet again, she said the ankle felt more stable. Next I had her bounce lightly up and down, not leaving the floor, just bending knees and learning to come downward lightly, with shock absorption, and healthy ankle placement. It may seem like a lot for the first try at rehab, but the idea was to learn how to step down without turning, jolting, or overpressuring the injured ankle—and the uninjured one, too. The idea was to decrease harmful strains, not increase them. Everything we did took about 20 minutes. I asked them to start with this, to ice it after work, and check in with me each day because it should get better, not worse. I told them that as it got better doing each of the skills we covered, to work up to light jumps, hopefully within the week. After all, you have to step up and down stairs, walk around, and carry things in an ordinary day. The ankle had to know how to do that safely.

Dr. Tom knew muscle physiology. He asked me what I thought of the studies that showed that tendon and ligament tensile strength after injury was at its lowest around the three-week mark. Should she be doing all this three weeks after the sprain? I agreed with him that in school, we learned not to do this and to keep someone braced until well after the three-week mark. The problem was that it wasn't working. People were getting repeat trouble. Limiting the use of a weak ankle only makes it weaker. Healthy movement helps healing. The rebalancing skills were precisely what was needed to keep the ankle from turning and stretching past its fragile, decreased ability.

Keep Ankles in Healthy Position

It is important to retrain your foot positioning when you stand and walk. Many people let their feet flop into any position, thinking it is their shoes—not their own muscles— that are supposed to "support" them. Your muscles hold you in healthy position, no different than not letting your shoulders round in a slouch.

Some people let their ankles tilt outward (Figure 6-3). They may be more likely to roll over their ankle, spraining it. Like car tires that tilt, it reduces shock absorption and creates extra wear on the structures.

Some people allow their weight to fall inward on their arches so that they sag flat (Figure 6-4). This condition is called "acquired flat foot." Think of a beginner on skates. They often let their ankles sag inward until they learn to hold them straight. In the same way, you can learn to hold your ankles and feet straight. You don't need inserts in your shoes. It is positioning, not unavoidable flattening.

Look down or look in a mirror and see if your feet tilt inward, or if you let your weight flatten your arch. Alternate pressing and lifting your arch while keeping the sole and toes on the floor. See how your muscles work on the inside and outside of your leg to either hold your arches up, or allow them to flatten under your weight. Make sure to straighten the whole leg in a healthy manner—not strain the knee or hip to straighten the foot. Make sure not to roll to the side making you roll to the outside. Most people find they have arches, and when they stand well the strain is less—not more—on other areas as well.

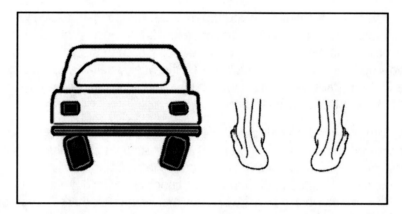

Figure 6-3. Your ankles are like car tires. Both can have posture problems in three directions – caster, camber (how much arch), and of course, toe (which direction the toes face). Tilting outward too much (camber) can make them wear out too soon.

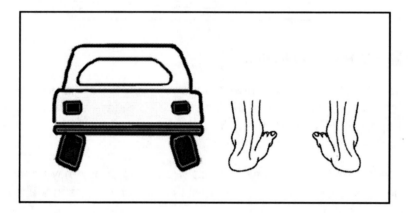

Figure 6-4. Ankles, like tires that tilt inward, can put extra wear and pressure on the inside. The cure is not changing the tires, but straightening the alignment.

- Stand on both feet using leg muscles to create healthy arch space. Don't let feet and ankles roll to the inside or outside. Use your foot and ankle muscles to hold straight.

- When you can adjust foot posture to have healthy arch space when standing on both feet, practice standing on one foot keeping healthy positioning. At first you may drop your weight back on your arch, but then learn to use leg muscles to keep healthy positioning, distributing weight on the whole sole of the foot and off the arch, with the foot and knee facing straight ahead

- The next thing to look for in healthy ankle positioning is to see if your toes point in or out. Practice walking with your toes straight ahead. That reduces much wear not only on the ankles, but also on your knees, hip, and lower back.

- When you can walk with healthy positioning, hop lightly in place, keeping positioning.

- As your ankle strengthens with combined strengthening and positioning exercises, progress to slalom hopping, keeping positioning

- Putting inserts and supports in your shoes doesn't always change bad positioning. Many people keep the poor position right over their inserts. Others never learn how to hold their own positioning and can never go without their special inserts or walk barefoot. The muscles that could hold their foot in good positioning atrophy. It's worth being able to hold positioning on your own. Chapter 7 provides more information.

Elizabeth landed with a pop from a round-off in gymnastics. She was not sure if she had turned her ankle, and it was not broken or sprained. But it hurt, and the outside of her ankle made a snapping sound. She had to move it back with her hands. In many kinds of ankle sprain, the tough bands (called ligaments) that hold the anklebones to the leg bones are stretched or torn. Elizabeth's ligaments were not injured. Instead, the tough "string" called a tendon that connects one of the lower-leg muscles to the outside of the ankle was so stretched by the injury that it moved over the side of her ankle bone with a snap. After that, it continued to snap and get stuck over the bone for the next many years when she tried to exercise.

Her doctor said she could have surgery to fasten the tendon in place so it would not shift, or she could just "deal with it." The surgery would involve weeks in a cast, then more weeks in a brace unable to do regular activities. It came with the warning that it could further injure the tendon, damage the nerves, become infected, or not work at all. When she said she could no longer run because the tendon would shift, the doctor said, "Don't run." He also told her to stop gymnastics and all other sports, which she did.

Elizabeth came to me years later. The problem was unchanged. Her doctor said she had peroneal tendonitis. The peroneal muscles are two muscles on the outside of the shin. The big shinbone is your tibia. The peroneal muscles attach from the smaller lower-leg bone, called the fibula, to the side of your foot. Their job is to move your foot to the side and downward. The bigger of the two peroneal muscles also attaches to the tibia.

Elizabeth thought her injury meant the tendon was "detached" letting it snap. I pushed and pulled her ankle in specific ways to see which area did not hold in place as it should. Nothing was detached or torn. A tear like that would leave the side of the foot flopping, without the peroneal muscles able to move the ankle properly. When you hear a word with "-itis," that means that the area is inflamed. Think of tonsillitis or laryngitis. Tendonitis occurs when a tendon is inflamed. Elizabeth's ankle was not swollen or inflamed, but the tendon still moved and snapped over the big, knobby bone at the outside of her ankle when she moved in certain ways. The knob is the bottom of the fibula, called the lateral (outside) malleolus—which means "little hammer," because of its shape. The tendons are supposed to lie snug in a groove behind this ankle knob. They are held in place by a small strip of tissue. Sometimes with injury, the tissue is damaged and lets the tendons snap around malleolus. Other times the tendon is overstretched. Sometimes both. Sometimes when the peroneal muscles are tight, the longer one (the peroneus longus tendon) cuts into the shorter one (the peroneus brevis tendon). The muscles can be tight and the tendons overstretched at the same time. In fact, when the muscle is tight, landing from a jump just wrong can overstretch the tendon.

The peroneal tendons help hold the back of the foot in place during weight bearing. They move your foot into an arch-downward position to resist the ankle from turning, the way it turns when you sprain it (inversion, described earlier). You don't want to land from a step or jump with your ankle rolling outward, which will overstretch the tendons. At the same time, letting the arch roll inward and flattened when landing from a step or jump stresses the tendons. Healthy positioning in the middle is key.

In the medical literature, peroneal tendon injury is known to be common, but is often considered "not clinically significant" because people can walk around. Still it was disruptive to Elizabeth who liked to be active and was being kept from favorite activities. She had taken up martial arts and was good at it, but her ankle periodically kept her from training. She was not able to do many moves without the tendon moving out of place with a snap. She could wear a brace to hold it, but that would create a negative cycle of atrophy of the muscles, because they wouldn't be doing the work, and more weakness and injury from the atrophy.

Retraining ankle positioning while moving and supporting body weight is important in stopping the effects of chronic lateral ankle instability. We started by having her rise on toe and not letting the ankle roll to the outside. She practiced keeping weight over the big and second toe. We moved to raising and lowering on toes, maintaining positioning. Then we practiced walking on toes with body weight over the big and second toe, keeping her foot from rolling toward the little toes.

Elizabeth said the tendon snapped out of place when she did certain things, she just wasn't sure what. When I moved her ankle up and down, the tendon did not slip over the knobby malleolus. That was good. Since maximal exertion on the peroneal muscles occurs with side-to-side movement and jumping, we needed to retrain positioning under increasing load. We started by having her take a medium size step backward, because that makes the foot bend upward, and the peroneal tendons, which work to move the foot down would resist this motion. She said she remembered that stepping back, a common move she needed in the martial arts, was one of the times it would snap out of place. Keeping the ankle well positioned let her practice stepping back without pain or snapping. The ankle positioning and loading during stepping back is also similar to the position she would need to run again without pain.

Elizabeth needed to stop snapping the tendon so that it could stop repeatedly overstretch and perpetuate the problem. I reminded her not to sit with ankles turned up, which stretched the sides, avoid pulling the ankles up to the side, or letting it turn when she walked. I showed her how she can stretch the front shin muscles by pointing her toe without letting the ankle turn. I told her to land softly from steps and jumps so that the entire leg decelerated her step, not just the peroneal muscles. I also gave her three exercises—rising to toe and lowering, toe walking, and stepping back to practice positioning and shock absorption—with the instructions to do them daily and report any change. With those exercises in place, we would move to small jumps to the back and the side, and pushing off to leap to the front. These exercises would increase stability the way she needed it for continuing in the martial arts, and to return to running if she wanted, without letting the tendon shift, and with increasing ability to sustain loads with bigger jumps.

Improving Balance

Cynthia called me to ask what she could do to get more mobile after falling and hurting her ankle. She had passed out on the sidewalk, fell in a hole, and broke her ankle. She already had surgery and her surgeon told her that there was little she could do to rehabilitate the ankle from there since "there was nothing left to rehab because she had torn the ligaments on the side of her ankle." Ligaments are the tough bands that that hold the foot bones onto the anklebones, like the latch on a briefcase that holds it closed. I asked her if she had ever fallen before.

"Yes, often."

"Have you been tested for anything that could be making you fall?"

"Yes, she said. She was involved in expensive and intensive testing for a number of things. It would be unfortunate if we devoted our time to balance training her ankle and body if the trouble came from a tumor of the balance centers of her ear, brain, or from seizures, or mini episodes of loss of consciousness.

The tests came back with good news and ruled out worrisome trouble. Cynthia's doctor told her to do ankle circles and to spell the alphabet, but nothing more to get her back on her feet. I asked her what she did to help her balance.

"I can't do that," she laughed. "I have terrible balance." I explained that balance is a fitness skill that you can train just by practicing balancing. Balance is a "lose or lose" skill no different than your strength or memory. You can make your arms stronger by using them and you can improve your balance just by practicing balance. Cynthia was delighted. She thought that she had to "live with being a klutz." I asked her to stand on one foot. "Oh, I can't even do that on my good foot!" Then she nodded and said that she realized that the lack of balance was not from the injury, as she had been told. She stood on the good foot, wobbled, but stayed standing, smiling.

"Money should be this easy," I said. "All you have to do is do it and get results." I told her to stand on one foot while brushing her teeth and the other while combing her hair every morning. That way she could practice while moving. It is necessary to do skills the way you need for real life—called functional exercise. She offered that she could practice balancing while talking on the phone and washing dishes. We worked on lunges (Figure 3-6), a combination exercise, when done right, for balance, strength, functional movement, and leg placement.

A few weeks later, I bumped into Cynthia in the supermarket. "I went to the art museum yesterday," she said, "and walked all over." She was standing straight and tall. She looked great, with rosy cheeks and happy eyes. Background music came over the supermarket loudspeakers playing a popular big band tune. She danced away through the tomatoes. I was happy.

Balance is an often forgotten aspect of fitness exercises. Good balance is key to preventing falls and the injuries that result from them. A vicious cycle develops when you get out of shape and decrease your balance skills. You become more afraid to fall, and start cutting back on activities requiring balance. You do less, lose more balance skill, and so on, losing more and more independence. Many people become housebound or even chair-bound—terrified of falls.

Balance Exercises

"I want tai chi!" Edna was adamant. Her senior group told her that tai chi would help her balance because it did something magical that nothing else could do.

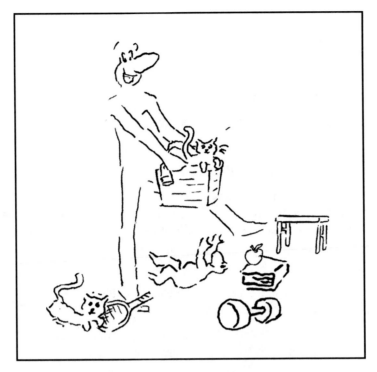

Figure 6-5. Balance is highly trainable. Ankles need exercises that train knowledge of positioning (proprioception), motor control, and balance awareness. Then you can better handle situations where you might other wise fall or get injured.

I said, "Edna, many exercises help your balance the same way."

"No! Tai chi!" she said. "I don't want to fall again."

I didn't blame her for wanting something magical to help her not fall. I asked her to show me if she could stand on one foot. She looked at me in disbelief and raised her voice louder so I'd understand that she couldn't do that because she had bad balance and that was why she wanted "the damned tai chi." I agreed with her again that it was a good idea to do something to get better balance. I told Edna that in tai chi they would have her stand on one foot. She didn't believe me. I told her that learning how to balance on one foot and shift her weight from foot to foot was a big part of how tai chi helps her balance.

Good balance exercises combine balance with positioning skill development. Balance skills are different when practiced slowly and quickly. Practice both for all the real-life situations where both are needed. Following are a few examples. Practice them keeping safety in mind.

Start at the Beginning

- Put on your pants, skirts, shoes, and hosiery standing up.
- Walk lightly.
- Get out of your chair without using your hands.
- Repeatedly throw an object in the air and catch it.
- Throw and catch a ball thrown against the wall and ceiling.
- Walk on a line. Walk backward. Walk sideways.
- Do tai chi or, if you don't have access to a class, try the ancient magic technique I learned in China from high-ranking tai chi masters, roughly translated as "imitate (or follow) tai chi." Shift slowly from foot to foot in each direction, pausing with weight on each foot. Follow your foot motions with your hands and body, as if pretending to do tai chi.
- Go ballroom dancing. Take tap dance lessons, Latin dance, or other styles. Put music on in the living room and dance.
- Stand on one foot while washing dishes, talking on the phone, or watching TV. Shift to the other foot. Hold each for increasingly long time.
- Lift weights while standing on one foot.
- Stand on a block of foam or other spongy surface that moves slightly underfoot.
- Try juggling. All the good bending to pick up the objects when they fall is good exercise, too.

Progress to Basic Balance Skills

- Get up from the floor without using your hands.
- Bounce and catch a ball while standing on one leg.
- Walk on a line while bouncing a ball. Walk backward. Walk sideways.
- Play games for balance, either commercial or invented. Check children's furniture departments for fun balancing things to sit, stand, and lie on. Check your neighborhoods and parks for parcourse. Parcourse is an outdoor circuit of fun exercise stations at distances apart. Walk, skip, dance, or run from one to the next to try specific activities. Some include balancing on a log, climbing a short incline, hanging from a bar, and stepping side to side among rocks or obstacles.
- Play physical arcade games like Dance Dance Revolution where you move your feet from spot to spot, depending on directions on the screen.
- Stand on a balance device. This action can be as simple as standing on a big pillow. Progress to standing on a board (or book) on a rock, ball, balled up shirt, or throw

pillow. Stand first on both feet, then on one foot. Various commercial products are available to practice walking and moving on unstable surfaces. Depending on your level, get or make your own increasingly wobbly surfaces. Practice balance with the idea of increasing skill, not injuring yourself.

- Do small knee bends while standing on one foot. Keep your heel down and the knee back over the foot. Don't stick your hips out in back.

- Do squats (Figure 2-8) and upright lunges (Figure 3-6) with both feet on a balance board or any wobbly surface. Practice moving in ways that simulate sports or motions you need in real life.

- Stand with each foot on a separate balance board, or two objects (even two rocks) that wobble differently. Move in ways that simulates your real life activities.

- Juggle while standing on one leg.

- Stand on a post or other small, raised surface and do stretches.

- An exercise ball is often used in ways that do little for balance. Many people just sit and lie on it, with as poor posture and little use of muscles as they do in their chair. To get balance from this fun tool, sit up straight and raise one foot from the floor, then both. Lie back keeping your body straight, not draped over the ball. Kneel on the ball. Put your hands on the ball and your feet on the floor, or another ball. Put your feet on the ball and your hands on the floor, or another ball. Have fun finding new combinations in safe ways.

When Strength, Mobility, and Balance Progress, Try Intermediate Skills

- Hop on one foot along a line on the floor. Hop side to side to along the line to "slalom" the line.

- Hop backward on one foot. Hop over things. Hop on things. Hop from one mark, crack, or designated object to the next. Use your muscles to land lightly with shock absorption; don't just come crashing down on your foot. Bend your knee when you land.

- Jump up to land with one foot on a post. Stretch one leg holding straight back positioning while standing on the other leg on the post.

- If hopping is too much, work up to it by leaping softly. Push off one foot and land lightly at a designated spot on the other foot. Leap backward to the first spot. Use muscles to decelerate your landing; don't come down heavily. Use balance and muscles to hop and jump lightly. Change sides. Try this in all directions—forward and back, sideways, and diagonally. Aim for landmarks, such as cracks in the sidewalk or floor, stripes in the carpet, or markers you place yourself for fun. Land lightly.

- Participate in recreational sports such as ice skating, roller skating, skateboarding, skiing, and windsurfing.

- In a safe, soft place, stand on a medicine ball or other wobbly object. Don't do this without medical clearance that you will be safe if you fall, and practice in safe falling techniques.

One clue that you may have poor balance is walking heavily. Many people walk like bricks, letting their feet flop down heavily in any position in which they fall. Walking heavily is hard on the joints and can contribute to a lot of aches and pains. The feet get a pounding but never any exercise. Walk lightly using your muscles for shock absorption. Your joints will thank you and your muscles will get free exercise.

My husband Paul and I spend much time in Asia, teaching and studying. We were traveling to a small, southern Thai island by wooden supply boat. The boat docked at the cement pier high above the water. There was a two- or three-foot gap between the swaying boat deck and the pier. I stood, gauging the changing gap and the long drop to the water. I figured I could probably jump, and my knapsack wasn't that heavy. An elder Thai woman brushed past me, wizened from sun and burdened under a wooden yolk on her shoulders with two overflowing baskets of goods to sell on the island. She easily leapt the gap, landed softly on the pier, and ambled off, baskets swaying with each step. She did this almost every day—lifting, bending, carrying, and balancing.

Achilles Tendon Pain and Tears

Joni came to me after suffering Achilles tendonitis that started in step aerobics class nearly seven years before. It was painful and limited her from doing physical activity, even walking. She said her tendons felt so stiff and "crackly" in the mornings that she was afraid they would tear. She tried sleeping in an orthopedic device to stretch the Achilles. She didn't like it because it was like sleeping in a cast and was difficult to walk if she wanted to get up in the night. She had gone to trainers who showed her gentle Achilles stretching, icing, massage. Nothing seemed to help so she remained sedentary and was gaining weight.

When Joni came to me, she had just started working out again, mostly riding a recumbent stationary bike and lifting weights. I explained that step aerobics aren't damaging when you don't do dumb things. During "repeaters," don't bang your foot down to the back, which suddenly yanks the Achilles tendon under all of your weight. Instead, hold your body weight up using the leg still on the bench and touch the floor with the other. Doing so gives better exercise for the leg still on the step. Joni was stepping up toes first. I showed her how body weight needs distribute to the entire foot with weight back toward the heel. Going up toe first, she kept the Achilles in a shortened position and was not using thigh muscles. She was throwing her weight on her front knee.

Joni had faithfully done the common "lean and lunge" stretch for the Achilles (Figure 6-6). I explained how that doesn't stretch the Achilles tendon as much as other stretches, and depending how it is done, sometimes not at all. Although she was spending much time doing an Achilles stretch, she had not been getting any stretch. Joni also kept her back foot turned out in class. In fact, she walked like that too. Without keeping the foot straight, she was not stretching the Achilles during each step she took, or even when doing a stretch specifically for the Achilles. I showed Joni a better Achilles stretch of pressing her foot to a wall, keeping both foot facing straight, not turned out, before and after step class and other activity (Figure 6-7).

It took only a week or so for the pain to be gone enough to go back to exercising as much as she wanted. A year later Joni checked in that the pain had not returned. Her weight had dropped. She was walking with both feet facing straight, for a natural Achilles stretch during ordinary walking. She was getting a better workout now that she was using her leg muscles instead of slamming her body weight down on her Achilles tendons.

What Does the Achilles Tendon Do?

Your Achilles tendon attaches your calf muscle to your heel. It is the "string" (or cord) you can see and feel at the back of your heel. When you contract your calf muscle, it pulls the tendon, and the tendon pulls the heel. Your heel comes up and that moves your foot and toes down. You use your Achilles tendon to point your foot down, which means you can stretch your Achilles tendon when you pull your foot back. It also means that normal walking with your foot straight gives your Achilles a nice stretch with each step. When you walk with your feet turned out, the foot doesn't pull back and stretch when walking. Turning the feet out also encourages rolling downward on the arches. The Achilles and the bottom of the foot don't get a normal stretch and can tighten. When it becomes very tight, just walking is too much pull, causing an inflammation of the fibrous fascia connecting the foot muscles—one way to start plantar fasciitis (covered in Chapter 7).

Walking with feet pointed outward can make the Achilles tendon and the calf muscles shorter because they no longer get normal stretch from walking. In turn, tight Achilles tendons and calf muscles encourage the feet to turn outward with walking, because they are too tight to stay straight during the push off and, instead, pull the foot outward. When bending the knees, tight Achilles tendons can make the foot turn out so much that it rolls downward on the arches, pressuring the ankles and the knees if they turn inward with everything else. Tight calf muscles and Achilles tendons can make you take shorter steps than normal. Tightness can lead to Achilles pain, tendonitis, knee pain, and foot pain. If the Achilles is very tight and is put under a sudden forceful pressure, like landing from a jump or pushing off to run or walk quickly, it can fray, and even tear.

Moe walked like a funny toy penguin, rocking from side to side. He picked up each foot then placed it down not much farther in front of the other, in the same position as he lifted it. "My doctor. She says she wants me using this cane."

"Moe, why does she want you using a cane?"

" I don't walk too good no more."

"Moe, why not?"

"The doctor, she checked me out. Says I've got the arthur-ritis."

They had made sure Moe didn't have more difficult conditions like Parkinson's disease, but even if he did, we would still work on balance. It was also important to get his ankles able to move up and down. The ankles were a main reason for his block-like gait. His ankles didn't bend enough so he rocked to lift each foot. We started with rising up and down on his toes, which started out barely raising his heels from the ground.

"Moe, go for the jump shot!" The idea of basketball didn't get his heels off the ground. When I mentioned jitterbug, the light smiled in his eyes. He grabbed my elbow and twirled me with a strong push. "Okay, Moe. It's jitterbug every day for you. You need to move again." We slowly triple-stepped around, his head at my neck height, tipping side to side like dancing penguins. After a few twirls, he was warmed up and inspired enough to try rising up and down on his toes again. From there, we stood on a board (a book or curb will do) with his heel off, rising up to mobilize the ankle and strengthen the leg, and all the way down to stretch the Achilles. Up and down. I told him to move his foot with his hands, too, every day.

He pointed at his shoes. "If I could reach my feet, I wouldn't need no stick to put 'em on." With that, we identified another easy, functional skill that would give balance and flexibility exercise by doing a normal activity. I told him he was to put his shoes and socks on every day by balancing with his ankle bent over his knee or by lifting his foot to his hands. I asked him to walk, watching himself in the mirror. The rocking surprised him. "Like a damned old man!" he muttered. We practiced standing on one foot to work the side-leg muscles, too, so that he didn't need to rock so much. Along with simple ankle flexibility to practice every day, and watching himself more often, he improved his balance and retrained a more normal gait without needing a cane.

Achilles Tendon Stretches and Strengtheners

On a Step

- Carefully stand backwards on a step with one heel off the step. Let your body weight press the heel downward. Rise up to toe, and down to stretch, to simulate regular movement by lengthening and shortening under moving body weight. This stretch prepares the calf and Achilles for lengthening under moving body weight without strain.

- Rise up to toe and down with your leg bent and straight. Roll onto the ball of the foot and back to move the stretch along the whole foot. It is important to stretch in the way you need to move. One of the reasons why some studies are showing stretching doesn't prevent injury is that people aren't stretching the way they need for real life. Stretching can help, when done in the way you move.

Standard Achilles Stretch Using a Wall

The common stretch associated with Achilles tendon stretching puts the hands on a wall while lunging. This stretch is not highly effective, even when done well, and is often done in ineffective ways, which is one reason why Achilles tendon stretching doesn't seem to be cutting down on injuries as hoped. To get the stretch as intended:

- Stand facing a wall (or imaginary wall), one foot in back.

- Keep the back foot straight. If it turns out, little or no stretch is accomplished.

- Stand up straight and lean your hips inward toward the wall. Don't lean the upper body forward.

- The key is not letting your hips stick out in back or the back foot turn outward. Doing either of these will prevent getting the stretch.

- Instead of rounding your back, keep head and back upright. You can always round over your computer if you want to round your back in bad posture.

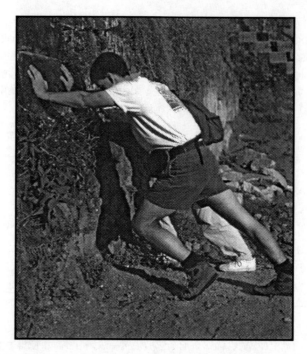

Figure 6-6. This Achilles tendon stretch is commonly done in ways that don't stretch the Achilles much, or sometimes not at all. It is one of the least effective of all the Achilles tendon stretches.

Lunge

Another reason the standard Achilles wall stretch (Figure 6-6) is not as effective as hoped is that it is done in a still position, while the Achilles tendon must stretch during movement. A better Achilles stretch than the standard stretch is the lunge (Figure 4-6). The lunge combines stretching with strengthening and functional movement the way you need for many dozens of daily chores. It is a built-in strengthener and stretch.

Downward Dog

Downward dog stretches the bottom of the foot, Achilles tendon, calf, hamstring, back, and shoulders at the same time. It is an effective, multi-joint stretch (Figure 6-7). You probably have seen dogs and cats stretch this way.

- Put your hands and feet on the floor, hands far forward of the feet like starting a push-up, with your weight mostly on your hands.
- Keep your feet where they are and lift hips high in the air, pushing backward. Relax your heels to the floor.
- Relax your head down.
- Straighten your back rather than letting it round or hunch.

- Keep feet straight, not turned. Keep weight on soles, not arches. Let heels come down to or toward the floor as much as you can.

- Push your fingers forward with straight—not locked—elbows. This motion pushes you back and is the key to getting the stretch on the back of the leg.

- Distribute weight on your whole hand so you don't pressure the wrists.

- Keep your hands far forward of your feet, with weight on your arms. Supporting body weight on hands lets you stretch the back without pushing the discs outward with forward bending.

- If your hands slip forward or your feet slip backward, use more muscles to pull inward. Don't flop your weight unsupported so that you slip.

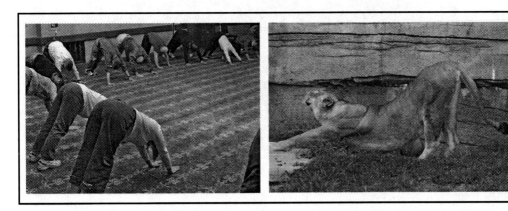

Figure 6-7. Downward-dog stretch is a good stretch for many areas at once. Keeping weight on your hands strengthens the arms and prevents forward-bending pressure on the discs.

Squat Sit

It is common in Western countries for people to squat on their toes. Toe squatting pressures the knees and doesn't stretch the Achilles. In many Eastern countries, squatting with weight on heels is the normal way to do daily activities from talking on the phone, to eating meals and doing household chores, to waiting for a bus. It has been found that in populations that usually sit this way, incidence of Achilles pain is low. People at every age, up to the oldest elders, often sit this way.

- Keep heels down and feet parallel to keep compression off the knees. Squatting on toes pressures open the knee joint as the thigh presses against the calf. This "nutcracker" effect is greater with heavy legs.

- Don't let feet turn out, which throws your body weight on the inside of the arch and knee joint.

- If your Achilles tendons are tight, you won't be able to squat fully with heels down. Hold onto a counter or other support with relaxed straight arms. Lean back and it will be a nice stretch.

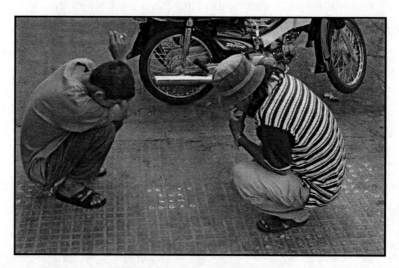

Figure 6-8. A common way to sit in much of the world, the full squat on heels (not toes) stretches the back, calf muscles, ankle, foot, and Achilles tendon.

Foot-on-Wall Achilles Stretch

This Achilles stretch is quick and highly effective (Figure 6-9).

- Stand about arm's length in front of a wall with both feet facing straight forward, not turned out.
- Place one foot flat against the wall around knee height. It will feel as if you're standing too close, but this distance is correct.
- Press the heel against the wall.
- Don't round the back or hip, or the stretch is diminished or lost. Don't let the standing foot turn out (left). Lift the chest to feel the calf and Achilles stretch (right).

Regular Bending

- Even without sitting in a full heels-down squat, when bending knees to pick something up, keep heels down and your weight back toward the heel.
- Good bending keeps body weight on the leg muscles and off the knee joint, stopping a lot of knee pain. See Chapter 5.

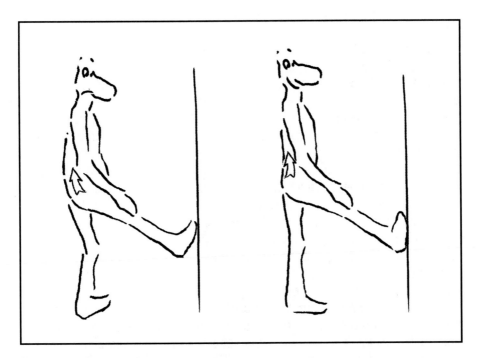

Figure 6-9. Wall Achilles stretch. Press your heel against a wall at knee height for a quick, effective Achilles stretch. Don't round your back or turn the standing foot out (left). Keep the foot of the standing leg facing straight ahead and your back straight (right).

- Keeping heels down when bending is the normal, healthy way to bend. It gives a natural stretch to the Achilles and calf every time you bend. Taking the stairs or using a stair machine also keep heels down and use thigh and hip muscles to power the push, instead of pressing with toes and using your knees to push. It is better exercise, healthier for the knees, and stretches the calf and Achilles with each step. Just walking toes forward, not turned out, gives a natural, small, but needed stretch with each step.

Hamstring Stretch

Stretching hamstrings can help stretch the Achilles and protect it from too much force during running. When the hamstring is tight, you take smaller steps when running because your leg doesn't straighten as much. The bent knee makes the ankle have to pull back harder, putting more stress on the Achilles when landing from each step. See Chapter 9 for hamstring stretches. When you do these hamstring stretches, for example, when lying on your back with one or both feet up, pull your toes back to add more stretch to the bottom of the foot and Achilles tendon.

Arana had multiple sclerosis. Many (multiple) small, hard, or sclerotic areas formed in her nervous system, giving her difficulty in moving and change in her vision. As walking became harder, she started using a wheelchair. By then, the weakness of lack of using the body was hard to tell from the issue of the sclerotic patches slowing the nerve signals to her legs. Deconditioning from lack of movement causes serious injuries to the body that are not from the original disease—which is called secondary injury. Arana could shift her legs when lying down, but not lift her feet enough to walk. I examined her legs. When I asked her to move her feet, the leg muscles that move her feet were activating. Why weren't her feet moving? The Achilles tendon had become so stiff from lack of movement that it was tightly holding her heel, preventing her from standing with heels on the floor. It was too much to stand and walk on her toes, so she sat. We needed to stretch her Achilles tendons so that she could try to stand. The simple fact of not being able to stand up causes too many other physical injuries to allow it to be lost without a good try. Besides Achilles stretching, her entire body needed to be moved through its whole range or risk losing many functions—just from stiffness and disuse, not the MS. If you take a healthy joint and put it in a cast, it is not long before it comes out weak, atrophied, and stiff. If you prevent joint movement long enough, you can permanently damage it. Not standing can cause major changes in the heart's ability to pump enough blood to the head to be able to stand and move. Movement is fundamental to health and recovery. We started with passive movement. I pulled and pushed her arms, legs, and back though normal ranges, showing her and her family what to try on their own. As much as she could, she was to push and pull her own weight and use as much extra weight (like lifting household items) to fight the loss of strength and bone density that comes from not moving. Not enough is known about multiple sclerosis (MS), making it hard to know what to do to stop it. Population studies show that sunshine is helpful to recovery, and that incidence of MS is higher in areas where people do not get enough sunlight. Every day she was to get outside and stand up, with whatever help was needed, to get as much weight as possible on her feet. The combination of movement and exercise, starting with stretching her heels enough to stand again, helped her prevent further loss and start making gains.

If you have any condition that limits movement, work to move. The disease makes it even more important to work your muscles and move your joints. Don't wait until you are in a wheelchair to strengthen your muscles and keep them moving through a range that you need to have an independent life. If you have any neurological condition that leads to loss of muscle use to raise the foot, a condition called "foot drop," stretch the Achilles daily to prevent tightness that further limits walking, even ability to rise from a chair.

Enrique tore his Achilles tendon. He was surprised since he wasn't doing anything strenuous. He was just going for his regular run. It was a partial tear, not torn completely through, but the pain and swelling still made walking or movement of the foot difficult. I explained that Achilles injury is common in the Western world. He wasn't taking antibiotics or steroids that can weaken the tendons. I sent him for a cholesterol screen. High cholesterol is sometimes found with Achilles tendon tears because high cholesterol can stiffen the area and predispose it to injury. Even if this not always the case, it was a good idea to check. Enrique asked why the cholesterol went only to the Achilles tendon. I told him it didn't; it clogs things all over.

"Where all over?" He seemed suddenly interested. "You mean like if things don't flow when they're supposed to flow?"

I understood his question. "Yes. Decreased blood flow to the genitalia is something you can tell your doc about, to check what's going on with your blood fats. You want to do this because that can save your heart, too." Enrique was able to bring his cholesterol down by eating fibrous fruit and vegetables, nuts, whole oatmeal, and less junk food. Whole grains contain fiber and niacin among other substances, which reduce cholesterol without the flushing and blood-sugar side effects of niacin pills.

Even if cholesterol hadn't affected Enrique's Achilles, improving his diet was healthy for his Achilles and the rest of his body. During this time, we exercised his Achilles because movement and resistance help healing more than keeping it in a cast or immobilized. We retrained his muscles to stop walking duck-footed. A negative cycle happens when feet face outward. The back of the legs don't get their normal stretch. The Achilles and calf get tighter and predisposed to tears. When the Achilles are tight, people tend to walk toe outward. We wanted to change that to a positive cycle. Stretching the calf and Achilles lets you walk with toes forward. Good forward toe walking stretches the calf and Achilles with each step. The Achilles no longer gets tight and pulls the feet to walk toe outward.

You can't just say, "Walk straight." If the calf muscles or Achilles are tight, the first time the person tries to run or jump with straight feet, he can pull or strain something from the new extra stretch. Enrique already had a tear. We worked on healthy, easy stretches and keeping the area moving until it was loose enough to allow healthy walking with toes straight forward.

What Else to Check

Your doctor can check for high cholesterol and hypothyroidism—both hidden factors in some cases of Achilles tendonitis and rupture. Several drugs are common contributors to tendon injury. Anabolic steroid use can strengthen muscles faster than the supporting tendons and ligaments. Sometimes tendons rupture with hard training. Long use of antibiotics like Cipro, Floxin, and Noroxin (fluroquinolones) increases risk of tendon or ligament tear or rupture.

Many common prescription drugs have a common side effect of joint and muscle pain, including the various statin drugs to lower cholesterol, Accutane (isotretinoin) to treat acne, anti-anxiety drugs, some prescription allergy medicine, and some prescription sleep drugs. It is not necessary to take drugs that cause more problems. Check with your doctor for healthy ways to stop the cause of the problem, to reduce the need for medicines.

What to Do Every Day to Keep Ankles and Achilles Healthy

- Ankles have posture that you can control. When you stand and bend your knees to pick things up, keep body weight on the soles of the feet, not leaning inward on the arches. Keep knee over your feet, not tilting inward. Use muscles to hold healthy positioning.
- Walk with feet and knees facing straight, not turned in or out.
- Do balance exercises to retrain knowledge of positioning at the same time that you strengthen the ankles. Strengthening alone is not enough to prevent repeat sprains. Have fun doing inventive balance exercises (safely).
- When coming down the stairs, land lightly and bend the knee lightly as you land, using muscles for shock absorption. Walk lightly all the time.
- Keep a healthy diet and do fun exercise to avoid cholesterol from clogging and hardening your arteries and tendons.
- Exercise frequently to keep ankles and Achilles used to movement.

What to Avoid

- Don't let ankles sag inward when standing, bending, or moving.
- Don't turn your ankle up sideways when sitting cross-legged. Keep the ankle straight and get the stretch from the hip.

- Don't deliberately stretch the outside of the ankles. Ligaments are not supposed to stretch. Once they are forced to lengthen, they don't hold the anklebones in place
- When coming down the stairs, don't land heavily, which forcefully lengthens the Achilles tendon. Keep the heel on the upper leg down as you step down, stretching it with each step. Don't let your ankles turn inward, flattening the arches when stepping down
- Bifocals are a hidden source of poor balance because of the different visual fields. Avoid them on the stairs.

When to Notice Ankles and Achilles

- A common time that people sag the ankles inward is when bending for something.
- Check your ankle positioning when sitting cross-legged to make sure you're not turning the ankles up sideways.
- When you bend knees to pick up something from the floor, can you keep both heels down and knees facing forward? If not, your Achilles tendons are too tight.

How to Get Natural Achilles and Ankle Improvement during Daily Activity

- Walk with both feet facing straight, not turned out, to stretch the Achilles tendon and bottom of the foot with each step.
- Go up the stairs with heels down. Keep your body weight back toward the heel of the foot as you press upward. This movement is healthier for your knees because it puts the exercise on the muscles and takes the force off the knee joint. Keeping heels down gives a nice stretch to the Achilles and calf muscles with each step.
- Some people walk lifting the heel almost as soon as the foot hits the ground. Early heel lift looks bouncy, almost like toe walking. Don't let the heel lift up right away. Roll from heel to toe, keeping the heel down until the whole foot lifts to take the next step.
- For all the many times a day you bend to reach or retrieve things, bend correctly using legs instead of bending over at the waist. Bend both knees keeping heels down on the floor. Good bending prevents back pain, is free leg exercise, and stretches the Achilles tendon with each bend. An average person bends several hundreds of times a day. Imagine the back pain you can prevent and the benefit to your legs just by bending right, as you know you should anyway.
- For natural balance, strengthening, and fun, pick up small objects or clothing around the house with your bare foot to transfer it to your hand.

- If you squat to sit, keep both heels down on the ground. Don't lean forward on the toes. Keep heels down when rising from a chair.

No More Ankle and Achilles Pain

Good balance and healthy leg positioning during your ordinary day prevents ankle sprains and supports your ankles more than high top shoes, supports, orthotics, and bracing. Weak ankles and relying on external supports are helpful clues that you need better ways of moving and holding your body weight. Fix the cause and you can fix the pain, stop recurring injuries, and create a healthier life at the same time. Instead of doing a bunch of ankle rehabilitation exercises then going back to injurious habits, you can naturally stretch your Achilles tendons, improve balance, and strengthen your ankles by using healthy ankle and foot positioning during everyday activities.

7

No More Foot Pain

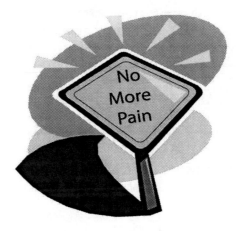

- Flat Feet and Pronation
- Duck Feet and Pigeon Toes
- Heel Pain
- Plantar Fasciitis
- Funny Toes
- Bunion
- Skewfoot and More

Feet need exercise like the rest of your body, but are often overlooked. Tight, weak feet are more likely to cramp, hurt, strain, and develop fasciitis—an inflammation of the tissue stretching across the bottom of the foot. Toes need to be straight and strong for balance and healthy gait. Weak, squashed toes—unused for balance and normal walking—easily deform and curl. Allowing your arches to roll in and flatten can cause foot pain. When one arch rolls down more than the other, which is common, it can create a leg-length difference. This difference is not in the bones, and can easily be corrected by not letting your feet just sag any which way under your body weight.

It used to be thought that feet were hard to exercise because they are already accustomed to holding up body weight. But walking and holding up your weight makes them easy to condition when you use healthy movement forces. This chapter shows how common habits can injure or deform feet and easy things to prevent and stop pain.

Flat Feet and Pronation

William came in with some very flat feet. His feet turned out like a duck and he rested his weight heavily on his arches, which flattened to the floor.

I asked William to rise on tiptoe. His arches appeared. When he came down, he flattened his feet against the floor again. I asked him to put his feet parallel—not turned out—which he did. I explained that his legs and ankles have posture, and that he controls this posture. I showed him how to rock weight on and off his arches. He realized that it was up to him whether his arches flattened against the floor, or whether he held his body weight on the soles and off the arches.

He patted the sides of his legs and said he could feel the muscles working when he stood correctly. He said he never saw arches in his feet before. He thought he never would since all his family stands with their body weight on their arches, and his doctor told him he had a foot condition that could not change.

At first he rolled so much to the outside so that his lower leg tiled outward. Then he straightened his leg, still lifting his arches. He looked in the mirror at his now-straight legs and new arches.

He said, "That's it?"

"Yes, that's pretty much it," I said.

"Okay, then. Thanks," he said. He started to leave. "Wait!" he said. "It doesn't stay like that." He pointed at his arches, once again flat on the floor.

"You just need to hold them in place" I said. He moved his feet back into position and his arches reappeared.

"Oh! Okay, that's easy." He walked around the room with his new gait. He said, "Hey, it feels different. My feet don't hurt." And that was that.

William reports in every now and then that everything is fine. He told me some months later he tried to show someone else the same success, but they argued with him that they didn't want to hold foot positioning themselves, and instead got a set of $395 orthotics to do it for them. "I saved a lot of money," he told me. "Thanks."

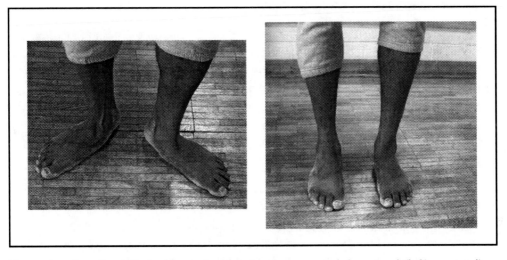

Figure 7-1. Standing with feet turned out and arches pressed downward (left) or standing with feet parallel and weight off the arches (right) is up to you.

Is correcting flat feet or the related problem of pronation really that easy? Sometimes it is. Many people have never been told that their legs have posture, just like their back and shoulders. They think it is unchangeable. One man told me his doctor said there is nothing you can do to strengthen or change how you stand on your feet "because the muscles in the feet are too small." Other patients have told me they were told that only surgery could change pronated feet, and they needed to wear shoe inserts for the rest of their life. I was taught that in school, too, when I was studying orthopedic injuries. But it is just like a beginning skater who lets their ankles turn inward. Then they learn to control their positioning and hold their feet straight without sagging.

Try it for yourself and see that if you let your body weight slump in any way it happens to fall, you will usually not stand straight. You can voluntarily move your feet, ankles, legs, back, neck, and shoulders into the posture you want. You can often do the same with feet. Then, just like toilet training, you learn to hold it, even when you don't feel like it.

What is pronation? Pronation is one of the normal ways you move your foot as you apply weight while walking or running. As your foot strikes the ground, you strike from the outside of the heel first. This outward rolling is called supination. Then as you transfer your weight forward in walking or running, your heel and ankle roll inward, and your arch flattens a little. Some people let it flatten too much, which is commonly called pronation.

Technically, the problem is overpronation, but the term pronation has come to stand for the overrolling. When you overpronate, the arch remains flat, and the ankle rolls too far inward as the toes begin to push off, which increases stress on the muscles and other structures of the foot.

Just looking at the bottoms of your shoes for wear patterns won't tell you if you pronate. It is true that shoes can tell some things, for instance, if they are completely worn only on one side. But it is natural to heel-strike slightly to the outside then roll to a more level position. Shoes with slight wear on the outside heel don't always mean that you are not walking "squarely." To determine whether you are walking squarely, you need to watch yourself in a mirror or have someone else take a look from the front, sides, and back.

Gina was told that she needed orthotics—expensive molds for her shoes. She explained to me that she was told that her feet had a condition called pronation and that was why her knees hurt. The orthotics would hold her foot properly. "I'm a pronator," she said. I asked her if she were wearing her orthotics right then. "Of course I am." She was surprised I would ask. "I am not allowed to take them off or I'll pronate."

"So you can never go barefoot?"

"Oh, no. That's bad for me," she said. I pointed down at her feet that tilted inward, turned toe-out, with her knees sagging inward, and asked her why her feet still pronated (Figure 7-2). She was surprised.

"But don't the orthotics change that?" she asked. I told her that the point of the orthotics was to help bolster up the arch, but if you keep pushing inward against the orthotics, it was hard for them to do their job. She said, "So if I stand without pushing in on them, they will hold my feet up?" I replied that if she stood without pushing in on them she would be holding her own feet up, and may not need them at all. Then she could wear her sandals and go barefoot.

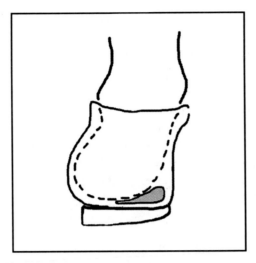

Figure 7-2. Some people roll inward, right over their orthotics.

Walking barefoot is not bad for you. Letting your feet slump when you walk barefoot is bad. The soles of the feet are built to bear your weight, but putting your weight on the arch overstretches and tilts the foot. That overstretching can happen with or without shoes and orthotics. I told Gina that all over Southeast Asia, the mountain guides wear flip-flops. I have found, especially after working with large numbers of patients and students, that it is simple enough to use your own muscles to get the same results as expensive special support shoes and shoe inserts.

I attend several sports medicine conferences every year, with lectures on evaluating and correcting many joint problems. In the foot lectures, you often hear that if the foot flattens so that the medial surface (the side with the big toe) turns downward to the floor, then you are a pronator and you need special shoes, arch supports, or orthotics.

One year I attended the foot pain lecture by a distinguished practitioner. I like this person personally and know that he knows far more than I do about feet. After his lecture portion finished, just before the practicum was starting, I asked him why pronation wasn't approached as a muscular issue, instead of something structural that a person can't change. He laughed and said that feet don't have posture. I pointed down at my own feet and showed him, by changing my stance, that it was easy to change from pronation to supination to other foot postures—both good and bad. He replied that a runner couldn't be expected to hold healthy position for the length of a marathon. He sat me on the examining table he used for the workshop demonstration, pulled off my sneaker and sock from one foot, and waved my foot in the air for participants to see. "Look," he said to the crowd. "A Morton's foot!" A Morton's foot is sometimes called a "Greek foot." The second toe is longer than the big toe. This situation is different from another kind of foot where the big toe (first toe) is longest, and the other toes shorter. Some foot specialists say that Morton's foot is more likely to pronate because it can sometimes be a more flexible foot. However, I have found that simple training can hold things in place, just as a dancer with flexible legs can position them wherever needed, with more strength and range than other people. A Morton's foot is not as bad as some people think. Most people with Morton's foot don't get the problems that are common to a stiff inflexible foot. "Look at the excess mobility," he told the crowd of practitioners as he wiggled and pressed my foot between his hands. "Look at that mobile ray!" A "ray" means the long bones of the foot.

A Morton's foot is thought of as an "older" foot. One explanation is that we developed from earlier beings who had a foot more like a hand, so that the "big toe" was more like a thumb. With later humans, the big toe lengthened and moved up toward the other toes. Some people have the earlier version before final lengthening occurred, and others have the later model with the big toe longest. Each is inherited from your parents who came before you, so it is in your genetic code. The presenter continued waving my foot over my head saying, "See? An unevolved foot! A throwback to primordial times of small brains and lack of capacity for rational thought." He was referring to my question that foot posture can be controlled.

The crowd of doctors laughed and waited for my reply. I patted my head and said, "I have a midsaggital ridge, too." This was true. A midsaggital ridge is a bony ridge along the top of the skull. It seems that I have several genetic markers in my bones of an "older model," most of which confer some physical advantage of sturdiness or speed, but also are good for jokes. He put my foot down and I stood up on the table. I showed them that while my foot was mobile enough to assume a pronated or flattened arch position when I allowed it to, I could also stand, walk, and run with a normal arch. You can too. Give it a try. If you have flat feet and want to change them, follow the guidelines presented in this chapter.

What to Do Every Day to Reposition Feet to a Normal Arch

Your feet have posture just like the rest of you. Many cases of flat feet are not unchangeable hereditary conditions—just poor foot and ankle posture.

- Stand facing a mirror. If no mirror is handy where you can see yourself full length, then stand up and look down at your bare feet.

- Let your weight flatten down and inward on your arches. You may already do this action as a habit. Now, pull your weight back off your arches and distribute it along the sole of your foot. You will probably find that you have arches.

- Don't pull so far that you teeter on the side of your foot.
- Keep weight on your whole foot and heel, not rocking forward to the toe.

Frank was an aerobics, yoga, and spinning teacher in his 40s. He came in with a long history of painful feet and continuing injuries. He wanted to ask about new orthotics. He told me how he started his athletic career as a distance runner in high school. In his first season, he got multiple stress fractures of the tibia (shin bone). Those injuries retired him from running in his first season. Looking for a substitute, he tried bicycle racing which he enjoyed for about five years. During his sixth year as a cyclist, he entered a triathlon. He thought his bones had become strong enough to endure the stresses of running. Not long after beginning running, he got new pains in his big toes, pain in both feet, and Achilles tendonitis.

When Frank was 22 years old, he went to a podiatrist (foot doctor) who told him symptoms were degenerative arthritis from overuse, bunions, and Achilles tendonitis. The doctor told Frank it was due to lateral (sideways) motion of the heel while running. The cause of these symptoms, he said, was pronation. He said Frank needed an operation to remove the bunions and "repair" the arthritic joints, and that he would need orthotic inserts in his shoes for the rest of his life. Frank had the operation, was fitted for the custom orthotics, and wore them religiously for almost 20 years.

Frank had tried to continue triathlons after the operation using orthotics in his running shoes, but the tendonitis continued and he couldn't run more than one or two miles without severe tendon pain and moderate, but nagging, pain in his big toes. He told me he had begun to think of himself as a debilitated, crippled has-been. He thought he'd never run comfortably or well in competition again. He retired from competitive athletics.

I checked his feet and found the cause of his pronation was not "fallen arches" as he had been told. His arches reappeared when I asked him to stand on tiptoe. He had no malformation—genetic or otherwise—of the bones or joints. He just allowed his body weight to slump inward on his feet, pressing on the arches, flattening them. The bunions, tendonitis, and pain were secondary symptoms.

We did gait retraining for Frank to feel proper foot posture without orthotics as he stood, then walked, and then, to his excitement, ran. He learned to begin each step on his heel, rock through his strides on the sole of his foot with "plenty of air" beneath what now looked like a perfectly healthy, arched foot. Rather then rely on his big toe to drive himself forward at the end of each step, he used all five toes.

Frank was thrilled to find he could use his own musculature to properly position his feet. The added benefit was that by using his foot muscles for the first time, his weak feet began to strengthen with all his normal activities. He no longer felt any pain, only strength.

Soon Frank could run, even box, without any foot pain, pronation, or stress fractures. He told me that his "revolution" occurred 30 years late. He said if he had know all this sooner, he probably would not have had the three stress fractures in high school, developed the arthritis or bunions, or needed the operations. He never would have needed the orthotics to prevent his "two flat tires."

About two years later, I saw Frank at a gym where we both taught classes. He wanted to show me that he was still bending properly from what I showed him about back pain for his students. He bent both knees with his back nicely upright. But his heels started lifting and both feet pivoted outward.

"Frank, what's up with your Achilles?"

"What do you mean?"

"Frank, do you see your toes facing outward? You're starting to slump inward on your arches again just from that turning out."

"What do you mean? I stretch my Achilles." He showed me the standard "lean and lunge" stretch with his back foot turned outward.

"Frank, the turned-out foot position prevents Achilles stretch. Walking like that also means your Achilles isn't getting normal stretch. No wonder it's gotten so tight that when you bend you can't keep your feet straight."

"What do you mean? I stretch."

"Frank you're spending time stretching and getting no stretch." I showed him the foot-on-wall Achilles stretch (Figure 6-9). He had become so tight that he couldn't put his foot on the wall and still stand up straight. He had to round his back and his standing foot pivoted outward even as he was standing on it.

"Frank, that's tight. Maybe start with downward dog." (See Figure 7.3.) Frank knew the downward-dog stretch and showed me. He even did downward dog with his feet turned out.

"Frank!"

"What??"

"All of this is going to drop your weight back down on your arches. Remember what happens with that?"

Frank said, "Oh, right. I'll work on it. It's never to late to start."

Pigeon Toes and Duck Feet

Turning your feet facing toe-out (duck-foot) or inward (pigeon toe) is a common habit. It is often ignored as normal or not changeable. However, they are both often easy to change and, by changing to a straight walking position, you can reduce or stop many aches and pains. It was once thought that walking and running slightly toe-out was desirable because that was thought to be the natural direction of the foot muscles. Now it is known that parallel feet position is a healthy and desired position.

Toe-out walking (duck-foot) strains the feet, ankles, knees, and hips. It contributes to pronation, bunion formation, and tightness of the Achilles tendon. It decreases the "push-off" phase because you press off the side of the big toe, rather than the ball of the entire foot and all toes. This habit reduces your speed and jumping ability, shock absorption, and the "spring in your step." Pushing off the side of the big toe pushes the big toe toward the other toes of that foot. Imagine pushing your big toe inward, step after step, for the thousands you take every day. Eventually, the big toe bones will obediently move. If you are already predisposed to bunion, you do not want to contribute further to the situation. Walking with your feet turned out is often mistaken for "flat-foot" because it often shifts your weight toward the inside of your foot, flattening your arches. Turning just one foot out can roll the arch down, making that leg length shorter than the other.

Standing and moving with your feet facing toe-in, often called pigeon toe, can strain the foot, ankle, knee, and hip, and affect normal gait. Keeping your feet toe-in can make you stand and move "knock-kneed," which is another bad posture—not a normal trait with which you happen to be born. Putting weight on the inside of your knees slowly pressures and strains them, wearing out the cartilage and interfering with normal muscle use and kneecap tracking.

What to Do Every Day to Reposition Duck Foot and Pigeon Toe

- Keep feet parallel and not turned in or out.
- Keep your body weight on the rims and sole of your foot, not arches, for all standing, walking, jumping, and movement.
- Make sure you don't always let your foot turn outward when stretching the back of your legs.
- Keep body weight over your whole foot including the heel when bending, not leaning forward on the toes.
- Make sure your straight-foot position is healthy and comes from straightening your entire leg. Don't just yank your feet straight from the ankle or knee, twisting them and substituting one problem for another.

Weak Feet: Walking on Bones

"It feels like I'm walking on bones." Anya wanted to know if she had growths in her feet. Each step felt like pebbles in her shoes. Instead of being padded with muscles, the bottoms of her feet were thin from lack of use, even though she walked daily. Wearing soft insoles wasn't helping much, because the shrunken, thin bottom of her feet mashed against her foot bones with each step, without soft tissue and muscle in between. Anya said she thought she was supposed to wear snug shoes to help her balance and support her foot. But because of the supportive shoes, her muscles never had to work, she never got practice in balance, and her feet became weak and unable to hold themselves up. Her risk of falling was higher from wearing the very shoes she thought would help her prevent falls. Loss of muscle in her feet—not extra growth of tissue—was the problem. She needed to use and develop her feet just like the muscles in the rest of her body, to prevent the loss that occurs with disuse.

I explained to her that muscle loss was not inevitable with aging, just with disuse. It was a simple matter of "use or lose." Although it is often said that shoes must support and hold up your foot, your own muscles that should do that. I explained, "You wouldn't put your head in a splint to hold it up, you just use your neck muscles." We started with barefoot walking to learn good foot positioning without the too-tight shoes. At first she walked with the same shuffle as she did with her shoes. Then she was surprised to notice that without being in the equivalent of a foot straight jacket, she could walk with less side-to-side waddle and a more natural, springy gait. She needed gait retraining to a more natural walk that would also uses her foot muscles. She also needed foot-strengthening exercises to give her more foot padding. We practiced rising to tiptoe and lowering, then walking on toes, and fun things like picking up objects with her feet and passing them to her hand. Anya joked that she would save her back from not having to bend over to pick up anything any more, just use her feet. I added that this exercise would give her better balance, too.

Feet Need Strengthening Every Day

- Rise to tiptoe and hold as long as you can. Keep weight over big and second toe, not leaning out to the little toes. Try for at least 10 seconds to start.
- Rise and lower on toes, maintaining positioning control. Keep weight over the big and second tow, not teetering outward over the little toes. Work up to at least 10 times with each foot.

- Rise and lower with speed and shock absorption so that you bounce up and down by bending your knees. Progress to small, well-cushioned jumps.
- Pick up objects with your toes.
- Practice walking lightly on the floor and stairs without making a sound.
- Walk on heels only, gently. Walk on toes only. Work up to at least 20 steps each.
- Press the side of your foot against a wall and push to build the muscles. Hold ten seconds. Do 10 times each side.
- Play "footsie" by pressing and pulling the sides, top, and bottom of your feet against an object or other person.
- Remember that it is your feet (not your shoes) that position your feet and how you walk. Don't let your feet slap down. Use muscular control whether you are wearing a running shoe with a special sole to help with the push-off, or a sandal. You can still walk normally by using your own foot muscles.
- Bounce up and down gently, maintaining healthy foot positioning. Rise as high as you can without leaving the ground. Progress to tiny jumps, so lightly that you make no sound. Progress to skipping, jump rope, and other movement using significant shock absorption to cushion all your joints. Don't let knees sway inward. Land toe first, softly lowering to heel and bending knees.

Heel Pain, Bottom of Foot Pain—Plantar Fasciitis

A fascia is a fibrous sheet of tissue, wrapping muscles and soft structures. You have fascia in several places—one is across the bottom of your feet. The term "plantar" means the bottom of your foot that you "plant" on the ground. Plantar fasciitis is when the fascia on the bottom of your foot is inflamed.

Your plantar fascia transmits your body weight across your foot as you move, and is a shock absorber for your entire leg. When you walk normally, you get a small stretch across the bottom of your foot. When you don't walk normally, your foot can get strained and, because it loses the normal stretch, it becomes tight. Every step you take on a tight fascia yanks on the heel where it attaches. Eventually the heel and bottom of the foot get irritated from the yanking and start to hurt.

Olaf came in wearing Frankenstein shoes. The shoes didn't bend, making him walk with a flat trudge. "I go clompin-clompin," he joked. He had gone to his doctor with painful feet. His doctor explained how the tight fascia was getting pulled on with each step, which made it hurt. Therefore, the treatment was to not let the foot stretch. Olaf was put into a stiff shoe that prevented his foot from stretching or moving at all when he walked. The pain was gone. It seemed simple. The problem was that the shoe did not solve the cause of the pain; it perpetuated it. The shoes prevented him from getting the natural stretch from walking that would lengthen the tight fascia so that he could walk without yanking. He could never go without these shoes. The shoes also changed his gait so much that it might begin to hurt his back and hip in the future. For people who want to be active again, tight shoes present a higher risk than before of injury, because the shoes have created an even tighter foot.

We needed to get him out of those shoes, and we didn't want him to have pain from the original injury, and his now-tighter foot from the shoes. We started with light foot stretches and training in normal foot positioning in walking. He stretched a little more each day, particularly in the morning and before bed, so that he wouldn't wake with foot pain. We added hamstring stretches because tightness keeps the knee bent more than normal when you walk and especially when you stretch your legs out to run, making you have to bend the ankle back more than normal, increasing the forces on the Achilles tendon and fascia as you land. I showed him to stretch his hamstrings with his foot turned in, straight, and turned out. I told him it was most important stretch his hamstrings without rounding his back. He was surprised to find how much he had been rounding his back before by sitting and leaning forward to touch his toes. He tried lying on his back with one leg up against the wall. With his back straight on the floor and not part of the stretch, he found that his hamstrings were tighter than he thought. "No vonder I vasn't getting no more stvetchable." His accent was fun.

He wore the shoes only to work, where he did a lot of walking. He wore them less each day as he increased the flexibility in the fascia, and the inflammation went down. Within a week or two he could walk without his Frankenstein shoes at all. No more "clompin-clompin."

Jeff also came to me with pain along the bottom of his right foot, more intense in the heel. He was active in martial arts, running, biking, and climbing. On exam, his right foot was considerably weaker than the left. He has seen a prominent foot doctor who gave him prescription anti-inflammatory medicine. I asked Jeff, "What exercises are you doing for it?" He said that he was shown some stretching, but had not done them because he "wanted to give it a rest." He was doing no physical activity except for an occasional bike ride and walk, which brought back the foot pain each time. I asked him if it came on suddenly during his physical activity. He said no, that it started 10 years before.

Three years before, it became so painful that he went to a podiatrist who made him casts and orthotics, which seemed to help. The casts prevented the foot from stretching, so it no longer pulled and hurt. But it turned out that "helped" meant that the pain was gone when he didn't exercise or do anything.

They had checked that an important nerve in the foot, the tibial nerve, was not making the pain. If the tibial nerve is pinched as it passes through a bony canal in the ankle called the tarsal tunnel, it can cause pain and numbness similar to the symptoms of fasciitis and heel spur. They tapped on the tibial nerve where it passes through the tarsal tunnel. This procedure is called Tinel's Test. They also put electrodes into the area to see if the tibial nerve was conducting properly. The nerve was fine. Jeff needed stretches and exercise for regular fasciitis.

The only exercise Jeff had done for his foot was to pull his toes back occasionally. He had given up running. He wanted to run again but was not doing what was needed to do that safely. "You've had this ten years? Has anyone looked at the way you walk or run to see if there is something you're doing to create the problem? If you continue the habits that caused the problem, you will not heal." He told me that he was doing something—giving up everything he enjoyed, and occasionally pulling his toes back, when he remembered. He also had many shots of cortisone into the area. I reminded him that while one shot may reduce inflammation, many could weaken the entire area.

I asked him to walk around for me so that I could see what might be going on, knowing that once someone is already injured, the injury itself changes their walk. You have to be able to differentiate the chicken from the egg at that point. It is a cycle of bad gait that injures, and injury that perpetuates the bad gait. He walked with both feet pointed outward like a duck, not just the sore foot. Because of the turn out, his big toe never bent much, so that the bottom of his foot never got the normal stretch that walking confers.

I bent his toes back gently. They bent easily so it was not another common problem of stiff toes preventing the bending that is needed. But the bottom of his foot was stretched so tightly you would think it would tear. This illustrated very well the problem that was going on inside. I told him that when he stretches, not to just pull the toes back, but to pull and stretch the whole bottom of his foot.

I explained to Jeff that when the bottoms of your feet get too tight, the tissues that attach to the heel can irritate the heel because they pull on it tightly with every step—which is how untreated plantar fasciitis can lead to heel spurs. Your heel gets so irritated with all the pulling that, like an oyster, it grows a pearl of a bony spur. I told him that it could be an easy matter of stretching the bottom of his foot, strengthening things so that they don't yank, and retraining how he walks and runs.

Jeff said that he planned to do more walking. When he got a chance. He corrected himself, saying that it was running and walking that made his foot hurt in the first place. So he may not do that. He said, "I have actually thought of having the foot cut off, and getting a titanium and graphite-epoxy prosthesis. Only the finest aerospace materials for me!" He waited for me to laugh.

"Yes," I said. "You'll do everything except stretch it. You need a structure of stretches and exercises specifically for what you are doing to injure your foot. Otherwise, it is a shot in the dark, and it is not likely that you will just hit on the right thing. Allowing 10 years to go by is working against yourself."

On follow-up a year later, Jeff said his pain was lessened. I asked how his running was going. "Oh, I had to give that up. I tried switching to martial arts but it flared up again, so I gave that up."

"Jeff, are you doing the stretches?"

"Well, no."

"What are you doing to help your foot?' He said had hoped it would just go away, and had gone to someone else who had told him to reduce his activity.

Martin had heel pain too. It almost sounded like fasciitis, but something was different. When I watched him walk, his feet turned out. Nothing unusual for fasciitis. But with each heel strike, he landed heavily on the inside of his heel. He had a heel bruise from walking turned out. It wasn't heel pain from fasciitis. He just needed to retrain his feet to not turn out when he walked and not to heel strike hard.

What to Do Every Day to Stop Plantar Fasciitis and Heel Pain

If your feet are very tender, simply do the following:

- Push the bottom of your feet with your thumbs to begin a gentle stretch.
- Some people enjoy rolling the bottom of their feet over a tennis ball to stretch it.
- When pulling your toes back, make sure to get the stretch across the whole bottom of the foot, not just the toes.
- Pull your foot and toes back with a towel while lying on your back.
- Stretch before going to sleep and first thing in the morning.

- Start gentle standing Achilles tendon stretches. Stand with the uninjured foot far in back to learn the stretch before trying it on the hurt foot. If they both hurt, do either one. Keep the back foot straight, not turned out, not even a little. Look at your back foot to see if it is straight. Bend your knees until the back heel lifts off the floor. Rock your weight toward the ball of the foot. Experiment with shifting weight forward and back to stretch where you feel the stretch best.
- Walk with feet pointing straight ahead.
- Stop letting your weight fall inward on your arches, straining the fascia. Keep weight on the soles of your feet, not arches.
- Avoid hard heel strike.
- Avoid striking on the bony inside or outside of your heel.
- When walking upstairs, keep your heel of the bottom leg down on the step as you push up. It will give the foot a nice stretch.
- Ice the injured area after exercising. Cold soaks are also nice.

As the injury recovers, add more weight during your stretch. See which of the following works best for you:

- Rise up and down on your toes.
- When the bottom of your foot can support rising to toe and lowering, stand on a book or board with heels off the back, stretching toward the floor.
- When standing with heels off the board is comfortable, rise and lower. Work slowly and carefully toward motion that is faster but still controlled by your muscles so that you don't strain the bottom of the foot, but support with musculature as you lower.
- Try the previous three skills, one foot at a time. Work to make strength and flexibility of both feet equal, but both better than they were before.
- Carefully stand backwards on a step, let one heel hang off, and press downward. Do this stretch with your leg bent, and with it straight.
- Stand facing a wall closely. Put the ball of your foot against the wall with your heel on the floor. Press hips forward to stretch the back of your lower leg and foot.
- After stretching the bottom of your foot, stretch your shins, too.
- Progress to small, then larger jumps, then pushing off as if for running.
- Exercise often to keep feet muscular and padded.
- Try the Achilles-tendon stretches in Chapter 6.
- Downward dog (Figure 7-3) can be a great plantar stretch if you keep your feet in healthy position. Get in push-up position, lift hips high in the air, and push back toward your heels, letting heels relax down to the floor. If you let your feet turn outward, you will lose the stretch. Keep feet parallel and weight on sole, not arches.

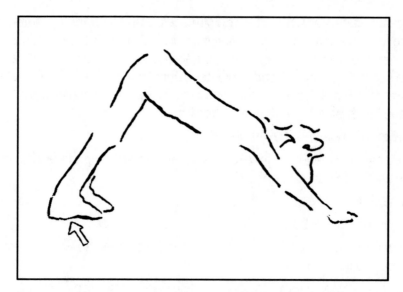

Figure 7-3. Downward dog stretches the feet if you keep feet both facing straight, not turned out, and weight on the outside rims of your feet, not arches. Keep hands far in front of feet and heels down.

Funny Toes—Bent-Up Toes

It is all too common to see toes that remain bent upward after taking off shoes—especially shoes with heels. You may put your foot on the floor, but the toes stick up off the floor. This result is not normal. It is tightness in the top of the foot. You can usually see the tight, string-like tendons on the top of the foot pulling the toes back.

When toes are held in one position too much, the muscles tighten and don't go back to normal length. Tight shoes push the toes up and sometimes make toes fold to fit. Many people do not use muscles in their feet or toes when they walk. The muscles that pull downward never work. The toes stretch up, but never down. Other conditions that hurt feet are diabetes and alcoholism, both of which can lead to nerve damage, furthering weakening the foot muscles.

Sometimes tightness progresses until the toes bend up then down again, sticking up in the middle, which is known as a hammertoe. Another problem, called claw toes, occurs when toes stick up in the middle and then curl down and under the foot. These deforming changes can be painful and make your toes rub against shoes—and each other—making corns and more trouble. Stuck toes get worse without treatment. Start now to prevent a cycle of toes so tight that it hurts to straighten them, and not straightening them only leads to more pain.

What to Do Every Day to Straighten Bent-Up Toes

- Stretch your toes with your hands several times every day. Stretch them apart, pull bent-up toes back down, pull bent down areas gently straight, and pull curled toes straight out to elongate them.

- Wear shoes with room in the toes. Snug shoes are not healthy. Unhealthy shoes are not beautiful.

- Support your feet by holding position using your own muscles, not a shoe "straight jacket" that lets ankles atrophy and doesn't let toes move, stretch, and straighten.

- Strengthen muscles that pull toes down by pushing against the wall or other heavy object with your toes. Try to push the wall away by pushing down on toes. Don't let toes fold, clench, or crumple. Push with straight toes.

Toes Misshapen and Stuck Together

Mrs. C had toes stuck together and bunched on top of each other. Her shoes were tight. She wore close-fitting hose over her feet all day and socks at night. Her toes fit together like puzzle pieces. She could not wiggle them or make them separate. I explained how toes are supposed to be separate and able to move. She didn't believe me, saying toes didn't do anything anyway. I told her that toes did many wonderful things for balance, walking, ability to jump and move quickly, for the shock absorption so important to her hip, and more. I told her that it was a common thought that shoes hold you up, but support should come from her own feet muscles. I pulled my own sneaker and sock off to wiggle my toes and show her. "Oh! That's disgusting! Your toes move!" She was aghast. I told her they are supposed to move. "It's like a monkey!" she said.

If your toes are bunched together, you need to stretch them apart. Take your toes in your hands and gently pull them apart. Some of my patients like to wear toe separators to bed, a soft foam device for separating toes for painting nails. Correct the problem with simple stretching before deformity progresses to the point where it is difficult to fix.

What to do Every Day to Prevent Misshapen and Stuck Toes

- Pull your toes away from each other with your hands.
- Straighten each toe gently.

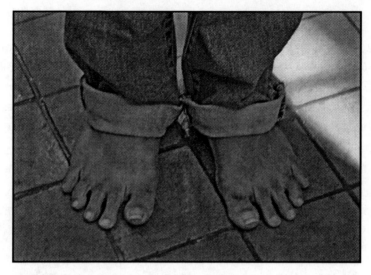

Figure 7-4. Healthy toes are straight, separate, and can move easily.

- Make sure all toes separate and can wiggle.
- Practice wiggling your toes.
- Don't wear shoes that push your toes together or keep them from moving.
- Avoid tight socks and stockings.
- When standing, don't tighten or clench your toes. Don't press toes into the ground to balance so much that they buckle and bend. Keep weight distributed over the entire foot, rocking weight back to the heel.
- Uncover your toes from shoes and hosiery and let them breathe often.

Stuck Big Toe—Hallux Rigidus

When your toes have normal flexibility and you walk with your feet facing straight ahead, the toes bend back with each step and you push off from the ball of the foot, the fleshy pad at the base of your toes. This flexibility is good. It is a nice stretch for the bottom of the foot and Achilles tendon. This built-in stretch helps prevent foot pain and fasciitis, and puts a "spring" in your step because of the push-off from the toes.

The medical name for your big toe is hallux. When the big toe is stiff and stuck and doesn't bend, it is called hallux rigidus, which means "stuck big toe." People with a stiff or rigid big toe will either have to take small, funny steps without bending their toes (and often having to lift their knees more than usual just to get their feet off the ground), or they will turn their feet out duck-style to walk without bending their toes.

When you walk with feet pointing out (duck-foot), your toes don't have to bend, and you lose your push-off and foot stretch. In a circular problem, one of the reasons that people walk with feet pointing out is that their big toe doesn't bend back enough, sometimes not at all. Turned out walking promotes tight toes. Tight toes promote turned-out walking. When the big toe joint doesn't bend when walking, it reduces the normal stretch on the bottom of the foot you are supposed to get just from ordinary walking, promotes bunion, takes away the springy "push-off," and changes how you walk. Your lower back often bears the brunt.

Keep your toes mobile by getting out of your shoes often and moving your toes freely in all directions. Stretch your toes with your hands. Walk normally so that ordinary daily activities keep them healthy. Don't force the big toe backward. Sometimes when people stretch a joint, they push the bone further against the socket and compress the joint rather than stretch the joint. Don't force your big toe back, jamming it further into the toe "knuckle" joint. Pull slightly outward when bending it back.

What to Do Every Day to Keep Your Big Toe Flexible

- If your big toe is stuck or not moving as much as it could, it is important to stretch and move it. Wiggle it gently up and down, and from side to side. Don't force.
- When stretching, pull the toe gently outward, instead of pushing it further into the joint capsule.
- Walk with feet as straight forward as possible to stop a cycle of tight toe and outward walking.
- Use shoes that allow your toes to bend normally when moving.

Bunion, Big Toe Tilts Toward Toes, Hallux Valgus

A related problem to stuck big toe is bunion. A bunion happens when the joint of your big toe enlarges, the bursa swells, and the big toe moves toward or over the other toes. A bursa is a fluid-filled sac that cushions the bone against pressure. The big toe bursa is on the side of the big toe bone. It swells when you pressure the side of the toe with tight shoes or walking with your foot turned so that you push against the side of the toe, instead of the bottom.

Many people walk with toes pointing outward putting stresses all over the foot and leg. This type of movement produces a variety of effects from corns to flattened arches to knee and hip pain. When you walk toe-out, the push-off place becomes the side of your big toe, instead of the ball of your foot. This squeezes the bursa against the bone, hurting it. Over years it can push the big toe over your other toes, increasing tendency to bunion.

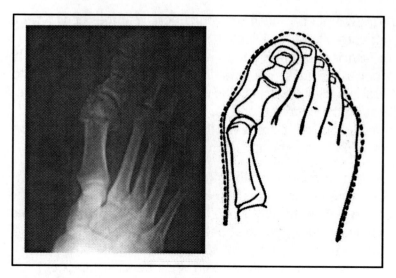

Figure 7-5. Bunion

What to Do Every Day to Prevent Bunion

- Stretch your toes with your hands, particularly your big toe.
- Stand with one foot behind you, and lift that heel as you do in walking, to bend the toes. Hold and repeat. Stretch your toes in the other direction by pressing the top of your toes against the floor behind you, or in your hands.
- Keep feet parallel and facing straight forward when walking and running.
- Practice using your own big toe muscles to move your toe to the outside. It is like opening your fingers wide. Open your toes apart using your toe muscles. Do 10 repetitions, many times a day.
- A tight Achilles tendon is one reason people walk duck-footed. Stretch the back of your legs with the stretches in Chapter 6.
- Change to shoes that don't push your toes into unhealthy position.

Skewfoot, Big Toe Tilts Away from Toes, Hallux Varus

Oren was in his 50s and was active until his doctors told him not to be. Over the previous four years, his toes had started moving away from their normal position. He was told to stop exercising to limit movement of his feet.

I looked at his bare feet. The big toe on each foot curved away from the other toes so that his two big toes pointed at each other. He had bilateral (both feet) skewfoot, the opposite of a bunion. With a bunion (hallux valgus), the big toe turns in. With skewfoot, or hallux varus, the big toe turns out from the foot and other toes. Sometimes skewfoot comes from overdone bunion surgery or trauma. Other times, like for Oren, the one side of his big toe was tight, pulling it away from his other toes. The other was weak and overstretched, letting it be pulled (Figure 7-6).

When Oren walked, he walked in a way that pushed his toes further sideways. As he put weight on each foot to take each step, the arch flattened, and the toes moved further out of place.

I examined his feet. They were soft and mushy. He hadn't exercised for a while and the feet had atrophied. The specialist at the university podiatry school told him he had "rolling pronation," and the only thing to do was wear orthotics for the rest of his life and have surgery. The specialist said that exercise is useless because the foot muscles "are too small to respond to exercise."

I asked Oren to stand and not to allow the foot to pronate and angulate. I asked him to use his foot muscles to pull his big toe and hold it in line intentionally. He was able to hold a straight position.

We were able to get Oren to stand normally without too much effort in about five minutes by having him use the muscles of his lower leg and foot. Then we would have the longer task of gait retraining for normal life, and regularly stretching the toe back into place toward the other toes. I made him a list of retraining exercises to do every day.

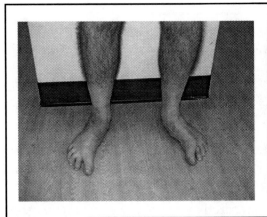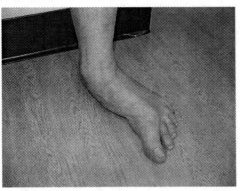

Figure 7-6. Tight muscles on one side of the foot pulls the big toes away from the other toes. Loose, weak muscles on the other side allow it, creating a skewfoot.

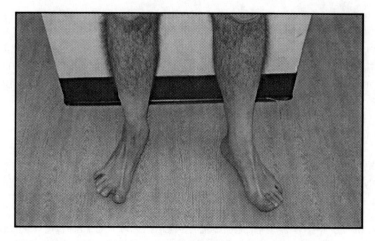

Figure 7-7. Repositioning, stretching, and strengthening can normalize a skewfoot.

Oren said he had an appointment at the hospital for orthotics. The soonest appointment he could get was almost five months later. For something they had told him was urgent and only fixable with orthotics, they didn't seem urgent about doing it. Orthotics could be used to aid his rehab training, since he needed something to hold his foot from getting worse while we made it better. Without access to them, we would control it ourselves.

Oren said everyone he saw insisted that no exercise helps foot disorders. I have heard this, too, but have found that people can often correct problems themselves without much difficulty—or any expense.

Skewfoot Exercises Every Day, Ten Times a Day

- For all exercises (except the last one), remove shows, socks, and look in a mirror.
- Normalize toe position as much as possible by shifting weight and using musculature. Make the foot position as normal as possible. Hold ten seconds.
- Stand on one foot and normalize toe position as much as possible by shifting weight and using musculature. Make the foot position as normal as possible. Hold for 10 seconds.
- Shift weight from foot to foot holding normalized toe posture. Hold for 10 seconds on each foot. Work up to faster pace.
- Pick up things with your toes and pass them to your hand. Ten times each foot.

- Pull a towel toward you with your toes by scrunching toes. Ten times each foot.
- Pull a towel weighted down with books or other heavy objects toward you with your toes by scrunching toes. Ten times each foot.
- Stand on your toes, making sure all posture is normalized. Raise and lower. Hold for 10 seconds.
- Press the side of your foot against a wall and push to build the muscles. Hold for 10 seconds. Do 10 times on each side.
- Put your toes under something steady like a door, or your other foot, and try to lift toes up. Hold for 10 seconds. Do 10 times on each side.
- You can still exercise when you are at work and wearing your shoes. Press your feet against each other—each side and top and bottom while sitting. Hold for 10 seconds. Repeat 10 times on each side. When walking, keep positioning to prevent further damage and get exercise.

What Else to Check

It is not common, but sometimes pain in the big toe is from gout. Gout is a painful inflammation from small, needle-like urate crystals that are thought to build up from the breakdown of purines. Purines are found in organ meats like liver, brains, and kidney, and fish like anchovies and herring.

More commonly, drugs to lower cholesterol called statin drugs have a side effect of joint pain, and sometimes, numbness or tingling in the fingers or toes. Other medicines with side effects of joint or muscle aches are prescription acid prevention medicine, some prescription allergy medicine, the calcium-channel-blocker drug, verapamil, the antibiotics erythromycin and clarithromycin, some prescription antidepressant and anxiety medicines.

Your doctor can check for foot pain from gout, various infections, worms, fungus, fractures, erythromelalgia, which is a skin condition on fingers or toes from dilation of blood vessels, cold injuries, autoimmune problems like Lupus, neurological diseases, damage from alcoholism and diabetes. With neurological injury and diabetes, good positioning and healthy use of feet become even more important and helpful.

What to Do Every Day for Healthy Feet

- Look in a mirror and see if your feet tilt in or out, making your arches too high or low.

- Practice pressing and lifting the arch while keeping the rest of the sole on the floor. See how the muscles work on the inside and outside of your leg to do that. See that you can position your own feet in healthy position, not too high or low.

- Don't let your body weight flatten out your arches. Foot positioning is a voluntary posture, like any other.

- Look in the mirror and see if your toes point in or out. Practice walking with your feet pointing straight ahead, parallel to each other, not toe-in or toe-out.

- Walk properly—an important and effective exercise. Walk and run by rolling heel first, through to the toe.

- Walk and step lightly, using muscles to decelerate and come down lightly. Don't just slap down your weight. Good shock absorption uses your muscles and burns more calories than sloppy walking habits.

- When going up stairs, step up on your whole foot, pushing through your heel—not just the ball of the foot.

- Take your toes in your hands and gently stretch them apart, up, down, sideways, and pull to straighten.

- When standing, keep your weight over the whole foot and heel—not leaning forward on your toes.

- Stretch the bottom of your feet, and then stretch the top, too.

- Wash your feet and between toes every day. Make sure toes are dry before putting on socks or foot covering.

- Get out of your shoes and socks for healthy exercise every day.

- Stay healthy and active to reduce chances of diseases that hurt your feet. Exercise also increases the circulation that helps feet combat the injurious effects of diseases like diabetes.

What to Avoid

- Don't clench your toes when standing.
- Don't wear shoes or socks that bend your toes against the shoe or each other.
- Don't keep toes squeezed in tight socks or hosiery all day and night.

When to Notice Feet

- Check your feet when standing on toes to prevent clenching and teetering on the little toes. Check when bending your knees to pick things up that you aren't pressing weight down on your arches. Check when walking and running that you are keeping both feet facing straight ahead.

- In the shower, can you easily wash between your toes? If your toes fit together or the big and little toe tilt toward each other, your toes are tight. This condition is usually from tight hosiery and footwear, and lack of use. Get bigger daily foot covering to allow straight toes. Stretch toes apart daily with your hands. Wiggle toes and use them to push of when you walk.

How to Get Natural Foot Stretch and Strengthening during Ordinary Activity

- Walk with both feet facing straight, not turned out, to stretch the bottom of the foot with each step.
- When going up the stairs, push off the heel for each step up. This action gives a nice stretch to the bottom of the foot with each step.
- With each step while walking and running, let the toes bend straight back. Don't push off the side of the big toe. Pushing the toe toward the other toes eventually moves it, pressuring the area when bunions form.
- For toe strength and mobility, pick up objects and clothing around the house with your bare foot. Transfer objects to your hand. Practice safely.
- Stand on toes to reach ordinary household chores. Keep weight distributed over the big and second toe, not tilted over the little toe, to strengthen feet while retraining healthy positioning.

No More Foot Pain

Your feet contribute to your overall body positioning, health, and shock absorption, which are important to preventing foot pain, and also back, neck, knee, and hip pain. Instead of doing a bunch of foot exercises or wearing special shoes, but continuing unhealthy habits for the rest of the day, you can easily change how you use and position your feet and toes for a healthier, more mobile, and comfortable life.

8

No More Leg and Foot Cramps

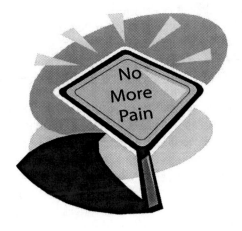

Dina came in to see what she could do about the foot and calf cramps she got almost every time she took yoga class. She said her doctor told her to eat more bananas but her yoga teacher wouldn't let them eat for two hours before class. Her personal trainer told her that cramps came from muscle fatigue after long activity, so she should rest more and drink more sport drinks, but her cramp often came on when starting a pose without having done much of anything before it. She said the pain was awful and her calf bunched in a ball and her toes pulled downward. The bottom of her foot felt like it was ripping. Her doctor told her it might be a vascular problem and that not much could be done for that without drilling open the blood vessels, taking medication, and exercising more. Dina said her yoga teacher had her do deep breathing "to get oxygen to the muscle" but that had never stopped the pain that made tears stream down her face. Her teacher told her that change is a necessary part of change—that she should work through the pain and welcome it.

I showed Dina where her calf muscle attached to her heel at the cordlike Achilles tendon. "A cramp happens when a muscle contracts and pulls whatever it is attached to. Your calf is attached to your heel and pulls your foot down like this." I pulled her heel up by the Achilles and her foot pointed down. Dina nodded. She had wondered why her foot pointed down during the cramp. I showed her where the muscles on the bottom of the foot attach from heel to toes and told her that when these muscles contract they pull the toes down too. She nodded again. I explained that unless you're ill or doing long hard exercise without food or water, cramps are rarely the result of needing food or water. Her leg and foot pulses were fine. When I squeezed her toes then let go, the blood refilled readily. I told her, "The most common cause of cramps is tightening the muscle so hard that it contracts and gets stuck. It's easy enough to give yourself a cramp just by clenching. That explains why it can happen even without doing a long race or fatiguing the muscle, even just turning over in bed." I asked her to show me the poses that cramped her legs. She sat on the floor with legs straight and together. She breathed in and out and pushed her fingers to her toes pointed in front. She said she could tell from what I told her that it was probably from contracting the calf and foot muscles so much when she pointed her toes. I reassured her it was common to get leg cramps that way. She realized that was probably why she got foot cramps at night turning over, too. She was tightening the muscles, instead of just using them easily to turn. You can contract your muscles—you need to use and strengthen them—but you don't have to force them into balled-up rocks.

Dina asked why she sometimes got the cramp in the top of her leg, too. I showed her how she was tightening her thigh muscles, the quadriceps, to help pull her body toward her leg. She was tightening the quadriceps because her hamstrings were so tight she couldn't lean forward to stretch otherwise.

I asked Dina if she ever got calf or foot cramps when standing. "Yes, when we balance on one foot in class, but I sometimes get them walking, too." She stood on one foot and put the other foot against the side of her standing leg. She stood there gripping the floor with her toes for balance. "This one kills my foot," she said. I showed her how to stand on one foot and shift her weight back to her heel to distribute her weight over the whole foot, instead of crashing forward on her clenched toes. "Hey, that makes the front of my leg feel better, too," she said. I told her this is the way to distribute body weight, not only for the occasional yoga pose, but when standing and taking the stairs. You don't want your body weight forced on the front of your foot, but distributed. Don't clench your toes when you walk. If your shoe is tight, the toes may already be pretty close to a position that is not advantageous for them. I showed her good walking gait and had her practice it with and without her shoes. A month later, when she called to check in, she said she no longer got leg cramps in or out of class. She said she was glad to learn that pain wasn't something that she had to have as 'a necessary part of change."

What Is a Muscle Cramp?

When you use a muscle in a way that makes it contract too tightly, too suddenly, it can go into an involuntary contraction—called a spasm—that does not relax again. That hurts.

What Do Muscles Do When They Cramp?

To understand muscle cramps, it helps to be able to picture what muscles do. The purpose of skeletal muscles is to move your bones. Each muscle attaches to a bone with a tough thick string called a tendon. When you want to move, you send a signal to the muscle to contract. As the muscle shortens, it pulls the tendon, which pulls the bone and moves it. Think of a marionette with strings. The strings are the tendons that hold the muscles onto the bone. The muscle pulls the string (the tendon) and the marionette's arm or leg bends.

Look for some of your own "strings." Look at the back of your hand and wiggle your fingers. You will see the strings that are the tendons of your forearm muscles. When you contract your forearm muscle, the tendon strings pull your fingers back (finger extension). Turn your hand over and bend your wrist toward you. See the tendon string of your arm muscle pull your wrist (wrist flexion). Now feel the sides of your bent knees for the tendons of the muscles in back of your thigh, called your hamstrings. When you contract your hamstrings, they bend your knee (knee flexion). Now feel for the string that is your Achilles tendon. Your Achilles attaches your calf muscle to the back of your

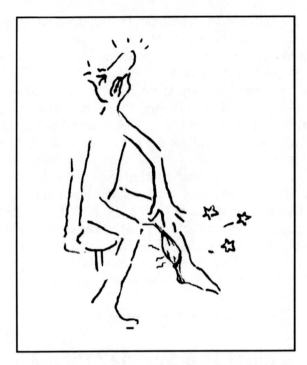

Figure 8-1. A cramp happens when a muscle shortens and won't stop shortening. In the picture, and in your own leg, find the tendon of the calf muscle, called the Achilles tendon. It is the "cord" that attaches to your heel. When the calf muscle cramps, it pulls your Achilles tendon, which pulls your heel up and your foot down.

heel. When you contracts your calf muscle, the Achilles tendon pulls your heel closer to your calf, moving your foot down—an action called plantar flexion. Plantar flexion flexes your ankle toward the sole, or plantar surface of your foot (the part you "plant" on the ground).

How to Stop Leg Cramps

A cramp can come on suddenly during activity, or just as suddenly in the night when all you did was turn over in bed. Even though the pain can be awful, it is easy to stop the pain quickly.

Leg cramps usually occur in your calf, foot, or hamstring muscles, but occasionally occur in the quadriceps muscles in the front of your thigh, or just about any other muscle depending on circumstances. Relieving a cramp can be easy and quick. A cramp is a contraction of a muscle. To release it, pull the muscle to lengthen it and the cramp will release.

Calf Cramps

If your calf muscle shortens in a cramp, it will pull your foot down. To stop the cramp, pull the top of your foot back to lengthen the muscle back to normal length. The Achilles tendon attaches to your heel. Bending the ankle and pulling the foot back lengthens the distance from calf to heel and stretches the calf muscle.

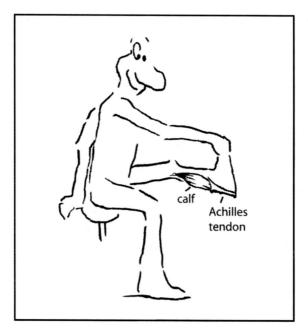

Figure 8-2. To stop a calf cramp quickly, pull your foot back
to stretch (lengthen) the shortened calf muscle.

Foot Cramps

Your foot muscles in the bottom of your foot run from heel to toe and, when they shorten, they pull the bottom of your toes and curl them downward. When these muscles cramp, they pull your toes, usually your two middle ones, downward toward the sole of your foot, painfully, and hold them there in spasm. To stop this, pull your toes back to stretch the cramping muscles on the bottom of your foot. Don't point your foot or start activity again too soon, or the muscle will likely cramp again.

Hamstring Cramps

A hamstring cramp will hurt in the back of your upper leg, and contract your hamstring muscles enough to make your knee bend. Straighten your leg and pull your foot back to stretch and stop the hamstring cramp.

Thigh Cramp

A quadriceps cramp will tighten the front of your thigh, causing your leg to straighten out, painfully. Bend your knee and pull the knee behind you to stretch the thigh.

Other Cramps

The principles are the same for any spasm your muscles may experience. Stretch the muscle to release the cramp. A common cramp is a "stitch" in your side, which can be from a cramp of the diaphragm, your breathing muscle. A stitch may occur during a run or other active sport. One way to stretch out a stitch is to take a big breath, and hold it while pushing against the held breath. The pressure stretches things a bit and often releases the cramp. Other people find relief by raising their arms and straightening up, changing from the bent-over position—which contracts the torso muscles—to a healthier muscle length.

Back spasms are also common. They can be ruinously painful, frightening, and hindersome to range of motion and activities. But they are just cramps like all the others and can often be quickly stretched out and relaxed with the proper exercises. They should not be left in spasm for any period of time. Like any other cramp, leaving it in spasm makes the muscle more ready to continue the cramp cycle.

Why Do We Get Cramps?

Land Activity

The most common reason for foot and leg cramps during activity is holding the foot, leg, and ankle muscles tightly, rather than letting them swing fluidly as you move. Tight shoes that restrict your toes or the natural range of motion of your foot when walking change the way your legs need to move, and can shorten the muscles into being more likely to cramp. Cramps in the bottom of the foot during exercise may come from clenching your toes against the floor, your shoe, or each other, during the effort.

Swimming and Finning

Calf cramps during swimming are usually caused by kicking with tight ankles, and holding the foot at a rigid angle. Cramps of the toes and the bottom of the foot during swimming or kicking with fins are usually from kicking with toes curled or clenched. Sometimes a swimmer will bend the knees too much or too hard while finning, over-contracting the hamstrings (the muscles at the back of the thigh) and causing them to cramp as well. In a pool, pushing too hard off the wall to do a start or turn can contract the calf muscle too tightly, making it cramp.

For calf cramps while swimming in shallow water, stop and stand on the non-cramping leg and stretch the cramping leg. In deep water, take a breath and float facedown to release the cramp. Remember not to point your foot right away, or resume the bad kicking that cramped you in the first place. The muscle needs time to settle down.

Sleeping

At night, a person may begin to turn over. They bend their leg, and the calf or hamstring cramps from the sudden contraction. These muscles seem to be more susceptible because in modern life, people keep these muscles shortened from sitting much of the time.

What About Walking and Pounding?

Standing up and walking around (or pounding the muscle) to stop a leg cramp is not effective, but can work coincidentally. Sometimes people with a calf cramp jump up and walk, which bends back the foot, lengthening the muscle enough to stretch out the spasm. Sometimes the pounding can push a muscle enough to lengthen it, but pounding is likely to make it contract more in sheer defense. Just stretch a cramp, and release the stretch slowly.

Should You Work Through Leg Cramps?

Don't ignore a cramp and allow it to continue cramping. Allowing a muscle to remain in spasm starts a vicious cycle. Spasm itself makes the muscle more "irritable" and ready to cramp again. In the moments after releasing a cramp, it usually feels like it wants to cramp again. For example, if you point your foot immediately after releasing a calf cramp, that contracts the calf muscle. Chances are that the calf will cramp again. Hold the stretch to release the spasm.

How to Kick Without Cramps When Swimming

The most effective prevention for leg cramps from kicking while swimming is not to kick with rigid ankles or curled toes. A good kick has loose ankles and floppy feet. It's easy to spot someone holding his ankles tightly while kicking in a pool. He barely goes forward when using a kickboard, no matter how hard he kicks. His legs often sink, and kicking is tiring.

An Exercise for Swimming Without Leg Cramps

The most common leg cramps are from holding your feet tightly. The best exercise to prevent this type of cramping is a drill to retrain your foot to be separate from the muscular control of the rest of your leg. It trains the ankle to flop loosely and not be rigidly connected to the up and down motion of the leg.

- Sit on a chair with your lower legs dangling. At a pool, sit at the rim of the pool, with your lower legs dangling free underwater.

- Grasp your lower leg near your ankle with both hands. Shake your leg up and down, paying attention to how your foot moves. It should flop freely as you shake it. Don't hold it rigidly angled at the ankle. Don't hook or curl your toes. This drill may take some work and practice. Let it be as loose and floppy as a rag doll.

- Carefully observe that as you shake your leg downward, your foot should flop upward, and as you quickly pull your leg up again, the water flops your foot downward. The foot and leg should not yank up and down as a unit. If you shake side to side, your foot should also swing freely. Make sure you use this relaxed ankle action for kicking when you get back in the pool.

The test of a good, loose kick is when you can go into a pool without fins, take a kickboard, and kick with easy, forward progress. People who have tight ankles make little, sometimes no headway. Those with tight, hooked ankles—who also use a large, deep swinging kick—can find themselves traveling backwards. Think of tight ankles, held rigidly at an angle from your leg, as airplane flaps. Trying to move forward with tight ankles is like trying to accelerate with your flaps down. With practice you can loosen your ankles, develop an easy, powerful kick, and stop most leg cramps while swimming.

What Else to Check

It is common to hear that not eating enough salt, or bananas, or lack of a specific food causes leg cramp. That situation is unlikely unless you are sick, have vomiting or diarrhea, or use diuretic medicines (water pills). An uncommon cause of constant, severe calf cramps is cirrhosis of the liver. A rare possibility is inherited disorders that specifically cause leg cramps. Sometimes the pain is not muscle cramps, but other conditions confused for cramps. Arteries of the leg can narrow for the same reasons as blood vessels anywhere in the body. Vascular disease is not just of the heart. When a person with narrowed leg arteries starts activity, the legs need more blood than can fit through those vessels, and the leg cries in pain for oxygen—which is called claudication, from a Latin word meaning "lameness." Those people at highest risk are sedentary, smokers, or fond of unhealthy diets. Another issue is pregnancy, which often presses on vessels exiting to the legs, causing leg pain and cramping.

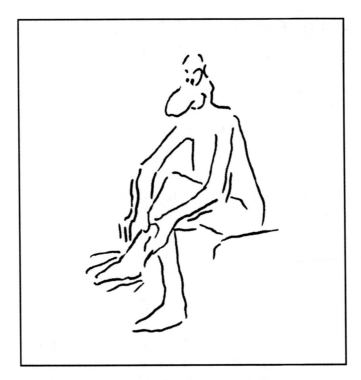

Figure 8-3. To retrain your ankles for swimming, practice this "floppy foot" exercise until you can flop your foot loosely at the ankle. Then use this loose ankle for flutter kicking. The rest of the leg still powers the kick, without the stiff ankle that slows the kick and causes calf and foot cramping.

What to Do Every Day to Prevent Leg Cramps

- Stretch the back of your legs. It has been noted by muscle physiologists that in societies without sit-down toilets, the habitual squatting stretches the muscles, making calf and foot cramps rare. See Chapter 6 on ankle and Achilles tendon stretches, and Chapter 9 for hamstrings stretches.

- Use healthy muscle motion for all activity. Don't do stretches and then walk around all day holding your leg, ankle, and feet muscles tightly.

- Make sure your feet can move. Don't wear tight, uncomfortable shoes, or shoes that you may think are comfortable but that restrict your toes or the natural range of motion of your foot and ankle when walking.

How to Get Natural Cramp Prevention during Daily Activity

- For all the many times a day you bend to reach or retrieve things, bend right using legs instead of bending over at the waist. Bend both knees keeping heels down on the floor. Doing so gives a built-in stretch to the back of the lower leg.

- When you squat down to sit, keep both heels down on the ground. If you are too tight to sit without raising your heels, the backs of your legs are tight.

- Sit up straight. Don't round your back and tuck the hip under when sitting, which can shorten the hamstrings.

- When you bend to sit in a chair, keep heels down on the way down. When rising from a chair, keep heels down on the way up.

No More Leg Cramps

Do regular, easy stretches for your legs and feet, and build up the muscles of your legs so they can handle exertion better, and so that they are not as likely to cramp. Learn easy cramp releases so that you don't have to suffer the pain of cramps, and can stop them easily and quickly.

9

How to Stretch Your Hamstrings

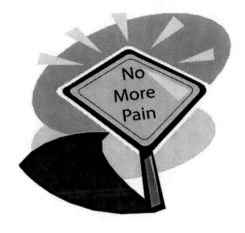

The Police Department Training Bureau phoned me. They had a candidate who had done eight of the nine months of the training academy. Stan was two weeks away from graduating but could not graduate. He had passed firearms and physical training and all his written tests with high marks. But he could not graduate to become a police officer because he could not pass the "sit and reach" test. The "sit and reach" test measures what people commonly associate with hamstring flexibility—how far you can lean forward when sitting and reach toward your toes.

The assumption behind the "sit and reach" test is that hamstring inflexibility is somehow related to getting lower-back pain. The department didn't want anyone out with back pain. So all candidates had to pass the test.

Stan couldn't pass the test and no one knew why. He had been sent for his tightness to the police doctor, then another doctor. He went for physical therapy, massage, and chiropractic treatment. He stretched every day. He had been to two personal trainers. They put him through workouts, warm-ups, and pushed and pulled his legs. He was ready to see a hypnotist next. Nothing was working.

I met with Stan. He looked strong and active. I asked if he wanted to graduate. Yes. Was he being pushed to graduate by family? No. Did he need any reason to get out of this? No. Did he want me to write him a note excusing him from testing? No. Everything seemed in order. The issue really was the "sit and reach" test. I asked him to show me how we was doing the test. He sat on the floor and reached forward. His hands hovered not much further than his knees. Not a passing score. Not close to a passing score.

I asked him what he had been doing to practice flexibility. He said that every day, he and the guys at the academy worked on it. He stood bent over and they pushed hard on his back. He said one of the guys told him to take two 50-pound weights and bend over with them, letting the weights pull him toward the ground. I told him those things could injure his back. He said, "You're not kidding. My back never hurt before until I started trying to touch my toes."

I asked him to show me how he would pick up something from the floor. He bent his knees in flawless lifting technique. I told him, "That's pretty good, most people bend over wrong at the waist or hip instead of keeping their body upright and bending their knees."

He said, "I *can't* bend over wrong. I'm too tight to reach the ground!" It was true. Stan's hamstrings were so tight that he had to bend correctly or not reach the ground at all. I asked Stan to sit on the floor again, legs out in front. He was able to do this by rounding his back and tilting his hip back (Figure 9-1).

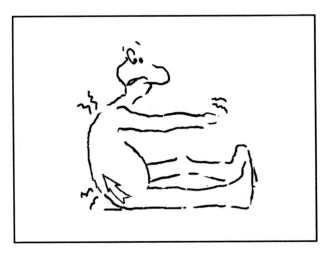

Figure 9-1. Doing hamstring stretches by rounding forward gives little hamstring stretch but reinforces poor rounded posture and adds outward pressure on the discs of the lower back and neck.

I asked Stan to tilt his hip so that it was straight up and down, not tilted back, sitting up on his "sit bones." He tried, but the hip didn't budge. That result is common with tight hamstrings because the hamstrings attach to the bottom of your hip bone, on the "sit bones." When the hip is tight, or the hamstrings can't lengthen, the bottom of the hip is held tightly pulled under when sitting with the legs out. You can't straighten your back to sit up straight. Your back and hip are pulled into a rounded position. The hamstrings stay shortened. It is a negative cycle of stretching wrong and staying too tight to get any stretch.

I had Stan bend his knees and sit cross-legged so that the hamstrings were no longer involved. I asked him to move his hip, and again it would not budge from the rolled-back, rounded position (Figure 9-2).

The answer was clear. Because Stan couldn't move his hip into a position that stretched the hamstrings, they never got much stretch—even when he was doing maneuvers that people commonly assume is a hamstring stretch—like touching the toes. He was rounding his back. He was craning his neck. He was stretching his arms. He was pulling his chin toward his toes. He was doing everything except moving his hip so that the hamstrings could lengthen enough to get any stretch.

I asked Stan to stand up again to make it easier for him to isolate the needed hip movement. I showed him how to tuck the hip under too much so that the bottom of the hip came forward, and then arch his back too much so that the bottom of the hip stuck out in back—like club dancing. At first nothing moved. He bowed forward and back from the waist, then tried bending from the hip—

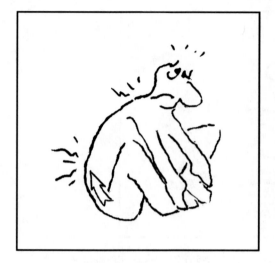

Figure 9-2. When hip and leg muscles are tight, the top of the hip tips backward and the bottom of the hip rolls under. The legs do not get the intended stretch and you sit reinforcing an overly rounded back and adding to outward pressure on the discs.

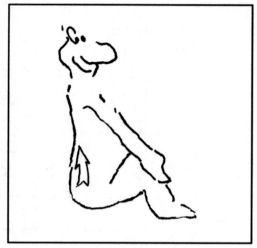

Figure 9-3. To sit straight, you need to be able to move the hip to straighten the lower back, by tilting the top of the hip forward. This movement stretches the legs and stops outward pressure on the discs.

like a formal Asian bow—but could not get his hip to swivel under and back. We practiced a bit until I thought I saw a glimmer of movement. We sat on the floor again. He tried sitting cross-legged again and moved his hip. This time he was able to move the hip enough to sit up straight (Figure 9-3).

I asked Stan to sit with his legs out straight again, rest his weight on his hands behind him, lift his chest so his body was sitting straight up, and straighten his back (Figure 9-4, right). His hip moved back and he looked startled. "What is that feeling?"

"Stan, that's your hamstrings. You never stretched them much before so you never felt them." The reason that all his stretching practice didn't improve his flexibility was that he never stretched what he thought he was stretching. His hamstrings weren't getting the intended stretch.

Where Are Your Hamstrings?

Your hamstrings are three muscles in the back of each upper leg. Each attaches to your hipbone on the bump at the bottom called the ischium—your "sit bone." The bump is called the ischial tuberosity. The hamstrings go from the ischial tuberosity down the

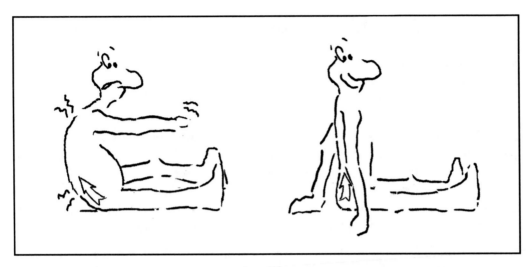

Figure 9-4. Letting the hip rock back (left) stretches the hamstrings less than sitting up (right). Try it yourself. Put your hands behind you to take weight off the discs, push to sit straight up, and get the stretch from the legs—not the back.

back of each leg and cross your knee to the top of your lower-leg bone. Two hamstrings cross the inside of each knee and the third crosses on the outside (Figure 9-5). You can feel the strings of the hamstring tendons on the inside and outside at the back of the knee. Hamstrings cross two joints—the hip and knee—which is why they can bend your knee and also help move your hip.

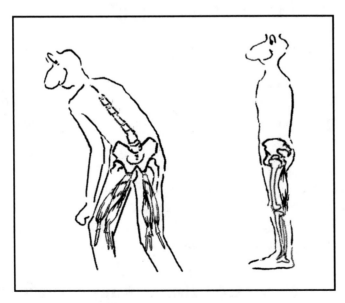

Figure 9-5. Hamstrings. Three hamstrings on each leg attach to the "bump" at the bottom of the hip, and the lower-leg bone below the knee.

Does Stretching Hamstrings Stop Back Pain?

Many people have heard that the hamstrings have something to do with back pain. It's a common extension of that assumption that touching the toes stretches the hamstrings and therefore will help prevent back pain. But what do hamstrings have to do with back pain? When hamstrings are tight, you cannot sit without rounding your back. The irony is that many people crane their neck, round their back, and tilt their hip backward, producing minimal stretch on the hamstring and great pressure on the neck, lumbar discs, and soft tissue of the back. Why do people round their back? Because it feels easier. In other words, it reduces the stretch. Rounding to stretch practices the already rounded posture that contributes to back pain. Even with flexible hamstrings, many people sit rounded, and the stretching didn't help either way.

One common hamstring-flexibility test measures if you have a minimum ability to raise one leg to 90 degrees straight overhead when lying on your back. Why 90 degrees? Because if you can't bend at the hip 90 degrees, you can't sit up straight without rounding your back. You hip needs to bend to 90 degrees to sit up with your back straight and your legs out.

You already know that sitting with a rounded back is poor posture. It is a common cause of back pain and pressures the discs of the lower back. It is just as damaging to stretch like that. Make sure that you stretch your hamstrings for the right reason, in the way that really does what you think.

How to Stretch Hamstrings Sitting

To stretch your hamstrings you need to lengthen them. Picture your hamstring muscles between the back of your knee and your sit bones. You need to make that distance longer. You can do that when sitting with straight legs by tilting your hip so that the bottom of the hip pulls back. Sit up and pull the ischial tuberosity "sit bones" back to do that. If you round your hip and back, you lessen the stretch (Figure 9-6).

Although the most common image of hamstring stretching is toe touching, you will lengthen the hamstring more by sitting straight when stretching, instead of letting the top of the hip roll back. Sit up with your weight on your hands in back. Feel the bottom of your hip, or "sit-bones," move back and the top of the hip move forward, until you can do this without resting on your hands. Instead of sitting rounded in your chair, remember to use healthier sitting position for all sitting.

How to Stretch Hamstrings Standing

Bending over from a stand is so damaging to the back that you already know not to lift

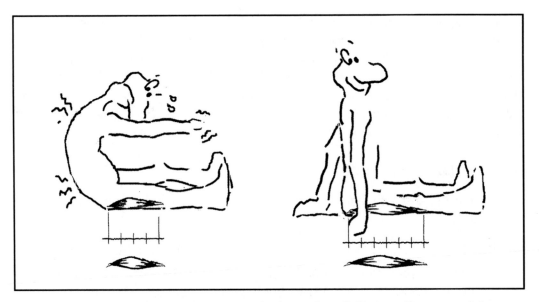

Figure 9-6. Letting the hip roll back shortens the hamstrings (left). Even if you spend time every day like this touching your toes, you will not get an effective hamstring stretch, but will practice the same rounded back that you already know is not healthy. Instead, sit up and tip the top of the hip forward to lengthen the hamstrings (right).

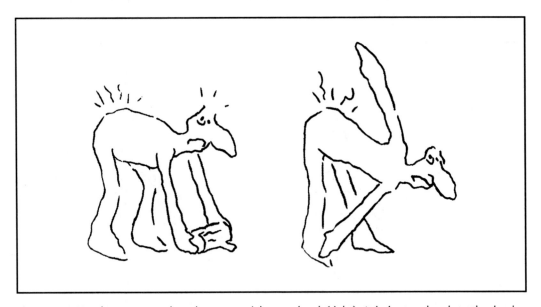

Figure 9-7. You know not to bend over to pick up a load (right). It is just as hard on the back to stretch this way (left).

packages like that. It is also damaging to stretch like that (Figure 9-7). With your back straight or rounded, different forces are on the lower back, but still not forces you want.

Bending correctly does not mean that you can't do fun or athletic things ,or that you must treat your back like you are an invalid—just the opposite. With healthy positioning you can do more than before. Lifting weights can be healthy. You just don't want to put that weight on the discs and joints of your lower back. For lifting things, keep the upper body as upright as you can and bend your knees, keeping knees over the feet—not slouching forward of the feet (Figure 5-4). More effective hamstring stretches are possible than simply bending over from a stand.

Standing Hamstring Stretch

A better hamstring stretch than bending from a stand is to stand upright and lift the leg (Figure 9-8).

- Prop one heel directly in front of you on a chair or other surface.

- Look down at your standing foot. If it is turned outward, even a small amount, the turn-out reduces the stretch. Move your foot to face the toes straight forward. The small change of facing the foot straight does much to change the stretch into one that stretches the hamstring.

- Keep your torso upright and straighten your back instead of rounding forward.

- Keep the stretched leg straight ahead not angled out to the side. Lift your chest, and pull the hip back to stretch the hamstring.

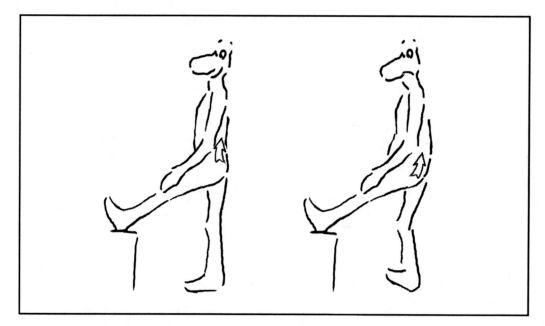

Figure 9-8. Positioning makes the difference between a good stretch and almost no stretch. Stand straight (left) and feel the stretch. Keep the stretched leg directly in front, not off to the side. Keep the standing foot and leg facing front (left), not turned out or bent (right).

- Don't "lock" the standing knee straight. Keep a small bend, with weight on the thigh muscles.

Standing Wall Hamstring Stretch

A quick, effective standing hamstring stretch is the wall hamstring stretch (Figure 9-9).

- Face a wall, standing with both feet facing straight ahead at about arm's length away form the wall. This position will feel too close to try the stretch, but it is about right.
- Look down to see if your foot is turned out. Keep your standing foot facing straight forward, not turned out—not even a small amount. Lift the other leg to about knee height and press the bottom of the foot against the wall.
- Stand with your torso upright. Straighten your back instead of rounding forward.
- Keep the stretched leg straight ahead not out to the side. Lift your chest and pull the hip back to feel the stretch in the hamstring. Don't "lock" the standing knee straight. Keep a small bend with weight on the thigh muscles.
- As you get better, raise the height of the stretched leg, keeping the standing foot facing straight ahead, not turned out.

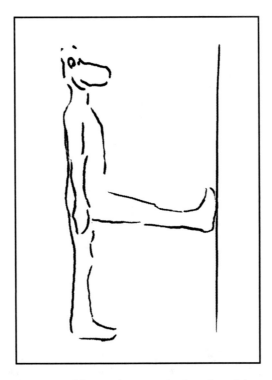

Figure 9-9. Wall hamstring stretch. Stand straight and push heel to wall for a quick effective stretch.

Standing Air Split

A fun way to stretch the hamstrings from a stand and improve balance is to tilt forward while lifting the back leg straight and high overhead.

- Stand on one leg and bring your hands to the floor. Lift the other leg straight and high overhead behind you.

- Instead of rounding your chest toward the standing leg, press your lower abdomen, keeping your back straight and chest up.

- Push your weight back toward the heel of the standing foot. Don't "lock" the standing knee straight. Keep a small bend with your body weight on the thigh muscles, not the knee joint.

- Keep the lifted knee facing down, not turned out.

- This stretch can also be done with the raised foot up on the wall. Push your weight back against the wall. Keep weight on the standing leg toward the heel. Relax your muscles into the stretch.

- To work on balance, do this stretch without hands. Keep body weight pushed back over the heel. Don't rock forward and round your back to keep balance.

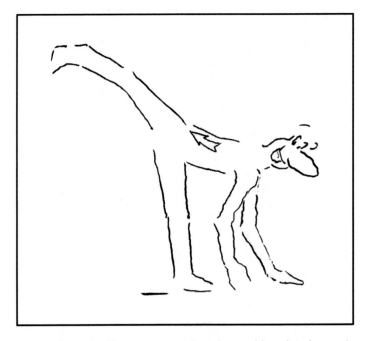

Figure 9-10. Standing air split is a way to do a forward-bending hamstring stretch without pressuring the discs or rounding the back. It also improves balance.

How to Stretch the Hamstrings Lying Down

A simple, effective stretch is to lie face up and stretch one leg overhead (Figure 9-11).

- Keep your head and hip on the floor, not rounding.
- Let your shoulders and head relax against the floor, not rounded upward.
- Keep chin in, not jutting upward.

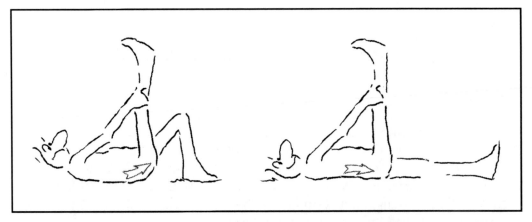

Figure 9-11. Bending the bottom knee reduces the stretch (left). Keep head and shoulders on the ground to practice healthy positioning. Keep the bottom leg straight (right). Doing so gives a better hamstring stretch and stretches the front of the hip at the same time, another needed stretch.

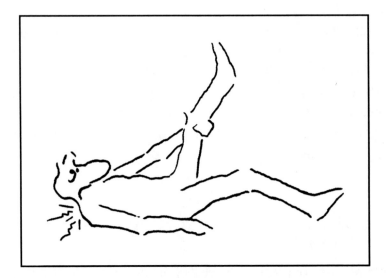

Figure 9-12. Don't let your other leg pull upward along with the leg you're stretching. This shows a tight hip. Get the free hip stretch by keeping the leg down straight.

- Don't round your back or let your hip tilt under. Keep both hips on the floor. Then the stretch comes from your hamstring, not the back.
- Keep the other leg straight on the floor, not bent at the knee. It is not true that you must bend the bottom knee to protect the back. Bending the knee perpetuates tightness and poor positioning.

When the front of the hip is tight, your hip will curl the under you when you raise your leg. This situation reduces the stretch, practices rounded posture, and increases pressure on your back (Figure 9-12).

Techniques to Increase Flexibility

PNF

One technique to improve immediate flexibility is called "push-pull," "contract-relax," "muscle energy technique," or "proprioceptive neuromuscular facilitation" (PNF). You can apply it to any muscle. The concept is to hold a maximum comfortable stretch, then push (contract) against resistance in the direction opposite the stretch for four or five seconds without moving the limb to fatigue the muscle. Then pull (relax) to increase the stretch. Use this technique slowly and safely.

- To stretch hamstrings with "push-pull" PNF, lie face-up with one leg lifted at maximum comfortable stretch. Shoulders, head, and other leg should be flat. Hold the lifted leg with hands or rest your heel against a wall or a partner holding your leg.
- Push the lifted leg downward against the resistance of your hands, wall, or partner. The resistance does not let the leg move, even though you are pushing. Push downward for about five counts to fatigue the hamstrings.
- Stop pushing down. Pull the leg gently toward your chest with your hands. It should gain a greater stretch.
- Repeat, pushing against resistance at the new stretch length, then gently pull in to the next greater stretch. Keep breathing. Repeat for three stretches on each leg.

Active Assist

Another technique for gaining greater stretch is "active assist." You use the opposite muscles to assist pulling the stretch.

- To use active assist for hamstring stretching, lie on your back, or stand, with one leg lifted. Shoulders, head, and other leg should be kept flat and straight.

- Don't hold your lifted leg with your hands. Assist the stretch of the lifted leg toward your body only using your thigh muscles. Hold in the air for four to five seconds, and then pull the leg further toward your body using your hands.

- Hold the new further stretch for four to five seconds, then let go of your hands and pull the leg further toward your body using your thigh muscles for four or five seconds.

- Try at least three assisted stretches on each leg.

Dynamic Stretching

Many people stand, sit, or lie still to stretch, then wonder why they pull or strain a muscle when they go do something. They were not training their muscles to extend and lengthen under loading. This lack of training is one reason why some studies are finding that stretching is not reducing injuries the way previously hoped. One reason is the way people stretch and then they way they more.

- Do lunges up and down in a wide stance (Figure 3-6).
- Stand with good back and body positioning. Swing one leg up with a straight—not locked—knee, high to the front. Make sure not to round your back or let the hip of the standing leg curl under. Do this motion slowly at first working up to faster swings. The idea is not to pull or strain a muscle, and to train the muscle how to exercise and stretch together in a functional, safe way. This method is also used for other muscles in other directions.

Rotational Stretching

- Turn the stretching leg inward then outward while stretching. Keep back and hip straight.
- Repeat ten to twenty times on each leg.

What to Do Every Day to Increase Hamstring Flexibility

- Stretch your hamstrings, keeping your back and neck straight. Relearn how to get the stretch from the leg not the back. When stretching one leg at a time, keep the other leg straight to get more hamstring stretch and add an important stretch to the front of the hip. Transfer this knowledge to healthy positioning during movement.

What to Avoid

- Don't let your hip roll under you, rounding your back when sitting, kicking, pushing things with your leg, ascending stairs, or stretching.

How to Get Natural Hamstring Stretch during Daily Activity

Instead of making your hamstrings tight all day with bad positioning then trying to undo the damage with a few stretches, it is healthier, easier, and smarter to live and move without making your hamstrings tight in the first place.

- Don't round when sitting.
- Instead of sitting in a chair when you watch television, lie facedown and stretch legs up to the sides or lie on your back, stretching legs up overhead and out to the sides in various ways—the way children do. It's better and more fun than shortening your hamstrings sitting in a chair.
- Try the "air split" (Figure 9-10) for picking things up around the house.

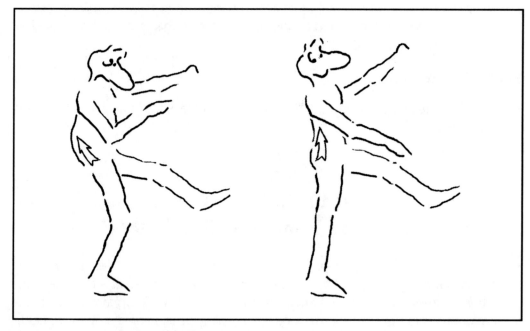

Figure 9-13. Letting the standing leg come forward when stretching or kicking the raised leg (left) is a bad habit that reduces stretch on the hamstrings. Many people do so because they are too tight to do it any other way. If you want to stretch to prevent back pain, don't add to back pain by stretching this way. Keep the back and the hip of the standing leg straight (right).

- When you run or step up high, don't let your back round, the hip tilt under, or your head come forward.

- Depending on your level, for fun try turning on light switches, even elevator buttons, or opening drawers with your foot. Remember that in some cultures (for example, some Asian areas), pointing at things—or especially people—with your foot is offensive. Know your locality.

- When you lift one leg to kick in aerobics, self-defense, ballet, tai chi, dance, or martial arts classes, or even to push a door open, don't let your back round and the standing leg bend forward. Keep the back upright, and the standing hip straight, not rounded under.

No More Tight, Painful Hamstrings

When you spend time doing stretches for your hamstrings, make sure you're really stretching your hamstrings. It is common to stretch everything except for the intended area. Don't hurt your back in the name of stretching your hamstrings, especially if you're stretching your hamstrings thinking it will prevent back pain. Lie or stand straight, and get the stretch from the hamstring, not by rounding the back.

One of the purposes of stretching is to lengthen the muscle. Check to see if you tighten your legs and body while stretching. Remember that lying still and stretching is not the same as using muscles for real activity. A main benefit of stretching is supposed to be that you apply healthy muscle length and positioning in daily life to prevent strains and pulls. Make sure that you don't stretch, then clench and tighten your muscles when moving in real life. Rethink your exercises to make sure your fitness is healthy. Instead of "doing a bunch of stretches," learn healthy movement from your stretches.

10

No More Wrist Pain

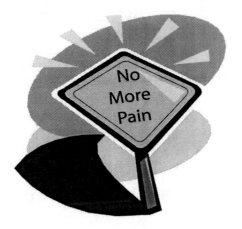

- Wrist Pain
- Repetitive-Motion Injury
- Carpal Tunnel Syndrome
- De Quervain's Tendonitis
- Weak Wrists
- Preventing Osteoporosis

everal things can make wrists hurt. This short chapter concentrates on the most common causes. Wrist pain can be easy to understand and to fix.

Is Repetitive Motion the Problem?

The most common explanation most people are given for wrist pain is overuse. They are told to rest the wrist, not bend it backward, and keep it straight, even in splints. Common treatments are medicines like pain relievers, muscle relaxants, cortisone shots, and surgery to widen the area. Luckily, these treatments are usually not needed, even though they are often used.

Pain that is usually thought of as overuse is frequently from not using hand and arm muscles to power the wrist. Weight falls on the joints of the wrist instead of being held up on the muscles of the forearm and hand. You can use your wrists all you want, at all kinds of angles, by healthy use of surrounding muscles.

What Are Carpal Tunnel Syndrome and De Quervain's Tendonitis?

Carpal tunnel syndrome occurs when a major nerve to the hand, called the median nerve, gets compressed at the wrist. The word carpal means wrist bones. The carpal tunnel is a small passage between the wrist bones. The median nerve and tendons that bend some of the fingers pass through this tunnel. Pain and weakness or tingling in the palm, wrist, thumb, or fingers can result.

De Quervain's tendonitis is named for Swiss surgeon Fritz de Quervain. Pain is on the radial (thumb) side of the wrist from pressure and swelling over two tendons that move the thumb (abductor pollicis longus, and extensor pollicis brevis). De Quervain's tendonitis is different from De Quervain's thyroiditis, a problem of low thyroid function also identified by Dr. De Quervain.

Osteoporosis

The wrist is one of three main sites of osteoporosis in both men and women. A fall on an outstretched hand should not break the wrist. A wrist fracture from a fall or impact that should not have otherwise broken the bone can be a sign of osteoporosis.

Exercise thickens bones from the physical pull of the muscles pulling the bones to move them and hold them in place against resistance. Lack of exercise is a major factor in osteoporosis, no matter how much calcium you eat. Without exercise, you "pee" the calcium you eat back out. You need to give calcium a reason to stick on the bones. Get sunshine. Calcium needs vitamin D to work to build bone through exercise. Exercising, even late in life, builds new bone and slows or stops loss. The kind of exercise that strengthens wrists puts weight on the wrists, either lifting weights or your own body weight (for example, holding a push-up position). Holding up your own body weight is a minimal skill to stay mobile and prevent being hurt by your own body weight.

Common medicines that decrease bone density are oral anti-inflammatory drugs called corticosteroids, often given for allergy, rheumatoid arthritis, asthma, pulmonary disease, and some pain syndromes. Most of the bone loss occurs within the first weeks of use. As a generality, it may take as many months or years to rebuild the bone density as the time spent on the medicine.

How to Stop Injuring Wrists

Carpal tunnel syndrome, De Quervain's tendonitis, and other pain syndromes that are lumped together as repetitive strain injury (RSI) or repetitive motion injury (RMI), all seem to be caused from not using the wrist well, rather than from using it too much. It is not repetitive motion itself that is the problem.

Wrists, like every other joint, need strong muscles to keep the joint in healthy position and do tasks. Splinting and limiting use weaken the wrists further. Like all joints, wrists need movement for joint lubrication and healthy muscle use. If you put any healthy joint in a cast or splint, it becomes shrunken, weak, and stiff. Any joint that is not moved enough usually begins to fill with stiff scar tissue, making movement more painful and difficult. The key with injured joints is making a balance between not injuring it further and getting the healthy motion it needs to heal.

To see the difference between bending your wrist back in healthy movement and squashing it, try the following:

- Put your palms and fingers together in front of you, as if praying.

- Use one hand to start pressing the other so that it bends backward at the wrist. Don't let the compressive pain start when doing this. Resist with the hand being pushed so that the hand still bends back the same amount, but the wrist joint is not compressed under the bend.

- Push hands back and forth strongly, so that you train moving the wrists backward, and become able to put weight on them without compressing the joint and soft tissue within.

Prevent Pain with Healthy Strengthening

Hand wraps and wrist guards are not needed for lifting weight or doing push-ups. Instead, retrain use of the hand, wrist, and forearm to power the wrist. It used to be thought that someone with wrist pain should not do push-ups or hold a push-up position. Then it was found that using and strengthening the wrists, even with push-ups, could fix many wrist injuries when done properly. Strengthening wrists by putting weight on them thickens wrist bones, important to osteoporosis prevention.

- Hold a push-up position. Keep weight distributed over the whole hand, pressing with fingers and using hand muscle, not just compressing the wrist. Keep body position from sagging (Figure 2-33). Don't "lock" the elbows. Keep them slightly bent to keep weight on the arm muscles and not the elbow joint.

- Hold a push-up position. Practice shifting weight from hand to hand.

Depending on your fitness level and goals, progress to the following. These activities are not necessary to stop wrist pain. They can be used to increase fitness while using the hands and wrists without injury.

- Hold the push-up position. Keep elbows slightly bent. "Walk" your hands and feet sideways, like a spider, a few steps, then "walk" back. Use hand and arm muscles strongly to cushion each "hand-step" instead of banging weight down on the wrists. Keep body weight distributed over the entire hand, not just on the heel of the hand, to strengthen the wrist without compressing the joints.

- Work up to holding a healthy push-up position with feet propped on a bench or other height. Increase the height of the prop until you can put most of your weight on your hands.

- Hold a push-up position, Turn your body and lift one hand so that you are standing on one hand and foot, facing the side (Figure 2-38). Keep body weight distributed over the entire hand, not just on the heel of the hand.

- When using band, strengthen in functional manner for your whole body while training good wrist position (Figure 2-41).

- Hang from an overhead support like a chinning bar or secure branch to get free traction for the wrist. Hanging is usually a good stretch for the whole body. Don't let body weight pull the wrist out of joint, use muscles to hold the wrist from being pulled too far. Increase time of hang to increase hand, grip, and arm strength. Begin doing little elbow bends, working up to pull-ups.

Prevent Pain with Healthy Positioning

When preparing food, instead of letting your wrist be forced back under the push of the knife or washing cloth, use hand strength to power the movement and hold your wrist. The wrist can bend back, but it is not angulated back under pressure. Use the muscles of the hand to push forward to prevent the wrist from angling back. This approach is the same idea as being able to extend your lower back backward for activities without compressing it under your body weight. Move the computer keyboard up and off the tray below the desk. Most ergonomic instructions say to lower the keyboard to prevent bending the wrists backward, but it is the low position that increases the backward craning, plus rounding at the shoulder that increases neck and upper-back pain. When lifting dumbbells overhead, don't let the weight crane the wrists backward. Use hand muscles to hold them straight, and to press against the backward push of the weight. When doing handwork like sewing, art, and home repair, use hand and finger muscles instead of letting the item you are working on press the wrist joint back. It does not mean that you should limit movement by holding wrists straight, but to use muscles instead of resting weight on the joint.

When punching a target or bag in martial arts, self-defense, and aerobic boxing classes, use muscles of the forearm to keep the wrist straight and the fist tight, and straight in line with the arm. Punching on a bent wrist—either up or down, or tilting to the side—are common causes of big injuries and aches. Keep impact directed through the first and second knuckle, not the side of the hand. Use arm muscles and keep the elbow slightly bent at the end range for shock absorption, don't just let the impact jar the wrist. For a sudden self-defense situation, it's better to use open-hand techniques, or use a rock or stick, than to use closed-fist punching. Without much training, and even with training, breaks and injuries to the hand and wrist from hand-to-hand fighting are common.

What Else to Check

Human growth hormone (HGH) is taken by some people hoping it will help their bodybuilding or make them seem younger. It can make the chin and forehead enlarge, and is a big hidden cause of wrist pain. Use of anabolic steroids, and long use of fluroquinolone antibiotics like Cipro, Floxin, and Noroxin, increases risk of tendonitis and ligament tear or rupture.

Your doctor can check for growths in the wrist like a ganglion cyst or metacarpal boss, tumor, infection, psoriatic arthritis that accompanies psoriasis, gout, thyroid problems, diabetes, and broken bones.

Common medications have the side effects of causing joint pain including cholesterol-lowering drugs called statin drugs, some prescription allergy medicines, stomach-acid inhibitors, prescription anti-depressant and anti-anxiety medicines, prescription acne medicines, medicines for irritable bowel, constipation, and Crohn's disease, some HIV medications, the calcium-channel-blocker drug, verapamil, the antibiotics erythromycin and clarithromycin, and others. Doing a few stretches and strengthening exercises does not stop this pain. In most cases, it is better to address the cause of the problems, rather than take drugs that cause other problems.

What to Do Every Day

- Stretch the shoulder with the pectoral stretch (Figure 3-3) and trapezius stretch (Figure 3-4) to restore healthy upper-body muscle length. Doing daily tasks with rounded shoulders can contribute to not using the wrists in healthy position, and can press on nerves that go down the arm, sending pain as far as the wrist and hand.

- Stretch hands and fingers back and apart.

- Wrap rubber bands around your fingers and open them against the tension of the bands.

- Hold one hand closed with the other and open fingers against the resistance.

- Get out in the sunshine every day. Lack of vitamin D can be a hidden source of joint and muscle pain, and is a large factor in osteoporosis.

- To keep wrist bones strong, load wrists through push-ups, weightlifting, and other exercise where you put weight on your hands and arms. Osteoporosis is not something that just happens to old people; it begins in youth. Your bone density later in life depends on what you are doing now.

- Hold a push-up position (Figures 2-33 and 2-35). Press with finger and hand muscles to keep the weight distributed over the whole hand—not compressing the heel of the hand and wrist.

- Hold a push-up position on your fingers. Increase ability of your hand to support your weight. Work up to push-ups and handstands.

- Rethink exercise as something that comes from daily healthy movement. Many people who exercise and regularly strengthen still have poor movement habits that create pain. While preparing food and cleaning surfaces, let the wrists move freely, and do not compress under the movement.

When to Notice Wrists

- Notice if you let your wrists angle back when preparing food, using dishrags, drawing, sewing, painting, assembling parts, typing, or driving. Use hand and finger muscles to power hand movement, don't just let the weight press backward on the wrist joint.

How to Get Wrist Strengthening during Daily Activity

Safely work up to doing more, not less. Wring clothes dry, give massage, knead bread, use hammers, pliers, and screwdrivers. Carry suitcases and buckets down at your side by the handles to strengthen hands. Carry bags and packages in arms using hand strength instead of letting the weight of the package push the wrists back. Snap sticks. Squeeze things. Work with clay. Open jars.

No More Wrist Pain

More use to strengthen wrists, not less use is often the answer for painful wrists. Weak, painful wrists can be a helpful warning to become more active with healthier habits. Instead of taking medicine and making wrists weaker and stiffer in splints, learn healthy use. Instead of doing a bunch of rehabilitation exercises then going back to injurious household and work habits, power all your hand movements with the muscles of the hands and arms, rather than letting the weight press and twist the wrists. Fix the cause and you can fix the pain, stop recurring injuries, and create a healthier life at the same time. You will be able to do more with less pain than before. You don't have to live with pain.

11

Multiple Pain–
When Everything Hurts

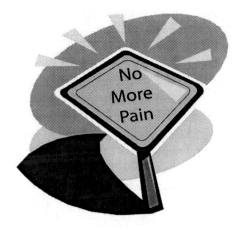

- Arthritis
- Fibromyalgia
- Mystery Pain and More

People often have pain in several places. Sometimes one pain is related to the other. Sometimes they are separate problems but both from unhealthy mechanical use. It is not complicated to apply healthy principles to rehab several problems or injuries at once. Other times more things contribute, like medicines that cause pain and feed into a cycle of doing less and hurting more. Many of the most common medications taken for pain, and even "health," are a surprising source of problems. The key is to treat the cause of the pain as directly as possible, not the symptoms with medicines, so that the pain stops at the source.

Von was an active salesman in his 50s. He went on travel often, always sending me word when he'd miss class. He was strong, cheerful, and worked hard. He started missing more often, until we didn't see him at all for a while. When he came back, he said he had hurt his shoulder on a shoulder machine. When he had brought the weight to his chest, the joint overstretched where his shoulder bone (acromion) joined the collarbone (clavicle). The joint is called the acromial-clavicular joint (A-C, for short). Von had an A-C separation. He was told never to bring a weight down to his chest, to cut back his weightlifting, stop doing push-ups, and take anti-inflammatory medications. The shoulder got somewhat better but continued to hurt when he tried weightlifting or push-ups. It ached combing his hair. I showed him that he could lift weight and protect the shoulder by not letting the weight press the A-C joint open. Joints need movement to heal and be healthy. When his arm lowered the weight, he would use the chest muscles more and not let the front of the shoulder come forward as the elbow went back. He could do the same with push-ups. I explained, "It's your muscles that are supposed to hold up the weight. I know it's easier to lever the weight the joint, but it's better exercise to use the muscles. Then the joint can move without being pried apart." The idea was to work on this until he could move the shoulder through full range, doing whatever exercise he liked to do, without prying open the joint. He left looking happy enough. We didn't see him again for a while.

When Von came to class, he didn't look like his strong, cheerful self. He told me he was being treated for flu or something else; no one was sure just what. He felt weak, he had body aches, and he had tingling in his fingers. Wow. Was the tingling from the shoulder injury? It wasn't along the usual nerve pathways that would be hurt or be compressed from something in the shoulder. I looked over his elbow and wrist, too. It didn't seem like it was from an injury but you couldn't be sure. Had he seen a neurologist? He had an appointment to see one. What about the body aches? Did he have fever? No. How long had it been going on? Months now.

I asked him, "Are you taking medicine?"

"No." "Are you allergic to anything?"

"No."

"Have you traveled anywhere with tropical diseases or unsanitary food?"

"No. Well, I had Mexican food at a restaurant here in town and got sick in my stomach and all over. My lips were tingling."

"Did you eat any seafood?"

"No, I'm allergic to seafood."

"I thought you said you don't have allergies. Do you take anything for allergies?"

"Flonase, but that's just for my nose."

I tried it a little differently. "Do you take glucosamine supplements?"

"Yes."

"Von, it could be the supplements. It is made from ingredients that people who are allergic to shellfish cannot take. You might have a low-grade anaphalaxis, which is an allergic reaction. It can explain the aches, the gastrointestinal distress, and the tingling. We hope it works for joint pain, many people are happy, but we don't know. Stop taking the glucosamine for a while and see how you feel."

Later that month I bumped into Von's doctor. He said I was nuts to take him off his glucosamine because he needed it for his shoulder pain plus all the other joint pain he had been developing. I said I thought he was having an allergic reaction. The doc told me I was wrong because Von could breathe just fine and it was no allergic emergency. I said it didn't have to be an emergency. A low-grade allergic reaction was making him feel not himself, hindering his life, ongoing, avoidable, and that was reason enough. He said, "That's not anaphylaxis."

A month later Von came in looking shaken. He had gotten faint in the gym and had been rushed to the cardiac ward. Because he was a man in his 50s, he was given a full battery of cardiac tests with radioactive contrast, plus tests and scans for cancer. He didn't have his results yet and it was on his mind.

"Von, what else are you taking?"

"Nothing."

"What prescription did your doctor give you?"

"Oh, well something for the joint pain, a kind of anti-inflammatory I think, and a prescription for my stomach, because that really acts up when I take the pain stuff."

"What do you buy when you go to the health food store?"

"Oh, well, you know, the usual." Von had been spending almost a hundred dollars a month on supplements that the clerks and magazines said would help. When he said "the usual," he meant "men's supplements" like saw palmetto, ginseng, ma huang, yerba, guarana, yohimbe, maca root, goat weed, energy drinks, and several others that contained central nervous-system stimulants. No wonder he looked shaken. He was shaking. He also looked a little red.

"Von, a lot of these things can raise your blood pressure. Especially when combined. Are you taking anything else?"

"No, I don't think so." He really couldn't think of anything, so we needed to go down a list, one by one. Von was surprised, saying he thought they were natural. I explained that being "natural" didn't mean they had no effects he didn't want. I told him that tobacco is natural. It wasn't so many decades ago that doctors recommended cigarettes after dinner for digestion, and prescribed them for many conditions. Their proof that cigarettes were "beneficial" was that without their usual "dose," people felt worse. I told him I thought that if cigarettes were discovered today, they would be sold as the magic, natural appetite suppressant and nerve-calming herb. Of course, they have unhealthy effects too. Many "energy" drinks contain large amounts of caffeine. Caffeine is natural but there are some commercial drinks with more than twice the caffeine of espresso coffee. Together with the other stimulants Von was taking, plus his usual coffee and soda during the day, he was getting unhealthy doses. Worse, he would become accustomed to high caffeine and start feeling poorly without them. That would make his life even more expensive and uncomfortable.

"Anything else you're taking?" He paused to remember and gave the name of one of the supplement powders.

He said, "It has sassafras."

Sassafras can be highly unhealthy for the liver, nerves, and stomach. It can give you a rapid heat beat. If you mix it with sedating products like St. John's wort, you can get overly fatigued and feel faint. "Von, the combination of those supplements can make you sick, jittery, weak, anxious, even depressed. Do you take anything for that?"

He looked surprised. He said he thought the supplements were supposed to give him a "pick-up" but he was taking St. John's wort and Zoloft. What about licorice? Niacin? Yes, and yes.

"After the cardiac ward, I thought I better take some stuff for my heart."

"Von, niacin may help with cholesterol when you eat it in whole food, but it can make your skin flush in large-dose supplements. The licorice root, in addition to raising blood pressure, can lower libido—although the Zoloft may be doing more of that.

"That's why I'm taking those other supplements," Von said. His doctor said they could raise the antidepressant dosage if he didn't feel better and that it takes time to feel better.

"Von, if it is making you depressed, that is not the answer, either. Supplements, like saw palmetto, and antidepressants can upset your stomach. The selective serotonin reuptake inhibitors (SSRIs)—like Prozac, Zoloft, and Paxil—can increase risk of a stomach bleed, especially if you're taking them with anti-inflammatory drugs."

Von said he said he had stomach pain but thought it was from the anti-inflammatories he started with, and besides that, he had acid-reflux disease anyway and was always burping up a bad taste.

"Do you take any antacids?"

"No, my doctor gave me something about a pump."

"A proton pump inhibitor"

"Yes."

Proton pump inhibitors (PPIs) are prescription medicines that block acid release in the stomach and intestines—including medicines like Aciphex, Previcid, Nexium, and Prilosec. Other products like Carafate, Pepsid, Zantac, and Tagamet block stomach-acid production by blocking H2 (Histamine-2) from making acid. They work a little differently, but both kinds can cause stomach upset and nausea—the opposite of what was hoped.

"Von, several of the things you are taking have the side effect of heartburn, gas, and abdominal pain—including the PPI itself and the glucosamine you started with. Even a lot of vitamins and mineral supplements, like iron and zinc, can make your stomach hurt. You're taking a lot of them together. Pain from anti-inflammatory medications is not an acid problem. Even though the whole reason that acid-prevention medicine is often given is in hope that it will protect against anti-inflammatory agents, you need that acid to protect your stomach from the anti-inflammatories and from bad germs. You need the acid to digest food. That may be why you're burping, uncomfortable, and gassy. Food is rotting in there. You can't absorb the vitamins and minerals you need. When you said you took the anti-inflammatory for the joint pain, you meant your shoulder, right?"

He said no, that he had started aching all over. The acid medicines and the antidepressant both seemed to be making his body ache, which is not uncommon.

Von needed vinegar, not acid prevention. The plan was for him to stop the all the prescription medicines and supplements. It sounded drastic, but we carefully decided on this remedy after seeing that staying on them was more drastic. He was to drink a little apple cider vinegar in water, and squeeze lemon on his food to stop the unpleasant burping. He got some fresh ginger in the grocery store. He grated a small amount over food and into his tea. His stomach pain started decreasing, so he didn't need stomach medicine. I asked him to try cabbage to help heal his stomach. He later told me he was surprised how good a little cooked cabbage tasted and, luckily, it didn't take much because it was also pretty gassy food. Once he stopped blocking his stomach acid, the burping, hard swallowing, and reflux decreased. I asked him about his nasal symptoms and he said he thought it could be milk so he tried stopping milk products and it seemed to help. He bought an inexpensive new pillow because dust mites live in pillows and if they were causing symptoms, it was cheap and easy to try a pillow without the mites. By some estimates, a high percentage of the weight of a two-year-old pillow can be dead mites and their droppings. Von said he had started taking some of the "men's" supplements because he was going to the bathroom several times in the night and was worried it was prostate trouble. It turned out that he was eating late and drinking fluids before bed. It was easy to see why he was getting up in the night. Without the stimulant supplements and the other medicines, his blood pressure started coming down. The body aches started lifting. I told him if he wanted some energy supplements to have an orange and raw pumpkin seeds—ordinary food. He felt better not taking the supplements, and saved a good deal of money. He started feeling hopeful and said that without the antidepressant he could function better. He hadn't needed it because the depressed symptoms were from other things. He said, "I'm in sales. I should know better about all that great sounding advertising."

Jan came in with neck and upper-back pain. She was slim and young and worked as an aerobics instructor. She worked out regularly at the gym doing all the usual machines and classes. She had been told by more than one person that the reason for her pain was that she was large-chested. "They all said the same thing, so it must be so," she said. "It's because my big chest pulls and makes my neck hurt." I told her that was a common myth. Her forward head and rounded shoulders were just the way she was standing, regardless of weight distribution.

"You can hold yourself straight, whether holding a handbag or yourself. Men get the same pain from her forward head and round shoulders." I first checked that her bra straps were not making red ditches in her neck. I showed her how to check if she were standing upright using the wall stand (Figure 1-7) and how to restore the resting length needed in the chest and neck muscles using the pectoral stretch (Figure 1-9) and trapezius stretch (Figure 1-10). Then it would be comfortable to hold herself from slumping forward, and she wouldn't get the neck pain. It was important to apply this approach to everything she did in the gym. Many common exercises are done with round shoulders. I asked her to stop furthering the rounding by stopping the common gym stretch of pulling the arm over the body in front (Figure 3-13). "I call that one the round-shoulder stretch," I said. She said she did that stretch in the beginning and end of every class she taught. She said never realized it was doing the opposite of what most people needed. She said most of the students already have round shoulders, and she hadn't known that it wasn't normal body shape. I told her there were far better core exercises than crunches. It wasn't necessary to curl the body forward to exercise the abdominal muscles. By relearning how to hold the spine straight and not let it sag into an arch, you could get an abdominal workout and stop lower-back aches at the same time (Figures 2-31 through 2-39 and 2-41). She was interested. Although she hadn't mentioned it, she now said she got achy in her low back now and then, but thought it was normal. She seemed smart and that she would be more aware of no longer doing things in the name of health that aren't healthy.

When she came back a few months later, she said she only got the neck pain when she sat or exercised with the forward head and round shoulders, or went back to her crunches. She protested, "But everyone wants crunches." I told her to teach them the new exercises I taught her instead. She said she would when she had a chance, but was worried about a new problem. She had been to her doctors for many tests. She was vaguely uncomfortable and swollen, with a strange, achy pressure. She was worried that she had ovarian cancer and was glad they found she didn't have evidence of cancer.

Jan claimed she ate healthy. "I eat lots of lean meat and pork." She said her nutritionist had given her many products to help.

"Is it helping?"

"I don't know, maybe. Not yet, I have other things that scare me."

"Like what?"

"Well, I wake up starving and when I go to the bathroom in the morning it looks really strange and streaky. He's giving me things for my hypoglycemia."

"Let's back up. You're saying a lot of things. Who is this nutritionist? Are you paying him? Does he sell these products? What products are you taking?" Jan repeated that he was a nutritionist and she liked him because he was going to keep her from needing the doctors. She wasn't sleeping well. I told her that anyone can call himself a nutritionist. You can take as little as a one afternoon course if you want a certificate. I have five or six of these nutritionist certificates myself. I keep taking these courses to see what they have to say. I've taken graduate courses in nutrient metabolism. But it is not the same as a dietitian who has a university degree in the field. Plus, dietitians will not sell you stuff; that's a conflict of interest. It's true that a big problem going on now is people flocking to any kind of cures because they are not feeling listened to. Jan said that she bought about a hundred dollars worth of products at a time from the nutritionist. Before bed, she was drinking a large soy shake and flax-seed oil for constipation.

"Jan, eating right before bed can make you hungry in the night and can stop you from sleeping well. All that unfermented soy will make you bloated and gassy. You're drinking oil! That's why you're pooping oil. You can't absorb your vitamins with all that oil in the intestines. Why are you drinking oil?" She said that her nutritionist said it was good for her. She needed omega-3 oils to lower the "bad omega-6," and that it would help her constipation.

"Jan, how much is this flax-seed oil?"

"Twenty-six dollars a bottle."

"Jan, a pound bag of plain flax seeds costs less than a dollar. You don't want to drink oil unless you're being punished. Oil goes rancid after pressing anyway. Keep the oil fresh in the seed. Throw some seeds in a blender drink and on food. The whole seed has fiber and other nutrients missing in the oil. Eating peas, nuts, lentils, oats, and sesame seeds gives you plenty of protein instead of all that meat, and should solve the constipation."

I sent Jan to an endocrinologist friend of mine who checked her blood sugar over a week using home testing. She didn't have hypoglycemia. Next, Jan said her nutritionist said she should get colonic irrigation—a procedure of introducing a long tube up the rectum to pour quantities of fluids into the large intestines. The chances of infection or perforation were small, but the intestines don't just transmit waste, they absorb fluid and minerals for the body to use again. Irrigations can disturb electrolyte balance. Sometimes herbs or chemicals are injected up with the fluids, which are absorbed too much too fast. The main thing was that she didn't need it to stop the mechanical distension and discomfort of unhealthy eating. I asked her if she had heard the joke about the vegetarian bathroom. There are no magazines, only flash cards. I tried to give her some ideas to use. "Instead of expensive soy powders, drinks, and bars, have tempeh or miso soup. The powders and other products are unfermented soy, which does not have the benefits of fermented soy, and you don't need that much. Without so much meat pushing up your omega-6 ratio, you may not need as much omega-3. Check if you get bloated or uncomfortable after eating wheat. Snack crackers, cookies, and refined wheat products seem to contribute to this kind of problem. Both junk food and health powders can have sugar substitutes like sorbital that can make you bloated and gassy."

Jan said her nutritionist said she should not eat proteins together with carbohydrate. I told her that I had heard that advice, too, but it was more likely that foods work better in combination, both for providing and absorbing nutrients, and for combining to provide the energy to exercise. It took some convincing for Jan to think about how to stop being unhealthy from her "health" foods and practices. I think she is still spending money on various products and still having uncomfortable symptoms, going from one doctor to the next alternate cure. My greatest wish for these people is for their fitness to be healthier.

Doreen asked me to show her abdominal exercises. She wanted exercises to help her get ready for, and recuperate from upcoming fibroid surgery. "Doreen, that's huge, difficult surgery. Have you been able to find anyone to help you avoid it?

"Oh, my doctor's good. We tried everything. I will stay a week at a spa after the surgery. They already warned me that I won't be able to do much for myself for six to eight weeks after."

"What is everything?" I asked her.

"Oh, we tried medicine and I'm exercising."

"Are you sure you need this surgery?"

"Oh, the doctor says it's necessary and nothing else can be done. My periods are heavy and hurt and come every three weeks. Look how big I am." She pointed to a cute little belly.

"Doreen, this is not my field and I don't have experience with fibroids. But a doctor who says there's no other way is only admitting that they don't know another way—not that there *isn't* one. This surgery is the most common surgery for women in the United States. Some professionals say it is the most unnecessary. Others say that it is only common because it is so expensive. I keep hearing some of the same things from people who come to me and mention they are all taking some of the same estrogen promoting supplements."

Estrogen-promoting supplements are soy, black cohosh, dong quai, primrose oil, damiana, red clover, kudzu, wild yam, chasteberry, St. John's wort, pennyroyal, and several others. Some people take estrogen-promoting supplements thinking it will boost their natural levels for various health effects. Others say that the plant-based forms (phyto-estrogens) are supposed to be a weaker form that bind to estrogen receptors and block the stronger forms from promoting estrogen-dependent tumors like fibroids. But what seems to be happening is so many people are eating so much of them that the opposite may be happening.

Doreen was taking many phyto-estrogen supplements, including large amounts of unfermented soy in the form of protein powders, bars, drinks, pills, and using soy flour, soy milk, and all the many soy products from cookies to imitation hotdogs and burgers. I asked her about hair products with placenta and estrogen. She wasn't sure, but when I asked her if she used any hair growth products, she said that she had been using them since childhood. I told her that people with a tendency toward estrogen-dependent tumors like fibroids, cystic ovary, and endometriosis probably want to avoid these supplements and products, and to talk to her doctor.

A week later, I called her and found that she said she had checked with her doctor and stopped eating all the soy and thrown out all the supplements—"cold-turkey." I asked her to keep me posted. Two weeks later, I called again and she said that her period, that had been early for years, seemed to have waited to a more normal time. Plus, she was saving money by not buying the supplements. She wanted to know if she would hurt her workouts not eating all the soy bars. I reminded her that most of them are filled with hydrogenated fat, corn syrup and other refined sugars, fillers, dyes, preservatives, processed heat-changed ingredients, and unfermented soy, which does not have the benefits of fermented soy. Some of the bars are little more than expensive candy bars. I made sure her doctor knew and was willing to see what happened in the next month. Five weeks later, all seemed better. Her surgery date was that week. I told Doreen, "I know it's a long time to wait until menopause, but that will shrink fibroids away. You don't have to go through such rough surgery."

"But the surgery is already scheduled."

"You can cancel it and go another time if you want."

"But I already booked the spa."

"So go. You don't need an excuse to do something healthy for a week instead of something that will harm your health for at least the next two months—and for many people, more. Health care is supposed to be healthy."

Mary Frances came into my stretch class. She said she had fibromyalgia and her doctor said a stretch class would help. She only wanted stretches for fibromyalgia. "It all goes right *here*," she said, stabbing the air at the back of her neck, lower back, and knees.

I explained that the places she indicated didn't seem to be the usual distribution of fibromyalgia and that I work with mechanical pain and could look into what else may be going on. She cut me off, "No, no, no. I have fibromyalgia! That's what I have. I know it and the doctor told me so."

I told her, "This stretch class will help."

She sat down on the floor and rounded her back forward to reach her toes. I thought this time would be perfect to show her a concept and asked her if she bent over her desk with her back so rounded, would that be a good thing? I asked her if she would practice sitting up straight until class started. She was angry that I "wouldn't let her do her stretches to get better" and besides that, why was I telling her to do anything when class hadn't even started yet. She seemed proud and worried at the same time that she had some disease. I explained that the word "fibro" referred to the strong fibrous body areas, and "myo" meant the muscles, and "algia" meant pain. The word "fibromyalgia" only means that the muscles and attachments hurt. Not much is firmly established about fibromyalgia. Sometimes it's thought of as an autoimmune issue. Sometimes people are just given this name when they have pain but don't have an obvious strain or fall identified. Many are prescribed antidepressants, when it seems that a more effective intervention is vitamin D. All too often, the pain is from the same mechanical causes as anyone else who moves in painful tight ways. No matter the cause, strengthening and reeducating movement patterns stops pain for many.

In the class we don't just stretch. I work on dynamic range of motion that people need in daily activities. Many people use no muscular control and simply flop their body weight on their joints, walking heavily, unable to support their body weight. They move stiffly. Many can pass a flexibility test, but have no idea how to use their body in daily life. They lock up segments together (for example, their shoulder goes up and neck forward with each arm raise). No wonder they have pain in the back of the shoulder and upper back. They may bend badly all day, making tender points in their back.

I asked the students to just hold a push-up position. Mary Frances went immediately to a "girl's" push-up position on hands and knees. Her back bowed like an old horse. Her arms shook and elbows hyperextended under her weight before she flopped to the mat. I asked her to hold a real position. A "real" push-up position simulates holding your body straight under the pull of your own body weight. If you can't hold yourself straight, then it is likely that you will sag badly when walking around all day. She was so weak she couldn't do it—couldn't even approximate it. It wasn't the fibromyalgia that was making her weak, it was her inability to hold up her own body weight during daily life that was causing so much pain.

I explained that when she stands and walks all day, her own body weight needs to be held up against gravity, and since her muscles are too weak to do it, her joints and attachments protest loudly. Big realization came into her eyes that she does not have some incurable disease; she can strengthen and learn how to hold her body so her muscles won't hurt and her joints won't be battered by her body weight pounding on them with no muscular support. I showed her the pectoral stretch (Figure 1-9) and trapezius stretch (Figure 1-10) so that she could stop some of the main causes of the upper-back, neck, and shoulder pain. She was to hold a push-up position every day to strengthen and learn how to hold up her own body weight straight without sagging. She fussed that it was advanced and said she was afraid to get hurt doing it. I told her that this is a bare minimum needed to stop squashing yourself under your own weight. She would hurt more by not getting stronger. I told her that all my oldest patients do this. They find they regain ordinary daily life abilities like walking without canes, and opening jars, and carrying their own packages—all without pain. Each week she came in we worked on holding body weight up – holding push-up positions on the front and side (Figures 2-31 through 2-39 and 2-41). She learned how to stand without letting her legs flop to poor position (Chapter 5) and be able to balance without the same happening (Chapter 6). She learned how to strengthen her core and abdominal muscles (Chapter 2, section on lordosis) and stretch her hamstrings (Chapter 9) without the forward bending that increases neck and back pain for so many. We do all this in my stretch classes. Her doctor was glad that her stretch class helped.

Artie was a psychologist and told me, "When I'm under stress, my gums bleed." Artie insisted it was stress. I asked him how he knew that. He told me that when he was unhappy he got bleeding gums—especially when his taxes were audited. I asked him what else he did when his taxes were audited. He didn't know what I meant. I asked him if he chewed his pencils, was grinding his teeth, ate or drank anything differently, or took medicine or herbs. It turned out that he usually took supplements of garlic, ginkgo biloba, vitamin E, GLA oil, and fish oil, all of which have the effect of "thinning" the blood, making it less likely to clot normally. When he was unhappy, he added St. John's wort. When his taxes were audited, he added a prescription antidepressant and a glass of wine with dinner. These substances all have blood-thinning effects. He nodded, adding that he just realized that he also bruised easily.

Other "blood thinners" are policosanol, selenium, lemon balm, primrose oil, devil's claw herb, bromelain, many over-the-counter and prescription anti-inflammatories for pain, aspirin, and medicines that contain aspirin like cold medicine and stomach and cramp remedies—even estrogen.

Artie was lucky that the bleeding was no more than in his gums and a few black and blue marks, as far as we knew. Taking blood thinners can put you at risk of stroke, or bleeding in the eye or brain from an accident or fall that wouldn't otherwise harm you. It put you at risk of dangerous bleeds when going into medical or dental surgery. Make sure to tell all doctors, dentists, anesthesiologists, and the staff administering any invasive tests or treatments of every supplement you take before any procedure—large or small.

Christopher had worked as a bouncer and security escort for years in some seedy environments. He got in plenty of fights—sometimes against armed opponents. After years of being bashed around and training in the martial arts, Christopher developed severe joint pain in his knees, shoulders, elbows, neck, and back. By the time he came to me, he said his pain was 15 on a scale of 1 to 10, and he was a tough guy who knew pain. Several doctors had told him over many years that he would have crippling arthritis for the rest of his life and that he would have to learn to live with it. They put him on medication. Still, some days he could not get out of bed without pain that made his eyes sting. His joint pain was so severe that he was missing work and valuable training hours at his martial-arts training school. Every three to six months or so they were giving him something stronger.

How did all this start? He began training in the fighting arts when he was 12. When he was 16 he was diagnosed with floating kneecaps. The orthopedist said that strengthening the muscle around the kneecap would prevent them from floating, which caused them to lock or give out. The doctor gave Christopher exercises to do over the summer and said that if they didn't work that he would do surgery. Christopher was given prescription ibuprofen for the pain. He spent the summer doing the exercises. They didn't work. He wore knee braces from the time he was 16.

When he was 17 or 18, Christopher dislocated his elbow wrestling in a high school tournament. He put it back in himself. Tough guy. The orthopedist told him he chipped it when he put it back in. By the time Christopher was 20 he was taking ibuprofen regularly. He was also on medication for what he was told was a hiatal hernia. By the time he was 25, one of his doctors told him that if he didn't quit the martial arts he was going to suffer debilitating arthritis his entire life.

At age 29, Christopher was taking the prescription Naproxin, the equivalent of three Aleve tablets, twice a day. By the time he was 30, he worried that the doctors may have been right. He had just earned his black belt in a martial-arts style called Kagedo. He was not able to train much of the subsequent year due to debilitating arthritis, spending days in such pain that he could not get out of bed.

In February of 2004, Christopher was taken to the emergency room for abdominal pain. Tests were done, but the doctors found nothing conclusive. They diagnosed him with a spastic colon and put him on Bentyl, Nexium, Zantac, and one other prescription he couldn't remember.

In the summer of 2004, just after turning 31, Christopher went to see the doctor again. The pain in his joints and stomach was too much. He would wake in the morning and lie in bed for over an hour trying to move enough to get out of bed. He hurt so much that he could not bend his knees, and barely his elbows. His shoulders ached constantly. His neck and shoulders were grinding almost all the time. He was in so much pain that everyone tried again to convince him that he might never be able to train in the martial arts again. He was starting to believe it himself. The new doctor prescribed Neurontin, a nerve pain medicine, and Tramadol, a painkiller.

In November of 2003, I briefly met Christopher and his teacher Master Sean at the Eastern USA International Martial Arts Association's annual black-belt event. Christopher didn't mention to me that any of this was going on. I was impressed with their fun loving nature. I noticed that Christopher moved oddly, but everyone was throwing everyone around that weekend, and everyone goes home walking funny from some of the better seminars. I asked Christopher how he was and he gave a jovial reply that I think I remember involved a string of obscenities. It sounded so funny the way he said it that I took it as a joke. The following year, we all met again at the same event. I was giving a seminar for martial-arts athletes on core training without back pain. Christopher and Master Sean were giving a seminar right after mine, on the Kagedo style that Master Sean developed. They were stuck there, so they attended my seminar. I thought they were just being polite. After my seminar, Christopher didn't mention his situation, just said something funny about feeling a (string of obscenities) difference in his pain. The room full of big, strong guys were all saying the same, minus the funny words, so I still didn't catch that there was more to it. I remember looking around at all the big, strong martial artists, thinking they were all living a fun life breaking boards and being stronger than the next guy. What fun to be a young, strong, carefree man who can do whatever we wants, I thought.

After the conference weekend, Christopher casually e-mailed what was going on. He said he had days where he was physically not able to bend his knees because of the joint pain. If it rained, it was a pain-filled day. He said that on many days, even after taking top doses for pain that "wreaked havoc" on his stomach, he could still only move from the bed, to the couch, to the bathroom, and back—and that was still too much.

I was startled that he didn't say something at the conferences. It was my turn to say the string of funny words you shouldn't say. I asked him if he wanted to fix it up. I started with basic questions: Where does it hurt? When? What are you already trying for it?

We checked everything else that might be causing or adding to pain from sexually-transmitted polyarthritis on down. His docs had been good and had already checked him for everything possible, which was good since they ruled out a list of things that were not the problem. "Christopher, you have a bad case of good insurance. You are seeing lots of doctors and taking many interacting medications that add to cycles of pain. We can do a few simple things to stop the mechanical sources of the pain so you don't need the medicines in the first place."

I gave Christopher things to try after explaining the concepts so he'd understand what he was doing and not just go through the motions. He had already attended one of my seminars so he knew how to start. Christopher was good as gold and read my books and Web articles—doing everything. After a week, he said he noticed enough improvement to try going without his arthritis medicines, which was a turning point. He felt better. The pain in his joints was reduced more by the retraining exercises than his medicines. By stopping the medicines, the stomach and body pain he got from the medicines would stop, and he wouldn't need the other medicines to combat those side effects. After another 10 days, he stopped taking the four medications prescribed for his stomach and gastrointestinal problems. He ate cabbage and ginger root, which helped bring down more of the stomach symptoms.

What specifically did we do? Christopher had worn orthotics since first or second grade and he walked pigeon-toed. This condition was made worse by training in Kune Tao—another martial art that required a pigeon-toe stance. He used it even for normal walking. His feet pointed inward and he leaned inward on his arches, adding to pain in his knees and ankles. I told him to make sure that his feet pointed forward—neither out nor in. The knee pain reduced, and the ankle pain was gone. He learned to hold his own arches up and no longer needed the orthotics.

Christopher was used to hunching over a computer desk all day, then driving home in a contorted position. When he walked, he hung his head forward hunched his shoulders. We realized his arthritis was not getting worse; his positioning was. He stopped letting his head hang forward and much of his shoulder pain stopped. He used the pectoral stretch (Figure 1-9) and trapezius stretch (Figure 1-10) several times every day to help reposition his head, neck, and shoulders, alleviating the upper-body pain. He used the hip-tucking method taught in Chapter 2 (Figures 2-23, 2-24, 2-27, and 2-28) during all activity to stop the lordotic arching that was making his back hurt so much. He didn't round his shoulders in ways that twisted his elbows anymore. He was happy and thought these improvements would be all he needed.

Then things took a back step. The day before Thanksgiving he got in a dangerous street fight. He was attacked by two thugs in a PCP drug rage. One had a piece of pipe. Christopher won, coming out of it with a broken nose, swollen cuts all over his mouth and face, a bruised jaw ligament, and an inability to close his mouth enough to chew. He had a 6 a.m. flight out of Pittsburgh to New Hampshire on Thanksgiving Day.

The emergency room doctor would not clear him to fly unless he agreed to take pain medication, which he tried to refuse. He was put on Amoxicillin, ibuprofen, and Vicodin. He couldn't eat solid food or stand or sit up straight. After two days, he felt worse. He was in pain and his stomach was not happy.

Christopher e-mailed me to let me know what happened. He thought it was the end of all the progress. I told him not to worry. Not only would he heal but he wouldn't starve. I knew he mostly lived on junk food. All he was eating since the fight was mashed potatoes. I told him to try putting raw nuts, spices, and fresh fruit with the seeds, pulp, and skins in a blender or food processor. Christopher wrote me excitedly" "I discovered a whole new world of healthy food. Fruit is my new sugar fix instead of my daily pile of junk food. I traded my two bottles a day of soda for water or healthy blender drinks. I feel better." To start eating soft food again, instead of greasy fast food he made thick lentil and leek soups and steamed his favorite vegetables in soy sauce and balsamic vinegar, topped with fresh raw tomato, crushed garlic, fresh green scallions, and cilantro. He found that healthy cooking could be quicker than frying, with less clean up. He didn't need a steamer, just a bit of water in his regular pot with the food, drizzle soy sauce and vinegars on top, put the lid on, and forget it for a few minutes. In two weeks, Christopher healed faster than expected and lost a few pounds. Once he could chew food again, he found that fresh raw nuts could be better than commercial roasted nuts. The oil in roasted nuts and commercial peanut butter quickly goes rancid and changes to less healthy products. Instead of juice, he used whole fruit in the blender for better nutrition and blood-sugar control. I told him that if he used a juicer, to mix the pulp back in. He told me he never noticed before that he spent so much time and money on junk food and unhealthy food preparation. Eating healthy could be cheaper and easier if you didn't fall for the hype about needing tedious preparation.

At his three-month follow-up, Christopher was writing a cookbook. He had returned to training for his second-degree black belt in Kagedo. He was pain-free—even with full contact martial arts. At his four-month follow-up,

Christopher said, "I have no pain except a few times I let my arches fall in and the knees started to hurt. I fixed that and that took care of that."

What he had never told me before this time was that when he first came to me, he had made the decision to leave the martial arts. He had tried his strongest all these years but was so wracked with pain that he thought he had to admit his doctors and family were right.

At his one-year follow-up, Christopher was still pain free. He was inspired by getting back to exercise and finding healthy food that he liked—and he quit smoking. Together with his martial-arts teacher and friends, he was planning to open a healthy café of the mind, serving his new, healthy, gourmet recipes.

12

How to Help Yourself Get Better

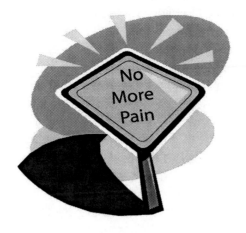

It's a shame when someone is considered "a good patient" when they accept limited physical ability and don't complain, while someone who wants to get better and says he doesn't want to give up activity or live with pain is told to accept and cope and not "be difficult."

Pain is not something you can't do anything about. Much pain is mechanically based and readily diminished or stopped with simple healthy movement skills. Feel reassured and empowered. Keep moving. Work the area that needs it. Make a knee work again, a hand, a neural connection that was damaged.

Many people who try the information in my books and articles write back in the next days saying it was already helping. Sometimes a postcard comes a year later from a far-flung place from patients saying they were doing wonderful things they thought they could never do, or never do again. Sometimes people write back a week or month after first contacting me, saying they have pain and ask what I can do to help them. I ask them what things didn't work so I can know what to try next. They tell me they didn't read it, or they didn't have time and would read it when they had a chance, or they tried one thing and not the rest, or they were doing exercises but then going back to every unhealthy daily habit that started the pain in the first place. I give them the date of my next workshop. I explain the goal is to fix their pain right at the workshop. Some say they won't try the workshop because they have their massage that day or that their back hurts too much to come. One man said his back surgery was coming up and he wanted to save his energy. Then there are the people who say, "I want to be better right now. When is your next class and what do I need to do?" These people come to the workshop or read this book, and do the steps to make sure they start getting better that day.

Judith called me for her ongoing back pain. When I arrived outside her home for her appointment, she was packing her car for a trip. She bent right over and yanked the bags to lift them. She arched her back to push them to the roof rack and then rounded over the trunk to lug the spare tire out of the way. She said she always did this because she was strong. I mentioned that this occasion was the perfect place and time for fun retraining in lifting and carrying. She said that, of course, she didn't need that "bend with your knees" stuff because her back pain was from stress and she wanted me in the house to show her the exercises so she could do them in the gym when she traveled.

It's important to think of exercise as normal, daily body movement—not something different and artificial. Fitness as a "lifestyle" doesn't mean working out at a gym or at home at specific days and times, then returning to real life of slouching, sitting around, bending wrong all day, walking heavily, and moving in unhealthy patterns. Strengthening and stretching are crucial, but alone will not change positioning or lifting habits, and so often fail in pain rehab programs. Some exercises even contribute to the original problems. Exercises are supposed to retrain how you hold your body all the time. Make healthy movement something you love to do.

Mr. Cahan came to me and said his doctor told him to ride a stationary bike or die soon of cardiac disease. I asked him if he loved it and he said he hated it but was motivated and was riding daily. He said his kids got him the bike. He was obese and moved stiffly. We talked a while about life. He said that as a young man he loved the snow and often went cross-country skiing. I told him to tell his kids to take back the bike and get him a skier, until he could get back out safely in real snow. He asked which machine was better. I told him: the one he loved.

My husband Paul and I were living and working in Japan. It was Paul's dream to study martial arts there, so I found work and we went. During part of our stay, we traveled to the central mountains and studied in a monastery. When we arrived, the old monk in charge met us, giving an indistinct greeting. I was not sure if he was speaking English or Japanese. He turned and hobbled off, leaning to one side. He indicated we should follow him to learn our way around. Each morning, he rang the waking bell at 5 a.m. with one arm, the other curled at his side. He toddled to morning prayers and smiled a crooked smile when we assembled. He spoke to us, and explained, "An-ur-im. An-ur-im." I realized he was saying "aneurysm."

"You had a stroke!"

"Hai, yes." He bowed crookedly. Each morning we kneeled with the monks in the darkened study hall. Our little monk chanted and waved his good arm over a leaping fire. After each morning prayer, he pushed a piece of chalk between his gnarled fingers and made a resolute mark next to hundreds of others to count his prayers. He needed ten thousand to thank the doctors who had treated him after his stroke. In the afternoons, Paul and I trained behind the monastery, where poles, climbing bars, and balancing posts were available. We could see the little monk in the Zen garden, raising and lowering his working arm in front of a tree. He was putting peanuts for the squirrel. I asked him about his curled, useless hand. He worked to enunciate. "Doctor say no good cannot fix. Always this way." His peaceful, little round face smiled on one side. His hand hung in a tangled ball.

When I try to learn a foreign language, I want to learn it the way the people of the country learned it. When they were children they grew up knowing regional toys, games, and songs. To share their collective memory of their country and language, I learn these things so I can see their life through their eyes. In Japan, I learned children's songs. One of the songs says, *"Mu-su-unde, hero ite, te-o ute! Mu-sun de."* It roughly translates as: "Open your hands, close your hands, jump up and clap! Open your hands, close your hands." I sang it for the little monk. His eyes brightened with a memory of a long-ago childhood. He nodded. I knew that I must not touch a monk, but Paul could. Paul took the monk's little fist in his giant, Western hands and began to gently work and pull and push until the monk's hand began to open. The monk looked at his newly opened hand, something he hadn't seen since the stroke the year before. He tried to move it. It weakly moved. He smiled. We smiled. He slightly opened and closed his hand again. We told him, "Every day." We bowed. He bowed. I was sad when it was time to leave the monastery. From time to time, we send a postcard that we hope gets to him up the mountain. We write: *"Mu-su-unde, hero ite, te-o ute! Mu-sun de!"*